STRAIGHT TALK ABOUT PSYCHIATRIC MEDICATIONS FOR KIDS

Straight Talk *about* Psychiatric Medications *for* Kids

FOURTH EDITION

TIMOTHY E. WILENS, MD
PAUL G. HAMMERNESS, MD

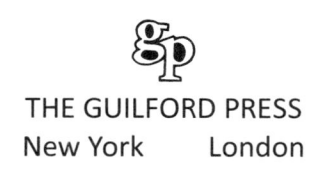

THE GUILFORD PRESS
New York   London

Copyright © 2016 Timothy E. Wilens and Paul G. Hammerness

Published by The Guilford Press
A Division of Guilford Publications, Inc.
370 Seventh Avenue, Suite 1200, New York, NY 10001
www.guilford.com

All rights reserved

The information in this volume is not intended as a substitute for consultation with healthcare professionals. Each individual's health concerns should be evaluated by a qualified professional.

Except as indicated, no part of this book may be reproduced, translated, stored in a retrieval system, or transmitted, in any form or by any means, electronic, mechanical, photocopying, microfilming, recording, or otherwise, without written permission from the publisher.

Printed in the United States of America

This book is printed on acid-free paper.

Last digit is print number: 9 8 7 6 5 4 3 2 1

FULL DISCLOSURE

Dr. Timothy E. Wilens has participated in, is a consultant to, and/or has received research support from the following: Bay Cove Human Service, Ironshore Pharmaceuticals, Major/Minor League Baseball (Therapeutic Use Exemptions), the National Football League (ERM Associates), the National Institute on Drug Abuse, Neurovance, Phoenix House, and Sunovion. Dr. Wilens also receives royalties from Massachusetts General Hospital, owner of a copyrighted questionnaire codeveloped with Dr. Hammerness that is licensed to Ironshore Pharmaceuticals.

Dr. Paul G Hammerness receives royalties from Massachusetts General Hospital, owner of a copyrighted questionnaire codeveloped with Dr. Wilens that is licensed to Ironshore Pharmaceuticals.

Library of Congress Cataloging-in-Publication Data

Names: Wilens, Timothy E., author. | Hammerness, Paul Graves, author.
Title: Straight talk about psychiatric medications for kids, fourth edition / Timothy E. Wilens and Paul G. Hammerness.
Description: Fourth edition. | New York, NY : The Guilford Press, [2016] | Includes bibliographical references and index.
Identifiers: LCCN 2015044848| ISBN 9781462519859 (paperback : acid-free paper) | ISBN 9781462525874 (hardcover : acid-free paper)
Subjects: LCSH: Pediatric psychopharmacology—Popular works. | BISAC: MEDICAL / Psychiatry / Psychopharmacology. | FAMILY & RELATIONSHIPS / Parenting / General. | PSYCHOLOGY / Psychotherapy / Child & Adolescent. | SOCIAL SCIENCE / Social Work.
Classification: LCC RJ504.7.W54 2016 | DDC 615.7/80835—dc23
LC record available at *http://lccn.loc.gov/2015044848*

Contents

Authors' Note		vii
Acknowledgments		ix
Introduction		1

Part I
What Every Parent Should Know about Psychiatric Medications for Children

1	The Preliminaries: Building a Foundation of Knowledge	9
2	The Psychopharmacology Evaluation: Finding Out What's Wrong	41
3	The Diagnosis and Treatment Plan: Laying Out a Strategy to Help Your Child	69
4	Treatment and Beyond: Collaborating in Your Child's Ongoing Care	98

Part II
Common Childhood Psychiatric Disorders

5	Attentional and Disruptive Behavioral Disorders	129
6	Anxiety-Related Disorders	141
7	Mood Disorders	153

8	Autism Spectrum Disorder	166
9	Schizophrenia and Other Psychotic Disorders	173
10	Disorders of Known Medical and Neurological Origin	178
11	Other Mental Health Disturbances Affecting Children and Adolescents	186

Part III
The Psychotropic Medications

12	The Stimulants and Nonstimulants for ADHD	203
13	The Antidepressants	230
14	The Mood Stabilizers	244
15	The Anxiety-Breaking Medications	255
16	The Alpha Agonists and Other Antihypertensives	261
17	The Antipsychotics	269
18	Medications for Sleep, Bedwetting, and Other Problems	281

Appendix A. Representative Medication Preparations and Sizes Used for the Treatment of Childhood Emotional and Behavioral Disorders	285
Appendix B. Medication Log	291
Resources	295
Bibliography	308
Index	321
About the Authors	342

> Purchasers of this book can download and print a larger version of the Medication Log at *www.guilford.com/wilens-forms* for personal use or use with individual clients.

Authors' Note

Medications have brand names and generic (chemical) names. In this book we've tried to use whichever name is most common but to give both in many places. (If the medication is still under patent, only brand-name versions will be available; once the patent expires, generics will also be available, and your child's doctor can indicate which is preferred.) Appendix A is a handy reference that lists both generic and brand names for the medications discussed in this book.

We have alternated between masculine and feminine personal pronouns throughout the book. Unless otherwise noted, all information applies equally to male and female children and adolescents.

All cases that illustrate diagnosis and treatment have been thoroughly disguised or are composites of actual patients we have seen.

Acknowledgments

Timothy E. Wilens:

My ability to write this book is a reflection of the environments in which I was raised and practice medicine. One does not simply wake up and find oneself a physician. That process is one that often begins early in life and is nurtured emotionally and intellectually. As you read this book, you will undoubtedly feel the influence of my now deceased parents: my mother, the liberal social worker, and my father, the conservative businessman-philosopher. I am forever indebted to my family, who have provided great support and confidence to me throughout my life. Their dissatisfaction with the status quo, future-oriented discussions, and intellectual curiosity provided the template in which I operate.

I am grateful to many colleagues who have so willingly shared their experiences with the sundry agents being used with children. I am honored to be part of the Department of Psychiatry at Massachusetts General Hospital (MGH) and am grateful to my colleagues for their longstanding support, both of my work in the field and in completing this book. Few professionals have the opportunity and supportive environment available to them to care for patients and conduct clinical research. I am particularly indebted to Dr. Joseph Biederman, Professor of Psychiatry at Harvard Medical School, who has served as my longtime mentor and colleague. His devotion, insight, passion, and thoughtfulness, which have guided the clinical research in this area, have profoundly impacted the lives of psychiatrically impaired children worldwide. I am also deeply appreciative of my close colleague who sits across from me from day to day, Dr. Thomas Spencer, whose friendship, originality, and keen and witty mind have been a great resource in our sharing of the unique clinical and research dilemmas so common in psychiatry. I also am highly appreciative of many colleagues, such as my coauthor, Dr. Paul Hammerness, who provide empathic and thoughtful care daily to some of the most ill children.

I also would like to acknowledge the very insightful comments from Chris Benton, who has provided valuable, thoughtful editorial guidance throughout the process of the original and revised versions of *Straight Talk*.

One of the greatest honors afforded in our society is being entrusted with the responsibility to care for others as a practitioner of medicine. My respect for my patients and their families is immense and is sprinkled with appreciation of their patience and trust, even after the eighth medication trial has failed. Through our collaborative relationships, I have grown as I continue to learn and study the safe and effective use of medications in children. I am also very grateful to the families who have participated in research studies at MGH and elsewhere to advance our knowledge in pediatric psychopharmacology.

Paul G. Hammerness:

I am indebted to my family for their love, support, and inspiration. I am grateful as well to my past and present colleagues, from my decade in academia at MGH to my clinical work at Newton Wellesley Hospital and my current position at Boston Children's Hospital. My experiences in clinical research, clinical care, teaching, and pediatric consultation have collectively shaped my professional life and aspirations. It has been a great privilege to work with my longtime mentor and colleague Tim Wilens on this edition of *Straight Talk*.

Introduction

Should you allow your child to be treated with medication for a mental, emotional, or behavioral problem? If you do, how will you ensure that your child gets the best possible treatment with the least possible risk? How can you be confident that your child has received an accurate diagnosis and that all available avenues of treatment have been considered? What do you need to know to monitor your child's care? If your child is among the estimated 10–20% of American kids—7.5–15 million all together—who suffer from psychiatric disorders, you are facing tough questions like these and many more.

In our years at the Pediatric Psychopharmacology Clinic and Research Program at Massachusetts General Hospital and Harvard Medical School—almost four decades combined—we have learned that considering medication for a child's psychiatric disorder is one of the most anxiety-producing decisions that many parents ever face, largely because so many questions remain unanswered. The parents we see do not want to be merely sent out the door of our offices with a prescription in hand. They want to understand their child's underlying condition and what causes it. They want to learn everything they can about what the disorder is as well as the current treatments and how helpful each alternative might be. They want to know how much hope they can have that their child's symptoms will improve and their family's well-being will be restored. They want to understand any risks posed by the treatment options, how to interpret what they read in media reports of research findings, and how to weigh the pros and cons of treating versus not treating their child. They want to be effective guardians of their child's psychological health and informed collaborators with their child's mental health practitioners. What they need is straight talk—honest and complete answers to the many complex questions that come up in the course of their child's treatment.

This book is an attempt to anticipate and answer all the questions you may have when your child has a mental, emotional, or behavioral problem that could be treated with medication. Since the first edition of this book was published more than 15 years ago, the field of child psychiatry in general and pediatric pharmacology in particular has seen remarkable advances. We have refined our diagnostic skills to better identify severe mood disorders in children, including bipolar disorder, and we have provided sufficient evidence to establish the persistence of attention-deficit/hyperactivity disorder (ADHD) into adulthood—to name two areas of diagnostic advancement. Government mandates and enticements have encouraged the pharmaceutical industry to better study the use of medications in children and adolescents, resulting in an explosion of new research. The pharmaceutical industry has come up with new forms of stimulants as well as nonstimulants and combined them to provide even more options for children with ADHD. We've had formal Food and Drug Administration (FDA) approvals for medications for pediatric bipolar disorder. Research into the genetic causes of mental illness and the workings of the brain continues to expand and be increasingly collaborative on the world stage.

Yet along with new answers have come new questions, which, not surprisingly, join some of the old questions that remain unanswered: What are the long-term effects of psychiatric medications on children? What happens to youth with bipolar disorder over time? As it did when originally published, this book addresses concerns that are likely to arise when you are just beginning to investigate what may be wrong with your child, all the way through psychiatric evaluation and diagnosis, treatment decisions, and long-term use of medications. The information offered in the following pages is derived from a wealth of scientific literature, ongoing research efforts in which we and our colleagues are engaged, and our own clinical experience. It represents the latest information available at the time of this writing, and to our knowledge is still, as were the first three editions, the most extensive layperson's book in print on the various medications used to treat children and adolescents with psychiatric disorders. Naturally, information in this field is only growing, making condensation more difficult. Nevertheless, we've made every attempt to keep the information and advice up to date, reflecting some of the most recent literature in the field. In most cases, this revision reflects many of the same tenets as the original publication; yet recent advancements have changed the way we conceptualize and treat some conditions (e.g., bipolar disorder, complicated ADHD, autism spectrum disorder [ASD]), so much of the information here has been revised.

Our goal is to offer everything you need to know to make the treatment decisions so important to your child's present and future well-being and that of your family. One of the first lessons we learned as child psychopharmacologists is that every child and family brings with it unique characteristics and response to treatment. This means that the care of your child will be an ongoing learning experience for you, your child and family, and your child's doctor. It also means that you are a crucial player on this team. You are in a unique position to observe your child, you understand your child better than anyone else, and the information that you can provide about what works and what doesn't, about the problems that arise during treatment and the solutions that work best, is invaluable to the practitioner you have chosen to manage your child's care. Many of our research group's findings and much of what you will read in this book, in fact, has been enriched and expanded by the experiences of parents and children we have had the privilege to work with over the years.

Our colleagues in the field of child psychiatry have found that, as time goes on, society in general and parents in particular are less and less willing to leave childhood mental, emotional, and behavioral problems untreated.

Not surprisingly, research has shown that the majority of major emotional and behavioral disorders in adults start during childhood or adolescence. Just imagine if these adults had been properly diagnosed and treated at the time they first started showing symptoms! It is increasingly accepted that psychiatric disorders affecting children are serious problems that demand attention, not just developmental phases, adjustment problems, or the effects of poor parenting. Many of these illnesses have a biological basis, meaning in part that the chemical messengers in the brain aren't functioning normally. Medications that affect neurochemistry can be critically useful in reducing symptoms and restoring children's ability to function. Pharmacological treatment is a firmly established option for parents whose children have psychiatric disorders.

That does not mean, of course, that medication is the only option. Psychiatric disorders in children can be complicated to diagnose and complicated to treat. Often the best solution for a given child is a combination of psychotherapy and pharmacology, and sometimes more than one treatment in each category produces the greatest improvement. Frequently only trial and error will tell what works best for your child. This book is by no means an advertisement for psychiatric medications, and we will frankly tell you what we know about adverse effects, limitations, and other problems related to the use of these drugs along with the success stories we have witnessed.

This book will supply the facts about common psychiatric disorders affecting children and the currently accepted treatments for them, with up-to-date details on the medications among those treatments. You and your child's practitioner will supply the other half of the equation—an understanding of your child—and the two of you will collaborate on a treatment plan. Throughout this revised edition, in fact, we will point out the expanded role of the parents in a child's mental health care. Since this book's original publication, it has become increasingly important that the parent participate in managing the care of the child. We think of parents of the children we treat as "saints"—they are tireless in their care of their child at home and are active in advocating within the mental health care process, from supervising the child's evaluation to monitoring treatment and coordinating the efforts of the mental health and educational team. The more facts you have at your disposal, the more effective the parent–practitioner collaboration becomes, the more fruitful the dialogue between you, and the more hope you offer your child. Hopefully you will find the information you seek in the following three sections.

Part I, "What Every Parent Should Know about Psychiatric Medications for Children," is the best place to begin if you need an overview of the issues involved in the medicating process or you have fundamental questions about that process. Part I addresses common concerns in the order in which you will probably encounter them, from the preliminaries to the evaluation and diagnosis of your child, to the creation of a treatment plan and your child's ongoing care. Part I is presented in question-and-answer format. Read it in its entirety or flip through until you spot the questions that have been on your mind (or use the index to find specific answers you need). The answers include some illustrative examples from our practice (either composites or well disguised to protect the privacy of patients and their families), although you'll find many more specific illustrations in Parts II and III. Interspersed throughout Part I are definitions of terms you're likely to hear often from your child's mental health practitioners. In this fourth edition we've added questions and answers on issues that have received great attention or about which more information has recently become available over the past few years, but we've also condensed some information, in the hope of making it easier than ever for you to become the best manager of your child's diagnosis and treatment that you can be—a collection of tasks that becomes more important with every passing year.

Part II, "Common Childhood Psychiatric Disorders," provides information on the common symptoms, biology, causes, and course (what happens to the disorder with time) of the major emotional and behavioral disorders that we see in children and adolescents. Each chapter ends with a review of the major medications and other interventions used in treatment. Diagnostic criteria and methods are always being reviewed and revised to reflect new research and clinical findings, and in this edition you'll discover what we've recently learned about bipolar disorder, ASD, ADHD, and other disorders for which new information has come to light. These disorders are grouped by related symptoms or by the problems associated with them. If your child has been diagnosed with a particular condition and you do not know which heading it falls under, check the index.

Part III, "The Psychotropic Medications," offers detailed descriptions of the major classes of medications used to treat psychiatric disorders in kids. Included are the common uses of the medications, areas of the brain and neurotransmitters affected by the medications, available preparations and strengths, dosing information, safe combinations with other agents, and extensive details on side effects. Questions and answers on typical concerns and problems raised by parents are featured throughout these chapters. Here, as in Parts I and II, we've updated the chapters to provide the latest information on new medications, new forms of older medications, and recent findings about the administration and effectiveness of these agents in children and teenagers. In some cases, major sections have been rewritten, and the order of use of certain classes of medications, such as antipsychotics, has been changed substantially, reflecting updated data on what works best and what is approved by the FDA, as well as any new longer-term safety issues—or lack thereof—of the various medications.

In discussing medications, we refer to each drug by its most commonly used name. In some cases this is the brand name, which is capitalized (e.g., Prozac or Ritalin). In other cases this is the generic name, which appears in lowercase letters (e.g., sertraline). A list of medications and their generic and brand names, as well as their suggested preparation and strengths, is available in Appendix A.

In discussing mental health professionals, we use various terms, from *doctor* to *practitioner* to *clinician* and other terms. Who provides what type of care for your child will vary, depending on your location, your health care plan, and the availability of specialists. We may refer to your child's pediatrician or prescribing physician when discussing a service that this particular professional is likely to offer, but in other cases, when you see the term *doctor,* please understand that it means the person responsible for the relevant facet of your child's care.

Likewise, we use the term *child* to mean anyone who has not yet reached adulthood. Where the subject applies exclusively to adolescents or younger children, we state that.

At the back of the book you'll find information on where to go for more information and for the support that many parents find helpful in meeting the challenges of raising a child with a mental, behavioral, or emotional problem. If you don't find what you need from any of these sources, don't forget the resources you already have—not only your child's prescriber, but all the other health care professionals at your disposal, from psychotherapists to nurse practitioners, from social workers to nurses, from your child's pediatrician to your family practitioner. Straight questions from you are the best way to get straight answers.

Part I

What Every Parent Should Know about Psychiatric Medications for Children

When your child has a psychiatric problem for which medication may be prescribed, a thousand questions beg to be answered. Parents come to us with an urgently felt need for information—and often more than a little anxiety as well. In this section, we've compiled the questions that come up—in our offices as well as at the talks we give for professional and parent groups in the United States and internationally—with the most current, complete answers that can be given in a book meant to speak to a broad cross-section of parents. The main goal of this book is to help you better understand the field of child psychiatry and the potential benefits of psychiatric medications for children, balanced with the known risks. In sharing these questions and answers we'll provide you with an insider's view. We expect that you will emerge more confident to embark on your journey.

As is stressed throughout the book, you are a key player in your child's mental health care. The importance of your participation in this process cannot be overstated. To fill that role optimally, you need to be well informed about your child's problem and the available treatments. The following questions, posed by hundreds of caring, concerned parents before you, will get you thinking as a proactive collaborator in the care of your child. However, remember that every child's situation is unique. The right answers for your son or daughter will come mainly from the cooperative efforts of you and the qualified professionals you've chosen.

The following questions and answers have been divided into four chapters, based on when in the diagnosis and treatment process they usually arise. Questions asked by parents who are just considering seeking help for their child come first. Next are questions and answers for those currently involved in the evaluation process. The third chapter addresses questions about the diagnosis and the treatment proposals that emerge from the evaluation. The last chapter addresses issues that come up when a child is already being treated with psychiatric medications.

Read all of Part I for an overview or turn to the individual chapters and questions within them as needed. Either way, we hope you'll find what you need to know. If not, please ask your child's practitioners—that's what they are there for. Finally, the Resources section at the back of the book includes websites and other contact information for mental health organizations that may provide further help.

1

The Preliminaries
Building a Foundation of Knowledge

It's never easy to face the fact that your child has symptoms of a mental health problem. A tough situation becomes harder when, like most parents, you know little about the subject of childhood psychiatric disorders and their treatment. It's even more difficult when misconceptions and myths abound.

Perhaps you've just consulted your child's pediatrician because your son or daughter has been behaving differently, and the doctor has told you that he suspects your child has a mental health disorder, for which treatment, possibly medication, may be necessary. Or you may be wondering whether medication could help your child now that a long-standing problem is worsening and no longer manageable by other means, such as psychotherapy or school services. Maybe you're just beginning to believe something might be wrong with your child, and what you've read about similar problems has left you confused and alarmed.

> **symptom:** A manifestation of a disorder. Cough and fever are symptoms of pneumonia; sadness and low interest are symptoms of depression.

> **disorder:** A condition characterized by a certain number of symptoms that occur at the same time and cause trouble with functioning in everyday living (e.g., an anxiety disorder, a mood disorder).

Remember, regardless of how you have come to this point, you're not alone. More and more people—parents and professionals alike—are realizing the importance of seeking psychiatric treatment for children and the potential benefits of psychiatric medications. The field of child psychiatry is not as young as it was when this book's first edition came out, and every year brings greater awareness and progress.

One of the major challenges is that while doctors look for commonalities, every child's situation is unique, complex, and evolving. A child psychiatrist's foremost role is to conduct a thorough evaluation of the child's problems and to thoughtfully consider a range of available solutions. As we will reinforce throughout this book, you have the right to seek a satisfactory explanation for any decision about your child's case from the doctor who has made that decision. Never be afraid to ask. You should have a good grasp of the conclusions your child's doctor has reached and the rationale that led the doctor to the recommendation before your child embarks on any form of treatment, medication or other. The entire evaluation, diagnosis, and treatment process should be a collaborative effort between you and your child's health care providers. Saying "I'm trying to understand how you came to that conclusion—can you walk me through it?" is one means of ensuring that the process remains collaborative.

In general, it's best to stay as open-minded as possible as you approach the issue of medications for your child. Objective information gathering will help you make the best possible decision. Try not to let fear of the unknown sway you before you tap all the sources of information available. Later in this chapter, we'll go into more detail about when medication generally benefits children and how it works. (For more specific information, consult the chapters in Parts II and III that cover your child's disorder, if it has already been diagnosed, and any medication that has already been recommended.) For now, view medication as one option for helping your child. Be prepared to balance its benefits against both the risks of the medication itself and the risks of *not* using medication.

Why does the pediatrician think my child needs medication?

Let's talk first about the practical reality. The pediatrician is most likely recommending medication because of concern about your child. The recommendation is based on the degree of emotional suffering (sadness, anxiety) seen or described. The doctor might also be recommending medication because your child has not responded to supportive efforts at home or school or to therapy. These are both reasonable considerations as long as the threshold applied to your child is the same as would be applied to another child in the pediatrician's practice. For example, anxiety that is present all day, every day, and is keeping your child from attending school is an appropriate threshold for medication, versus anxiety that is present only once a week, in certain situations. If you're uncertain, ask the pediatrician what he or she considers a severe enough problem to warrant medication. And ask similar questions about the other treatments your child has tried: Was it the right therapy? Did we try it long enough before turning to medication?

> **Always ask your child's pediatrician to explain what problems he considers severe enough to warrant prescribing medication.**

Another rationale for recommending medication would be to treat an underlying biological deficiency or imbalance, such as a low level of a brain chemical needed for healthy energy and mood. We hope that as our knowledge of child emotional health matures we'll be able to identify the specific causes of emotional and behavioral disorders in youth. Unfortunately, while we suspect a biological deficiency underlies emotional illness for many children, at present there is no blood test or brain scan to prove a medical etiology for a child's psychiatric disorder. In the absence of such testing we look for other evidence, and one place to look is in the family. If many members of a child's extended family have similar problems, the condition may have a medical etiology due to a genetic abnormality—that is, it might be a disorder passed down along generations. From a medical standpoint you can consider this evidence of an inherited problem.

Let's say your 10-year-old daughter has developed some unusual repetitive hand-washing rituals. As you talk about your concerns at a family birthday party, you're surprised to hear about a grandparent, an uncle, and several cousins in your family with "OCD" (obsessive–compulsive disorder). This "family loading" of a psychiatric condition increases the chance that your daughter's rituals will continue and develop into a full disorder because of an inherited condition. Compare this to your neighbor's child, who had a similar period of heightened focus on hand washing, without any family history, and it just passed without concern.

> **etiology:** The cause of a disorder, such as an abnormal gene that leads to an abnormal transmission of a brain chemical.

Attention-deficit/hyperactivity disorder (ADHD) is another well-known example of a psychiatric disorder that runs in families. Scientists believe that the impulsivity, short attention span, and other symptoms associated with ADHD are caused by a specific, inherited problem in the brain. Ongoing research is investigating the very specific pathophysiology of childhood mental health disorders like ADHD. Much of the attention is on the processes by which chemical messages are passed between nerve cells (neurons) in the brain. Possibilities include abnormally low levels of brain chemicals being produced in a neuron, so the message needed to control focus or to ignore environmental distractions is not sent to the next neuron, or dysfunctional receptors in a receiving neuron so the message is not received.

> **pathophysiology:** The actual disturbances in the body organs or brain (such as problems with neurochemicals in a specific area of the brain).

Even if a disorder has a medical or biological cause, such as abnormal brain messaging, the onset as well as the degree of any given child's problems may depend on environmental factors. Factors in a child's environment typically involve home and/or school stressors. In the case of 7-year-old Molly—whose parents both suffered from depression—feelings of sadness, isolation, and withdrawal began after the death of her grandmother, continued for 8 months, and were accompanied by failing at school and social withdrawal. We suspected that the stress of losing her grandmother had triggered in Molly a major depressive episode stemming from a biological predisposition (i.e., genetic risk) toward mood disorders.

Similarly, 12-year-old Joy had become withdrawn, apathetic, and listless for many months following her dog's death. A tendency toward depression that she may have inherited from her mother appeared to be activated by the trauma of losing her beloved pet. Joy's withdrawal from family and friends only served to increase the environmental impact on her psychological health by removing needed support.

Fascinating research suggests that environmental factors such as the loss of a loved relative (or pet) can cause brain changes that may be similar to inborn abnormalities. Medications may help to correct abnormal brain functioning regardless of the cause, inherited or environmental or, most likely, a mixture of the two.

We hope to offer more certainty about the causes of psychiatric disorders in the years to come, but at present your child's pediatrician is most likely basing his recommendation for medication on the perceived degree of suffering and/or lack of response to other treatments. In the future doctors may be able to prescribe a medication specifically targeting the known medical cause of your child's disorder, perhaps based on a blood test or a certain type of brain imaging.

> **pervasive:** Occurring across many settings, such as anxiety at school, at home, and at baseball practice.

It's also possible, however, that increased knowledge about the causes of psychiatric problems in the future could support recommendations for nonmedical treatments. For example, a brain abnormality could be found that indicated a need for a treatment other than medication, such as a certain type of therapy or nutritional supplement.

> **dysfunction:** The state of not working properly, such as not performing up to potential at school or having conflicts with friends or family.

Are there other options besides medication?

Yes, there is a wide range of nonmedical treatments. One primary form of nonmedication treatment is psychotherapy. Psychotherapy (informally called "therapy") is often an appropriate starting point for the treatment of mental health problems in children when the distress or impact on a child's day-to-day functioning is relatively mild. Many forms of therapy exist, so your child's practitioner should prescribe a *specific type* of therapy. Check the chapter in Part II that addresses your child's problem for more specific information on treatment choices.

These days, some child psychiatrists provide therapy alone or in combination with prescribing medication. This model of psychiatric care is typically found in "private practice." Commonly in private practice you pay the psychiatrist outside of insurance, meaning you pay the full cost of the session, not simply a copay. Some insurance plans may allow you to submit the bill, however, and you may be reimbursed for some portion of the session's cost. Appointments are typically 45–50 minutes long and can occur weekly, monthly, or less frequently.

In comparison, in a clinic setting, medications are usually prescribed by a psychiatrist and therapy is conducted separately by a psychologist, social

> **therapy:** An umbrella term that covers the broad range of "talking" therapies.

worker, or other mental health professional. Appointments with the psychiatrist are typically 15–30 minutes long and occur monthly or less frequently. These appointments are billed to your insurance, with you being responsible only for copays.

The many varied forms of therapy available for children and families include:

> **pharmacotherapy:** Treatment of a condition using medications.

- Interpersonal and dynamic-oriented therapies
- Social skills training
- Family therapy
- Cognitive-behavioral approaches

Regardless of the type, it's always important to understand and help to define the specific goals of therapy for your child. Therapies tackle the core issues of psychiatric disorders as well as the secondary effects.

> Any therapy or medication should be prescribed with specific goals in mind.

For example, a therapy may aim to improve a depressed child's way of thinking about himself and his future, help a child with Tourette's disorder lessen disruptive shouting out (i.e., tics), or teach a teenage girl with an eating disorder to regain the proper perspective on the role of food in her life. Jason, a 13-year-old with ADHD, had very few friends at school and fought with his siblings at home. Over time Jason improved his ability to be patient and a better listener in a form of therapy called social skills training. While not "cured," his impulsivity became more under his control. Family therapy, involving a fair amount of education for Jason's siblings and attention to consistency in his parents' parenting approaches, led to a calmer, less reactive household. Therapy and medications together may have a very powerful additive, long-lasting effect as compared to either treatment alone, but success depends on using the right kind of therapy and medication for the disorder and the specific, unique needs of the child, and often the family too.

Working with children and families in therapy provides the opportunity to move back and forth between what may be the central, initial "cause" of the family strain (e.g., a rageful depressed teen) and the "effect" on the family (e.g., parents yelling back or avoiding the teen).

Specific styles of parenting often develop partly in reaction to the hardwired personality (temperament) of a child, and those parenting styles may in turn affect the child's development. Therefore it's difficult to disentangle whether the child is acting a certain way based on a particular parenting style or whether the parent is reacting to the child's biologically based problem. In some cases, of course, the rageful depressed teen is reacting to parents who are highly conflicted and avoidant themselves.

A clear-cut case of confusion between cause and effect involved a 14-year-old girl whose severe OCD continued to keep the family awake at night despite 6 months of family therapy. Emily spent every night checking to be sure that doors were not left ajar and that all of the electrical plugs were pulled out of the outlets. The family felt frustrated and hopeless, and the therapist hypothesized that the family's anger was the cause of Emily's unusual behaviors. While her treaters were well intentioned, the problem began with a hasty discussion between parents and primary-care doctor and led to the wrong type of family referral. The inappropriate therapy referral led to the wrong therapeutic approach. Fortunately the therapist recognized this over time and referred the family to child psychiatry. After 1 month of medication, Emily's compulsive and ritualistic behaviors greatly diminished. Almost immediately, the family reported reduced conflict in the home, as well as improved relationships between the various family members and Emily. As is the case for many of the children we see, the child's emotional or behavioral state greatly disrupts the family, and positive interactions can become scarce. Education and therapy with parents and family members can significantly improve family relationships.

If you're not sure you understand why a certain type of therapy is prescribed, ask the practitioner to list your child's specific needs. Do you concur with the list? If not, review these needs with the doctor; don't hesitate to offer parental insight. Once you and the doctor agree on a list of needs, ask the doctor to outline the therapies that address each need before you agree to pursue one or more of them.

Could my child get better without treatment, medication or otherwise?

The good news is that a number of mental health disorders that affect children can improve with time. Separation anxiety can lessen with time. Children with oppositionality commonly outgrow their argumentative features as they mature. Another common example is ADHD, which is thought to lessen considerably into adulthood in roughly half of the children affected, particularly the hyperactive–impulsive symptoms of the disorder.

However, postponing treatment may lead to future problems born of years of demoralization and poor self-esteem. Justin, for example, had a social anxiety disorder and began avoiding social situations despite wanting friends at the age of 10. When he showed up at the office at age 17, he had so fully isolated himself that despite gains with medication and therapy, he remained socially disconnected and lonely.

In thinking about the natural course of psychiatric problems, the type of problem may be less important than the severity, in terms of predicting which child may get better over time without treatment. Children with more severe problems (or with more than one psychiatric disorder) are more likely to have continued problems without treatment.

You'll find more on this subject in the chapters on specific disorders in Part II, and your child's mental health care providers can tell you what the future may hold for your child.

The pediatrician said it seems my child has two problems and therefore may need two different psychiatric medications—or at least two different types of treatment. Is that common?

Many young people may have two or three different psychiatric disorders. Whether these disorders just happen to run together, as is the case for some children with bipolar disorder and ADHD, or one disorder leads to another, as may happen in children with long-standing OCD who develop depressive symptoms because of demoralization, is unclear. Whatever the suspected cause, the occurrence of two or more disorders together is called comorbidity. A child with depression and anxiety, for example, would be said to have comorbid anxiety and depression.

It's important to keep the possibility of comorbidity in mind because in many children new symptoms or problems surface once the diagnosed disorder is treated successfully. Fourteen-year-old Mike's severe obsessionality was greatly reduced when his OCD was treated with a selective serotonin reuptake inhibitor (SSRI), along with cognitive-behavioral therapy, but his academic problems continued. As it turned out, those problems were caused by inattention and distractibility related to ADHD, which had gone undiagnosed because of the severity of his OCD. The addition of a stimulant medication for the ADHD proved very effective, while not causing an increase in anxiety.

If you suspect that your child has more than one problem, be prepared to describe all the specific symptoms for the practitioner who ends up doing the evaluation. By carefully asking questions about common behavioral and emotional disorders in children, your child's doctor can disentangle the overlap of symptoms to make sense of your child's condition. Some commonly co-occurring conditions include:

- Depression and anxiety
- Substance abuse and depression
- Bipolar disorder and ADHD
- Tourette's disorder and ADHD

> **substance abuse:** A pattern of misuse of drugs or alcohol generally resulting in interpersonal, occupational, legal, or medical problems.

Won't medications just mask the underlying problem?

This concern is perfectly logical. Just as we wouldn't simply reduce a child's high fever with medication without treating the underlying illness (such as an ear infection), we would want psychotropic medications to treat the underlying mental illness, not just the symptoms. Unfortunately, we cannot yet identify the medical disturbance associated with most psychiatric disorders with certainty.

> **psychotropics:** Agents that affect the central nervous system, resulting in changes in thinking, behavior, or emotion. Synonymous with psychopharmacological and psychoactive agents.

Therefore, in general, we see medications as lessening the severity of disabling and distressing psychiatric symptoms. Another way to think about this, from an opposing viewpoint, is that medications may actually unmask the child's strengths and abilities. With less intensity to her sadness after 4 weeks on an antidepressant, Jane started to tackle some conflicts with her 11th-grade friends, and her interpersonal warmth returned her "to the kind and now more resilient Jane," said her mother. When effective, medication can provide the support needed for a child to make gains in coping, academic, organizational, and other skills.

Exactly how effective are these medications?

Psychiatric medications for children vary in effectiveness. Roughly 40–70% of children will respond favorably to medications for ADHD, anxiety, and depression. That is quite a range, and it's disappointing to know that some medications may not provide a 50% response rate. Yet this is a very rough summary estimate, with the additional caveat that the bulk of the literature regarding response involves short-term improvement (e.g., 6–12 weeks) in treatment studies. This response rate can be compared to how many children respond to a placebo. A placebo is an inactive substance given in treatment studies to provide a comparison to the actual medication. The presence of a placebo helps to determine whether the response is due to the medication or to the idea of taking a medication. In general, placebo response rates vary from 20 to 50%, with lower placebo response in ADHD studies and higher placebo response in depression studies.

The most consistently effective medications for children are stimulant-class medications for ADHD, with a response rate that may approach 75% of children (and a far lower placebo response rate as stated). Anxiety medications such as SSRIs may be nearly as effective as these ADHD medications; however, the SSRIs yield a lower response rate for depression, closer to 50–60%. Interestingly, placebo response rates for childhood depression studies are relatively high, in the range of 40–60%. In part, this makes it difficult for the medication to be proven superior. However, when medications for anxiety and depression are given in combination with specialized therapies, like cognitive-behavioral therapy, the response rate improves significantly and is typically clearly superior to placebo.

One final group of medications is worthy of note, the

> **SSRI:** A medication named for its action—a selective serotonin reuptake inhibitor. This class of medication has evidence supporting its use in depression and anxiety disorders in children.

> **cognitive-behavioral therapy (CBT):** Treatment in which the therapist is actively involved in helping the child face problems such as anxiety or depression. Research evidence supports the use of this type of therapy for depression and anxiety disorders in children, including alongside SSRI medications.

newer-generation "atypical" antipsychotics. Originally developed as new and improved medications for psychosis (as compared to the older "typical" antipsychotics), these medications have been shown to be highly effective for symptoms of aggression in bipolar disorder and in autism. Their impact on the depressive phase of bipolar disorder or other aspects of autism is less robust. See Part III of this book for more details on specific medications.

> **stimulants:** A class of medications—including methylphenidate (e.g., Ritalin) and amphetamines (e.g., Dexedrine, Adderall)—thought to activate select areas of the central nervous system involved in attention and behavioral control in order to treat ADHD.

How do the medications work?

Scientists have learned a lot over many years about how certain brain regions, shown in Figure 1, are involved in our emotional experience, our thinking (cognitive functions), and our movement (motor functions).

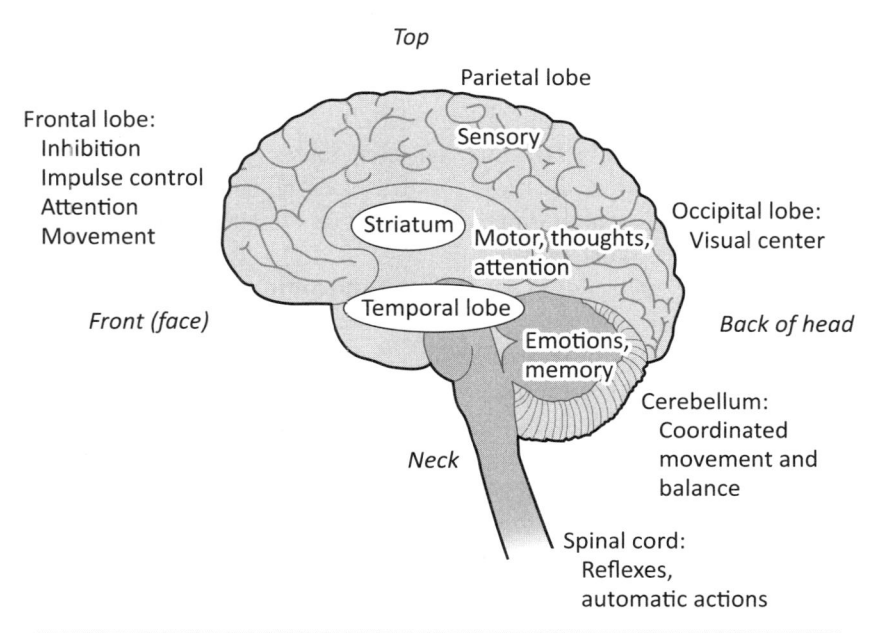

Figure 1. Brain areas relevant to neuropsychiatry disorders.

> **cognitive functions:** Activities related to the ability to take in and process information, reason, memorize, learn, and communicate.

> **motor functions:** Activities related to the ability to move.

Much of our emotional processing occurs deep in the brain, in the region referred to collectively as the *limbic structures*. Disturbances in attention or impulse control appear to be located to some degree within the frontal lobes. Another important structure in the brain, called the *striatum*, is critical to attention and reward. Such discoveries have guided researchers in where to look further for causes of psychiatric disorders.

Ongoing research is trying to determine what types of dysfunction in certain brain regions could be resulting in psychiatric symptoms in children (as well as in adults), and a lot of attention has been paid to the transmission of chemical messages. Studies have found, however, that what may be most critical is how these brain regions are connected. For example, symptoms of ADHD may be caused by problems in the front areas of the brain, or they may result from a brain chemical "signal" not being generated by another brain region as it is supposed to be, and/or not being transmitted correctly to the frontal region. Picture your flight from New York to Los Angeles arriving late. This could have happened because of problems in New York, Los Angeles, or anywhere along the route. The end result is that you were late.

This type of understanding has contributed greatly to theories about how particular medications (or classes of medications) exert their effects on certain symptoms and certain whole syndromes. But we have a long way to go. Most research is still at the level of studying dozens of children, looking for average differences or patterns of differences in those with psychiatric problems compared to those without such problems. So investigations continue into how brain structure (size of a brain region), brain function

> **syndrome:** A group of related symptoms and other objective findings. Posttraumatic stress syndrome, for example, is a group of symptoms that have been observed in people who have suffered a significant trauma.

(how that region works), and brain connections (how that region connects with other regions) may be related to response to medications.

Brain regions function and communicate with each other through nerve connections called *synapses*. The synapse is composed of three basic parts, illustrated in Figure 2: (1) the nerve cell sending the chemical signal (presynaptic neuron); (2) the channel between the nerve cells (synaptic cleft); and (3) the nerve cell receiving the signal (postsynaptic neuron). Chemical signals, or neurotransmitters, include dopamine, serotonin, norepinephrine, GABA (gamma-aminobutyric acid), and glutamine. The process of neurotransmission goes something like this: A molecule of a neurotransmitter is released from the sending presynaptic neuron, travels across the cleft, and is received by a postsynaptic neuron, which contains receptors, which catch neurotransmitters, sort of like a complicated baseball glove. When the neurotransmitter binds to the biological "baseball glove," the receiving neuron is activated. The neurotransmitter is then taken back up into the presynaptic neuron by a process called *reuptake*. Reuptake serves two major purposes: (1) to reduce the amount of neurotransmitter in the area between the

> **receptor**: A chemical structure on the surface of sending and receiving nerve cells that binds or catches the chemical messengers (neurotransmitters), causing other reactions in the nerve cell.

Drug effects

Stimulants release neurotransmitters

Antidepressants and stimulants block reuptake

Antipsychotics block receptors

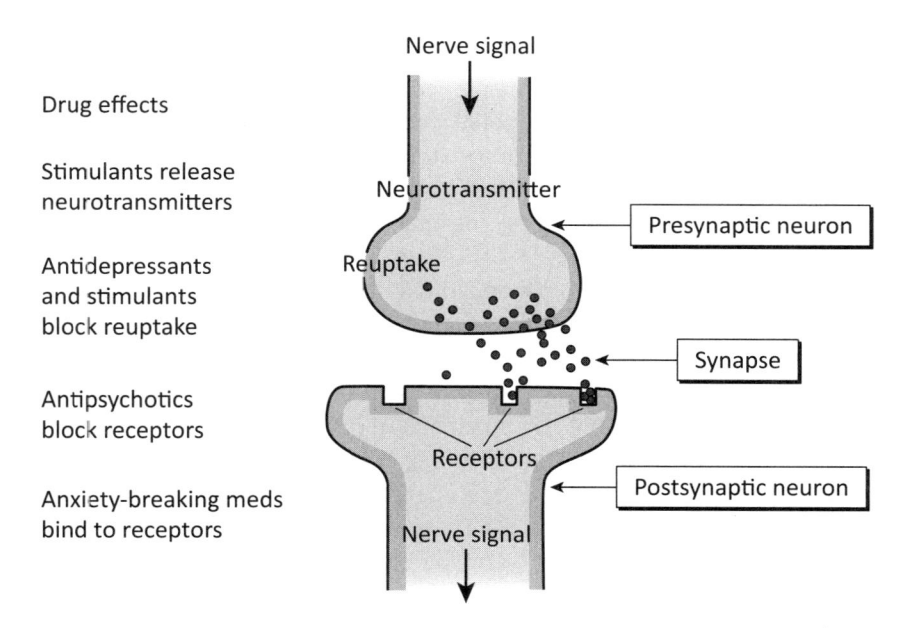

Anxiety-breaking meds bind to receptors

Figure 2. The nerve-to-nerve connection.

nerve cells (synaptic cleft) and (2) to conserve neurotransmitter, as it is broken down and reused. Not surprisingly, the brain is quite an efficient recycling machine!

With that background, we now return to the question: how do medications work? Many emotional and behavioral disorders are thought to be related to disturbances in the flow of neurotransmitters from one cell to another. Low or dysfunctional serotonin, dopamine, and/or norepinephrine activity in specific brain areas is linked to such problems as depression, inattention, and poor impulse control. This is not to suggest that the brain of a given child does not contain any serotonin or dopamine. Instead, the day-to-day amount of these chemicals may be lower than in a psychiatrically healthy child. Or, despite normal levels of neurotransmitters, they do not activate the postsynaptic neuron receptor in a typical manner. There are a host of possibilities for what may be "wrong."

Psychiatric medications can impact brain communication (and function) in many different ways. Some medications increase the release of neurotransmitters (stimulant medications for ADHD, for example) to increase the functioning of a brain area, for example, to increase a child's ability to sustain attention. Other medications (such as antipsychotics for psychosis) block neurotransmitter receptors to decrease an overactive brain area, for example, to decrease hallucinations. SSRI antidepressants block the reuptake of the neurotransmitter. Blocking serotonin reuptake results in a greater amount of the neurotransmitter in the synapse, making more of it available to activate the receiving postsynaptic neuron to increase the functioning of brain areas regulating mood, energy, and sleep.

Recent imaging and biochemistry studies have assisted us in better understanding what neurotransmitter systems are related to the various neuropsychiatric disorders (see Table 1). Anxiety and mood disorders in children appear to involve inadequate or dysfunctional serotonin systems, which may be corrected by SSRI medications. Medications that increase norepinephrine or dopamine are the most effective for the treatment of ADHD.

> neuropsychiatric: Related to the interface of psychiatry and neurology; referring to the set of mental operations that are related to both thinking/emotional states and neurological operations.

Unfortunately, the pharmacology is not as simple as it sounds. Not only is

Table 1. Brain Regions and Neurotransmitters Associated with Various Neuropsychiatric Disorders

Disorder	Neurotransmitter	Region
Alcoholism	GABA, glutamine, opioid system	Global, frontal lobes
Anxiety	Norepinephrine, GABA, dopamine	Amygdala, hippocampus
Attention-deficit/hyperactivity disorder (ADHD)	Dopamine, norepinephrine	Frontal lobe, striatum
Depression	Serotonin, norepinephrine	Frontal lobe, limbic areas
Drug abuse	Dopamine, opioid system, GABA, glutamine	Multiple, hypothalamus, tegmentum
Obsessive–compulsive disorder (OCD)	Serotonin	Striatum, cingulate
Psychosis	Dopamine, serotonin	Frontal lobe, striatum
Tourette's and tic disorders	Dopamine, serotonin	Basal ganglia, frontal lobe

there a large degree of overlap between the various neurotransmitter systems, but certain neurotransmitters may play a role in a number of different psychiatric disorders. To complicate pharmacotherapy further, neurotransmission in a certain brain region may be the cause of psychiatric symptoms but may also be involved in healthy body functions. So when a medication targets that region, it may cause unwanted effects (side effects or adverse effects) while it is alleviating the disorder. The striatum, for example, is the source of hallucinations but also governs movement. Therefore, while an antipsychotic corrects a disturbance in the perception of reality, it may also cause muscle dysfunction. At times doctors will take advantage of side effects, such as prescribing an anxiety medication that reduces anxiety but also causes weight gain or sedation (sleepiness) as a desired side effect in a slight child with significant insomnia.

Exactly how do these medications affect brain structure?

We do not yet know how medications may affect the actual structure of the brain. In other words, we don't know if medications change the size or shape of brain regions. Medications' impact on the function of the brain may be more important, although size and functioning may be related. A child with a small and low-functioning area of the brain responsible for paying attention may suffer from ADHD.

If medications can work so well in treating children with psychiatric problems, why do I hear such conflicting reports?

Conflicting reports abound mainly because child psychiatry and psychopharmacology is still a relatively new science, with a history that dates back only about 30 years. The 1990s, "the decade of the brain," saw a near revolution in thinking about children's psychiatric disorders. Not long before that, children's emotional and behavioral problems were thought to be rooted entirely in disturbed parenting.

> **psychopharmacology:**
> The study of compounds that affect the central nervous system, resulting in changes in thinking, behavior, or emotion.

Findings of genetics, neurobiology, and brain imaging studies began to lead mental health and other medical practitioners toward a new model. Individuals are now viewed as biological beings interacting with the environment, with each factor influencing the other. This perspective has transformed psychiatric views of cause and effect. Now an anxious child is likely to be viewed as having a nervous temperament (biology) that induces those around her to be overprotective (environment), increasing avoidance, limiting development of coping skills, and leading to increased anxiety and dysfunction.

As you will learn in Parts II and III, thanks to clinical research, many medications that had not yet been approved for anyone other than adults when this book was first published have now been approved for use in youth. Research has been stimulated in part by some important federal regulations. Beginning in the late 1990s, the U.S. Food and Drug Administration (FDA) Modernization Act encouraged manufacturers to conduct studies of medications in children. This was an important step in encouraging research on medications that were being used in children despite being initially studied and approved for adult use. In the past decade Congress has continued to support these efforts, including the Best Pharmaceuticals for Children Act and the Pediatric Research Equity Act. These laws now afford the FDA the ability to give incentives and the power to require pediatric assessments, such as safety studies of approved adult medications. For example, a company may be required to study the pediatric safety of a medication that is known to be commonly used in children (let's say an antidepressant approved for adults).

Despite these gains, child psychiatry and psychopharmacology remains a relatively young field. Uncertainty can be accompanied by fear and mistrust. The "case report" or isolated story of a bad outcome for a child remains a powerful influence. It's not unusual for families to come to us saying that a relative, friend, or coworker told them not to seek psychiatric help, and not to give their child medication due to some individual story. It's our job to present the latest understanding of benefit and risk based on the literature and to openly welcome any and all questions from families.

If child psychopharmacology is still fairly new, how can we be sure that medications are safe?

If medications are taken as prescribed, and communication with the doctor is good, psychotropics are considered "safe." However, all medications carry some degree of risk. The more sophisticated response is to say that "safety" means that a given psychiatric medication provides a greater chance of benefit than risk of harm. For example, we may tell a parent that a recommended medication reduces anxiety in 65–75% of children treated, but only 10–20% have side effects that would cause problems and lead to stopping the medication.

Many medications listed in this book have been used in children for over two decades. Some, such as the amphetamine preparations (for ADHD), have been used with children since the 1930s. However, because the use of most psychotropic medications in children is relatively recent, many of these agents have not yet gained FDA approval for pediatric use. Lack of FDA approval does not automatically mean a medication is unsafe for psychiatric use in children. By and large all of the medications used by child psychopharmacologists have FDA-approved indications, but they may be approved for adults and/or for a different condition than the one in question. A medication may have FDA approval for OCD in children but be prescribed for a child with social phobia or generalized anxiety. Or a medication may have FDA approval for a less relevant condition, such as a medication prescribed to a child with ADHD that has been approved for adults with hypertension (the link between ADHD and hypertension has to do with the regulation of adrenaline; reducing adrenaline lessens hyperactivity and decreases blood pressure).

> Parents—not children or teens—should always be responsible for safely storing children's medication.

We have more to say about safety of medications suggested for your child in Chapter 3.

In the meantime, the greatest danger of medications is an overdose. Although children with certain disorders such as depression are at risk for harming themselves, the bulk of lethal overdoses are accidental and occur in family members or friends, such as when a younger sibling thinks the medication is candy. It's important to remember that medications that are safe in daily administration can be very dangerous in overdose. That is why you have to designate a special storage place (locked cabinet) and policy for your child's medication. And remember: Parents or legal guardians—not children—should be responsible at all times for the medications.

What about all of the press on the use of medications in younger kids?

Considerable concern has been raised about the use of psychotropic medications in children, based on reports of increased medication use, including in preschoolers. Many parents are naturally alarmed by such reports when they provide little or no explanation for this practice. Over the years, a more balanced view of medication usage, including in young children, has emerged, based on the understanding that both overtreatment and undertreatment can be occurring at the same time. Or it may be that increased use of medication reflects increased detection of psychiatric illness in children.

We are identifying psychiatric problems earlier, thanks to refined evaluation and diagnostic methods. Therefore we are treating them earlier. But we are also treating them more intensively, because the earlier a problem emerges in childhood, the more serious and impairing the problem may be. Few in medicine would advocate that severe problems be left untreated without an intervention. For example, no one would consider allowing a preschooler with another brain-based disorder, such as seizures, to go untreated.

It's becoming clear to mental health researchers and clinicians that the earlier we intervene, the better off patients may be as they grow up (exhibiting improved self-esteem and less substance abuse, for instance). This is the principle on which we operate when considering prescribing medication to a younger child. It's also important to note that early treatment does not necessarily mean longer treatment. In theory, early intervention may shorten the course of medication and/or therapy that would be needed for an older child or teen who had suffered the harm of being untreated for a longer period.

> **We prescribe medication for younger children when there is reason to believe that early intervention will protect them from developing secondary problems like low self-esteem later.**

What do we know about the effects these medications might have on our child years later?

Unfortunately, children have not been taking these medications long enough for us to have much data on long-term effects. Concerns about the effects of medication on physical growth, the heart, and cognition are valid, as is the worry about the risk of dependence. Each of these concerns is quite difficult to study and requires public and political support to prioritize research funding.

Consider the challenge in trying to determine the influence of a medication on one growing child, in isolation from the complex array of genetic and environmental influences he carries with him. For example, how could we determine that a medication for ADHD taken by a boy who is currently relatively short for his age will affect his eventual height when he doesn't take the medication every day, the dose changes at times, his diet is variable, and his parents are not tall? You would need a very large number of children, half taking medication and half not, with a tremendous amount of detail about all the possible influences on height and with absolute confidence that you could monitor the medication exposure. Then you would need to follow them through development. Rest assured, just because this is daunting does not mean the research community has given up on answering these important questions.

For now, as a parent who will be responsible for the everyday monitoring of your child while she is on medication, it's important to recognize that some side effects are inevitable because of the way our current medications work in the brain. As explained on page 25, we have not yet reached the point where we can isolate a drug's action so that it affects only the targeted function within a brain region or the targeted molecules in certain neurotransmitters. Thus long-term side effects may be due to the medication's intended (less irritability) or unintended (weight gain) actions. You will need to be prepared to monitor your child closely for any side effects, short or long term, and discuss them with the child's practitioner.

> **neurotransmitters:** Chemical messengers that are the main communications link between nerve cells.

Aren't psychiatric medications addictive?

Addiction and *dependence* are different words with different meanings. We prescribe medications without general concern that children will become *addicted*. We do not expect that a child will get a "high" from medication or alter her behavior to get more medication. Addiction is most relevant in adolescents receiving controlled substances such as stimulants for ADHD and benzodiazepines for anxiety. Although there is potential for abuse with these medications, the overall risk that a teen will develop an addiction to medication is very small. Your careful management of your child's medication coupled with your ongoing observation will help prevent this problem or help you identify it quickly if it emerges.

> **controlled substances:** Medications categorized by the U.S. Drug Enforcement Administration as potentially addictive.

However, children and adolescents may become *dependent* on the medication, meaning the child does not want to stop the medication for fear that his symptoms will return. Most individuals receiving medications develop a trust that the medication is effective and safe and will help eliminate distressing psychiatric symptoms. We don't want children to feel hopelessly and passively "dependent" on a medication to function. We do want them to depend on themselves, to embrace treatment (including medication if necessary), and to work on handling stressors in their lives.

A poignant example of typical and reasonable dependency is Abigail, a 15-year-old girl who successfully battled substance abuse but still suffered from depression. Treatment with an antidepressant improved Abigail's mood, peer and family relationships, and school performance. She was very concerned her doctor would stop her medications now that she was feeling better. She didn't want to "go back to feeling bad" but was worried about her need for the medication. After a year of being symptom-free, she has done very well after having the medication tapered off slowly. Concerns about reliance on medication are common and can be dealt with by sharing them with your child's doctor. Teenagers can have quite thoughtful, reasonable discussions about their dependence on medications. Embrace this as a wonderful teaching exercise on how people make use of medications in their lives while remaining in or gaining control.

Won't taking medications lead to later drug abuse?

Many parents fear that taking psychotropic medications will predispose their child to taking "street drugs" (illegal drugs such as cocaine) later in childhood or adolescence. However, to date no long-term data support this concern. When such children do develop a later addiction to a street drug, it is likely the underlying disorder (e.g., depression, anxiety, or ADHD) and the environment in which they are involved that place them at greatest risk for addiction. Parents who are using or abusing illegal substances also put their children at risk through genetics as well as poor modeling.

You should also consider the possibility that not being treated for the disorder—optimally or at all—may lead your child to future drug abuse. The demoralization, distressing symptoms, and underachievement that can result from leaving a psychiatric or psychological disturbance untreated are known to place children at risk for later substance abuse. Think of this risk as reminiscent of the well-known medical risk of stroke following untreated hypertension. Although the hypertension may not be life-threatening, poor blood pressure control may show up as serious complications decades later. Similarly, your child's disorder may not seem very severe today, but leaving it untreated can subject your child to an accumulation of harmful secondary effects that may very well put the child at risk for adolescent substance abuse.

If the cause of my child's problems lies in the brain, how is it possible that intelligence isn't affected?

You're right—a child can have serious problems functioning in some areas but still be quite capable in others. Intelligence (i.e., IQ) tests generally measure specific kinds of cognitive aptitudes or capacities and not how well the child actually functions. The brightest child may perform poorly in the classroom or on homework due to symptoms of a psychiatric disorder such as forgetfulness or disorganization or depression.

One very important and very complex aptitude is organization. You may have heard about so-called executive functions in the brain and how psychiatric disorders often come with problems in these areas. Executive functions (think head executive of a company) include critical skills like planning and time management. Without proper executive function, children often have difficulties preparing themselves for the day, starting a homework assignment, allocating proper time for homework or other projects, and sticking with projects.

Executive function problems are commonly seen in children with ADHD and can cause greater problems into the middle school and high school years, when organizational demands increase. Although medications can greatly improve a child's ability to focus, to be less distracted, and to be calmer physically, organizational abilities can remain a problem.

Researchers are trying to build consensus around how to diagnose executive functioning, whether by a pen-and-paper report, a computer task, or other means. In addition, with the awareness that ADHD medications are not entirely effective for these complex cognitive abilities, there is much interest in models of therapy to help develop these skills. These models are based on cognitive-behavioral therapy and therefore include skill development in managing emotions, such as work on increasing one's ability to handle stress and frustrations. Having good emotional control ("emotional self-regulation") may be a very important part of executive functioning. An effective executive (your child) is calm and cool under pressure, thinking about solutions to the problem of his missing homework and how to avoid misplacing it in the future!

We really trust our pediatrician, and we're worried that we'll end up dealing with a new doctor who doesn't inspire our confidence. Can our pediatrician guide us through the whole process?

Assuming she has the authority to prescribe medications, your child's pediatrician (or family practitioner) is qualified to supervise a psychotropic medication trial for your child. (For more on choosing a doctor for your child's diagnostic evaluation, see Chapter 2.) See the box on page 32 for a list of those who can and cannot prescribe.

It's important to understand that the authority to write prescriptions is not the only criterion that qualifies a provider to treat a child for psychiatric disorders. Experience is critical. Many pediatricians are highly experienced and competent to treat a range of psychiatric problems. However, these primary-care clinicians vary widely in their experience and comfort with prescribing medications for mental health conditions in childhood. For children with serious behavioral and emotional problems, referral to a qualified mental health professional may be desirable.

> Parents often confuse child *psychologists,* who usually are involved in diagnostic testing and therapy but are not qualified to prescribe medications, with child *psychiatrists,* who are qualified to diagnose, treat, and prescribe medications.

We understand the difficult reality that many communities have few, if any, child psychiatrists. Increasingly, psychiatric access programs are being set up across the country, connecting pediatricians or groups of pediatric practices with one or more child psychiatrists for phone consultations and/or one-time in-person psychiatric evaluations. The intent is to support ongoing psychiatric care in the pediatrician/primary-care "home" with recommendations based on the phone consultation or in-person psychiatric evaluation.

I have a pretty good idea of what's going on with my child. Should we take him to a clinic that specializes in that type of problem for diagnosis and treatment?

In general, if your child has not had treatment before, it's not necessary to seek out a specialized clinic, which can involve longer waits and

> **Those who can write prescriptions include:**
>
> - Medical doctors (MDs): family practitioners, pediatric medical specialists, pediatricians, child psychiatrists, and child neurologists
> - Doctors of osteopathy (DOs)
> - Nurse practitioners (NPs)
> - Physician assistants (PAs)
>
> **Other mental health providers who *cannot* prescribe medications include:**
>
> - Psychologists, who may have a master's degree (MS or MA) or a doctorate (PhD, DSc, DEd, DPhil)
> - Social workers (BSW, MSW, LICSW, DSW)
> - Counselors, usually required to have a master's or education specialist degree to be licensed

possibly greater cost as well, particularly if it's a private clinic and not hospital based. However, if you're not making progress with a general pediatrician and/or child psychiatrist, it's quite appropriate to ask about specialty physicians or clinics in your area. Seeing a specialist can be a one-time consultation to ensure you are on the right track, that the diagnosis is correct, and the treatment path is consistent with the diagnosis. For some children who have not responded to many treatments, or who have a highly complex combination of problems, ongoing care with a specialist may be necessary.

If your child has not yet been evaluated and diagnosed professionally, however, be aware that these specialty clinics often pop up on an Internet search. This is why many parents ask us whether they are worth seeking out, even if there isn't one anywhere near them. We usually advise them that they might be better off saving their resources for treatment and support than traveling long distances to a specialty clinic. If you suspect your child has ADHD and you take your child to an ADHD clinic, guess what diagnosis you're likely to get. If your child does in fact have ADHD, your pediatrician or a local child psychiatry specialist could diagnose ADHD and prescribe medication, sparing you the travel expenses.

We've already been working with a therapist we all like, who recommends continuing with therapy, but our pediatrician keeps bringing up the fact that medication often helps with our child's particular problems. What should we do?

If you find yourself stuck between differing treatment opinions, you need to seek consensus. Work to understand the difference in viewpoints that may arise from different information getting to each member of the treatment team or may reflect one member's greater experience with the area of concern. Open and honest conversations about this can be very helpful—such as telling the doctor that the therapist has years of expertise with this kind of anxiety problem and has told you that she has seen progress over the last month and expects real improvement in the coming 3 months. Then you could go back to the therapist to say that the doctor understands and appreciates his perspective and suggests a follow-up appointment in 3 months to reconsider medication. You can help pass general information and recommendations between providers, but of course direct conversations are often needed between therapist and doctor in this situation, to develop a clear, mutually agreed-on treatment plan.

Disagreement about the course of treatment can also arise when one of your child's treaters does not have a solid working diagnosis or is approaching the problem from a very different viewpoint. It's quite reasonable and likely quite effective to ask each provider, "What are we aiming to do here? What is my child's main problem, and how do you think we can improve it?" When there is agreement on the diagnosis, everyone can proceed to use the most effective known treatment(s) to ease the problem. Also note that in Part II of this book we tell you which treatments are considered the best first and later choices for specific disorders.

But when there is fundamental disagreement about a diagnosis, understandably the treatment plan will suffer. You can look to a third party, such as a trusted pediatrician, or ask for a consultation to determine which direction to take. There are no easy right answers, but you must pick a path to follow. We recommend focusing on picking the diagnosis that feels most accurate to you. Then the treatment will follow. For example, in the example above, perhaps the therapist sees your child as primarily anxious and the doctor's view is that ADHD is causing the anxiety. Keep it simple and ask yourself, "What is the day-to-day issue my child struggles most with? Is my child basically an anxious child, or is she primarily unfocused?" As you choose practitioners for an evaluation, diagnosis, and treatment, keep your eye on the need to distill simple summary impressions to guide the process. Again, treatment should follow the "right" diagnosis—the one you have the most faith in.

If we start medication, will my child have to take it for the rest of his life?

No one knows how long your child will need a particular medication—or any treatment, for that matter. The only way to determine whether someone still needs medication is to discontinue it and see if the symptoms come back. For many children, it's prudent to reevaluate the need for continued medication following a positive response of 6–12 months, particularly for those with their first psychiatric illness (such as a first episode of depression) and first medication treatment.

Your child's doctor can work with you to decide when it makes sense to consider reducing and stopping the medication. In general, medications are reduced slowly (*tapered*) over a period of weeks if not months while watching for recurrence of the problem. More details can be found on page 121 and in Part III for specific medications.

If my child takes medications, everyone—teachers, relatives, friends—will know something is wrong. Won't this be hard for my son?

First of all, it's your right to share details about your child's medical treatment only on a need-to-know basis. Before you air any aspect of the subject, ask yourself whether this person needs the information to protect your child's well-being. If not, it's certainly reasonable to treat the information as private and confidential: Keep it to yourself. Advances in medications now allow for more discretion. For example, extended-release forms of stimulant medications used to treat ADHD mean that children no longer have to "announce" their problem through regular trips to the nurse's office at school for midday dosing of shorter-acting agents.

If anyone who knows about your child's treatment expresses undue alarm about it, share the information you've gathered about medication's role in treating this type of problem. Knowing that medication is one of the treatments of choice for many childhood psychiatric disorders often reassures people and prevents them from overreacting in ways that will make your child self-conscious.

There are people who will speak of your son's treatment in less than complimentary ways ("*Oh,* Johnny's on medication—*no wonder* he's so impossible"). There are also many people who harbor misconceptions about psychiatric disorders. You can't control other people, but you can go a long way toward protecting your child from the myths and prejudices fueled by ignorance.

Of course, you also need to be aware of any preconceived notions of your own and how they might affect your child. You may find yourself having difficulty accepting the fact that children can have emotional and behavioral problems just like adults, or you may face your child's problems with fear or even guilt. It may be easier to tell yourself that this is not a "true" biological condition, because accepting that notion implies that your child inherited it from you or your family. Yet from our point of view, the inheritance of a psychiatric disorder should not be cause for greater guilt than you'd feel if your child had inherited allergies or any other medical condition.

The most important reason to protect your child from misinformation about psychiatric problems is to make sure he doesn't view the disorder as some sort of personal failing or weakness. Explain, in age-appropriate terms, that he has a problem he can't help having. Say this problem is largely physical in the same way as Aunt Alice's asthma or Daddy's high blood pressure. You may have to offer these reassurances repeatedly. At the same time, try not to imply that the child's condition is something he is stricken with in a passive, helpless way, or that it is a weakness. Again, just as Aunt Alice can do things to help her asthma and Daddy can do things to help manage his blood pressure, your child has an active, powerful role in his own life.

How do I talk to my child about taking medication?

First of all, don't assume your child will have the same concerns that you, her other parent, her teacher, or her coach may have. As long as they haven't been influenced by myths and prejudices imposed by others, children are often the most prepared for and logical about taking psychiatric medications. Increasingly celebrities, from professional athletes to influential business leaders, actors, and politicians, are being open about using psychiatric medications. In addition, medications are becoming more commonplace in books, including children's stories whose main characters are taking medications for psychiatric disorders. A list of some that parents have found helpful is in the Resources at the back of the book. Your child's generation may be far more accepting (and knowledgeable!) about medication than yours.

Despite this remarkable progress, plenty of children resist taking medication, particularly every day. They may have a variety of reasons:

- They don't believe they have a problem requiring medications.
- They may blame teachers, parents, or others for their problems.
- They might not acknowledge a problem with their behavior at all.

If your child seems to deny that a problem exists, try to find some common ground from which to start a frank, nonaccusatory discussion. Capitalize on the moment when the child or teen expresses *any* frustration or pain about *anything* related to the psychiatric condition. Even if the complaint isn't related to your own primary concern about how the disorder is harming your child, it might open the door and get your child thinking about the reality of the situation.

For example, your main concern may be that your daughter looks remarkably sad and disinterested, but she may be most frustrated with her trouble sleeping. You might note that the medication may help with sleep or emphasize the relationship between sleep and sadness. This is not to suggest that you pass off an antidepressant as merely a "sleeping pill." Dishonesty will certainly lead to longer-term failure, where the child or teen is manipulated only in the short term and refuses to continue treatment over time.

Always couple the concerns with positive comments about the child, acknowledging the child's strengths. Comment that you know how hard your child has been working despite, or in the face of, the problems. Likewise, you need to keep reminding your child how much you love him. Say that you want to find out what's wrong and have it treated because you care so much. Although you may be angry or frustrated by your child's behavior, he is usually feeling even worse about it. Younger children in particular often harbor unspoken fears of being "different" or "not good enough" and consequently losing your love and approval. Children need your patient support to feel safe being honest about their problems.

Another excellent way to convince children that it's okay to admit to a problem and to get help for it is to offer examples of others who have benefited from treatment. Many children have had a friend or relative, including a parent, who has been treated for some type of psychiatric or psychological problem. Although you should exercise discretion in disclosing others' treatments to your children, by using such examples you can normalize the disorder(s) and make your child understand that there are others with similar problems. Likewise, by pointing out the other person's positive response to treatment, you can help reduce the hopeless and helpless feeling your child may be experiencing.

How do I talk to my teenager about taking medication?

Adolescents may pose unique challenges. Distrust of the parent or guardian or doctor is not uncommon among teens who feel alienated due to their condition and perhaps alienated in general. While teens are searching for independence and identity, they do want to fit in with their peers. Adolescents may be more likely than younger children to be worried that the medication will alter their personality. If your teen brings up an example of a friend who looked "drugged" on medication, comment that her friend may be taking very different medications for very different reasons. Reassure your teen that if such a reaction were to occur, the medication would be discontinued promptly. Medications should help adolescents (and children) feel better, concentrate longer, and be less angry or anxious. Medications should not change anyone's personality. You should contact your child's doctor if your teen (or child) manifests emotional states out of character while on medication.

> Contact your child's doctor if he shows signs of an emotional state that is out of character after starting a particular medication.

Remember, first and foremost, to listen to your teen. You may be surprised by your teen's reason for refusing medication. Julie, a 14-year-old with long-standing depression and anxiety, thought she would have to give up her skepticism toward life if she were started on medication. Although she was quite insightful about her depression and the impairment caused by it, such as having no friends, she felt as though her core image as a cynic would be tarnished if she were on medication. Some teens have been influenced by horror stories from their peers. Angie, a 15-year-old girl with trichotillomania (hair pulling) and OCD, was reluctant to take "drugs" because of concerns she had picked up at school about becoming a drug addict. Fifteen-year-old Samantha stopped taking the medications prescribed for her depression because she did not want to be like her estranged schizophrenic aunt. Seventeen-year-old Todd was so angry at his abusive, alcoholic father that he "wanted nothing to do with" anything his father recommended, including medication that would alleviate Todd's ADHD symptoms.

In cases like these, explore the teen's thoughts about other family members, the teen's problem, and the role of medication. Explain that your child is unique and describe how much her circumstances differ from those of any other family member she is identifying with. To prevent your teen from adopting a victim stance, stress the powers she has over her destiny and the need to work with the treatment to get better. Teenagers respond well to feeling empowered.

Keep in mind that you can inadvertently disempower your teen by using language that seems to take control away from him. Saying, for example, "We need to medicate him" connotes that you're *externally* imposing a medication treatment. It's far better to use language like "Tom chose to see if medication could help him," which supports the teen as an active participant in decisions about his own care. Medication is supposed to support your child's ability to control his own mood or behavior. Helping your teen maintain a sense of *internal* control is critical to self-esteem.

In some cases, it can also be helpful to tell your teen how effective the medications can be, especially if you know that the medication prescribed is considered the first-line treatment for the child or teen's problem.

Aren't medications really expensive?

Yes, medications can be expensive, but the expectation is that public and private insurance plans will offer reasonable prescription packages with reasonable copayments to ensure families can afford psychiatric care. Copayments for medication range widely but can be affordable, particularly when generic alternatives are available. Increasingly, 3-month prescriptions are available at a cost savings. This can be a helpful option once your child's medication dose is stable.

While some children require a brand-name medication, many children can receive similar benefit and tolerability with generic medications. It's important to keep track of changes in your child's medication, noting whether it is a generic or a brand name. If the pharmacy substitutes one generic medication for another in a given month, keep a log of this, so you can inform the doctor about any changes in your child's response or in side effects. The documentation of problems (i.e., lack of response or side effects) with a generic medication may result in your insurance company authorizing a newer or brand-name medication.

If you were to purchase the medication without insurance, it could cost in the range of hundreds of dollars per month. On average, it takes many years to study a medication in the laboratory and to test it in humans before a pharmaceutical company can bring it to market for public use. Current estimates are that it takes a staggering several billion dollars to take a medication all the way through this process. Companies then have a certain amount of time to sell the medication, to make back that money and to make a profit before other companies are allowed to copy it, as a generic substitution. Thus the high price of a new medication.

Where else can I find information about medications?

Important information is now easier to find. The American Academy of Child and Adolescent Psychiatry (AACAP) has a very comprehensive website, with information about psychiatric disorders and medications. In addition, just in this decade, the FDA has directed pharmaceutical companies to improve the information provided to consumers in the package inserts that come with prescription medications and in medication summary handouts. Safety warnings are more clear and easily identified than in the past. If you have any questions about information accompanying a medication prescription, ask your pharmacist as well as your child's doctor/prescriber about them.

As you read the rest of Part I of this book, you'll find more detail about what should be factored into the decision-making process. We can't emphasize enough how critical it is that you obtain the answers to your questions so you feel sure that a particular medication is the best option for your child. You should always start out with a clear understanding of what your child stands to gain:

- Which symptoms is this medication likely to ease or eliminate?
- Which is it unlikely to address?
- How long will it take for benefits to appear?
- Is this medication likely to treat the symptoms sufficiently on its own, or will more than one medication be needed? Why?
- Is this the best medication for the circumstances?
- Does your child have any preexisting conditions that would make this treatment a risk?
- What side effects occur soon after treatment, and which ones do you have to worry about occurring in the long term?
- Has any new research evidence been reported on this medication?

Before your child starts taking a medication, be sure you know the warning signs that warrant a call to the doctor and which signs should be considered emergencies. Package inserts list most likely side effects as well as other, less frequent yet concerning side effects. When you leave the doctor's office, you should have not just a prescription but also an understanding of what predictable side effects may occur and what more serious, albeit rare, ones you should know about.

> Before your child starts a medication, be sure you know the signs of adverse effects—and which ones warrant a call to the doctor versus a trip to the emergency room.

2

The Psychopharmacology Evaluation

Finding Out What's Wrong

Surgeons don't operate without having a good idea of what is wrong with their patients, and mental health professionals should not prescribe medication or suggest any other treatment until they have a handle on your child's psychiatric problems either. The only way to come to treatment recommendations is to begin with a thorough professional psychiatric evaluation of the child.

If your child is referred to a psychiatrist for an overall psychiatric evaluation, you can expect a comprehensive assessment and treatment recommendations, which may include medication, therapy, school supports, or even simply education and reassurance. Your child could also be referred to a psychiatrist specifically for a psychopharmacology evaluation, either because the child is exhibiting symptoms that may respond to medication or because a specific type of expertise on the psychiatrist's part seems likely to shed new light on a tough problem to diagnose and treat.

For example, your child's pediatrician may refer your child to a general child psychiatrist, asking for a "psychopharm eval" and saying, "This is a child who is well known to me, healthy, without significant home stressors, who has ADHD and no other problems, who responds very well to stimulants—but they all seem to suppress his appetite; any ideas would be appreciated." Such an evaluation may be centered primarily on ADHD and medications for that disorder, and the psychiatrist may have greater experience in ADHD than a pediatrician yet be fairly typical for child psychiatry. On the other hand, a child with ADHD, depression, tics, and OCD may be referred to a child psychiatrist known to specialize in psychopharmacology who has taught courses on psychopharmacology and done clinical research on new medications. In this latter case, the child with a very complex combination of problems may have already been seen by a pediatrician and a "general" child psychiatrist and referred to a psychiatry specialist because of lack of treatment response.

While both referrals may be considered "psychopharm" referrals, the evaluator's level of expertise varies. In addition, although each case is centered on a request for an assessment for medication, you can expect the evaluating doctor to be able to address questions related to a broad treatment plan. Either doctor in the scenarios above might conclude that a specific therapy is the critical missing element in the child's treatment, not a change in medication.

You may not need all the information in this chapter, but we've attempted to answer all the questions that parents ask us most frequently. These run the gamut from "How do we find the best doctor for an evaluation?" and "What does an evaluation involve?" to "How can we prepare our child for the evaluation?" and "What kind of conclusions should we expect?"

As parents, you're in a position to supply much of the information that an evaluation will take into account, so it's crucial that you provide the history requested. However, the evaluation is also a good place to start gathering expert information. Think of the evaluation as the beginning of your active collaboration with your child's mental health practitioners. We clinicians need you to provide clear and accurate information. You, the parent or guardian, benefit from our ability to make sense of that information, to bring it together into a "formulation" or summary of our clinical impressions.

The end result of a psychiatric evaluation is an initial diagnostic impression. An evaluation is often couched in the words *initial* and *impression* because diagnoses can evolve over time and there is no blood or brain test (yet!) to enable us to be certain. Yet you're free to ask the doctor to share her degree of confidence in the diagnosis. For example, a doctor might say, "From what you describe, Tim appears to have a very typical presentation of ADHD, and I don't see any evidence of a learning disability or other psychiatric problem . . . I'm confident in this diagnosis." In another case a doctor might say something like this: "Molly has sad and angry moods that are most consistent with depression, but a different kind of mood problem, bipolar disorder, remains a possibility... I'd like to speak to her therapist and see you back in a week to continue our evaluation."

A diagnostic evaluation typically takes place in one session, but it's not unusual for doctors to continue the assessment over subsequent visits before offering treatment recommendations. The doctor should then remain alert for new symptoms or other information over months or years of working with you and your child and be open to making changes in the diagnosis.

What should we look for in a doctor to evaluate our child?

Naturally you want a doctor who has the best credentials and experience. Don't be afraid to ask any prospective health care provider about her background. Professionals to whom you're entrusting your child's diagnosis and care should be more than willing to tell you about their qualifications. The following questions can help you get a synopsis of the professional's philosophy, training, and experience:

- "What is your training [medical school, residency, fellowship]?" This will clarify that the doctor is a psychiatrist—a medical doctor (MD)—not a doctor of psychology, or psychologist (PhD). Psychiatrists can prescribe medications.
- "Are you specifically a child and adolescent psychiatrist?" This will clarify that the doctor completed specialized training in child psychiatry after adult psychiatry. Some adult-trained psychiatrists will treat older teens or see younger children in consultation if child psychiatrists are not available.

In addition to college, American physicians complete 4 years of medical school and several additional years of residency training in their chosen field. Child psychiatrists typically have completed 3–4 years of adult psychiatry training during residency, followed by a 2-year specialized fellowship in child and adolescent psychiatry. Following completion of training, many doctors will take an intensive test created by the American Board of Psychiatry and Neurology to become "board certified." The national board test is intended to promote excellence in practice by testing doctors' specialized skills and knowledge. Passing the board is only one measure of a doctor's knowledge of the field. Inquiring about board certification may be more helpful if the doctor is not part of an academic or hospital-based clinic, which has its own in-depth process of review. For doctors who practice alone, asking about board certification may be helpful, but a doctor's reputation is likely far more important.

It's not uncommon for children with emotional/behavioral health concerns to be referred to pediatricians, developmental pediatricians, and neurologists in addition to child psychiatrists. Neurologists and pediatricians have completed medical training during residency, while child psychiatrists typically have completed 3–4 years of adult psychiatry training during their residency, followed by a 2-year specialized fellowship training in child and adolescent psychiatry. The younger your doctor is, the more relevant his training may be to how he practices.

Follow-up questions for psychiatrists:

- "How many years have you been in practice?"
- "How many children like my son [or daughter] have you treated before?"
- "Do you have an area of specialization?"

These questions help you understand the range of the doctor's experience in diagnosing and treating children and adolescents. Don't expect to hear that a child psychiatrist you've found has an area of specialization unless the doctor is at a large academic/teaching hospital. In these settings you may encounter doctors with specialization in areas such as ADHD, depression, bipolar disorder, OCD, or autism. Be aware, however, that "specialization" may have a couple of different meanings: The doctor may simply choose to treat primarily children with a certain disorder. Or specialization may mean the doctor has clinical, research, and teaching experience as a true local or even national expert in a certain disorder.

Seeking out a specialist is likely more important for a child who has not responded to standard treatments and may often occur at the urging of a general child psychiatrist. For example, the child psychiatrist you are seeing may say that one-fourth of his practice is teens with depression and recommend you go see a colleague whose practice is primarily adolescents with mood disorders. However, how long the doctor has been working factors into this equation as well.

> Be aware that some states, such as the Commonwealth of Massachusetts, allow patients access to doctors' license status and complaints lodged with the state medical board, including medical malpractice cases filed against a physician. If you want this information, contact your state's medical board or division of consumer affairs.

Now that you have a sense of the doctor's background, you can inquire about clinical experience in more detail:

- "What does your treatment plan typically look like?"

Evangelical or closed-minded responses about the doctor's preferred treatments should raise a red flag. Remember, medical practice is based on science and not philosophy or immutable beliefs. While there is room for individualism, you will benefit from a doctor whose assessment and language reflect mainstream medical knowledge—as this knowledge can then be more readily shared with others, including other medical professionals, as well as educators and others involved in your child's life. Therefore, you would expect the doctor to talk about the importance of education and general supports, such as school services, in addition to specific therapy and medication recommendations.

Even if you find a doctor whose qualifications seem suitable, keep in mind that certain attributes that may be more difficult to ascertain could be the most important aspect of an optimal evaluation (and ongoing care, if the doctor, as is ideal, can keep taking care of your child during treatment):

> A practitioner's thought and decision-making process is every bit as important as, and sometimes more important than, professional credentials and experience.

- Excellent listening skills
- Ability to pull together information into a compelling clinical "story" or diagnosis
- Flexibility in thinking
- Ability to incorporate new information and, when necessary, thoughtfully change treatment course

These attributes might not be easy to identify during preliminary conversations with practitioners you're considering for your child's evaluation, but picture what they might look like in practice. Let's say your child has already been evaluated, received a diagnosis of anxiety, and been prescribed medication. You go to an appointment and are asked about how the past month has been. After listening for 5 minutes or so as you describe how you think your son seems less anxious, the doctor asks a series of questions to get more details: "You said he was less anxious about making it to the bus in the morning—was that every day this week? . . . What do you think, Andy? Did you feel different? . . . What were you thinking as you headed to the bus? . . . About soccer after school or about 'Oh, no, am I going to miss it!?'" This is a nice little interchange that shows the doctor asking about the frequency of symptoms and, by knowing what the child's specific worries are, being able to make some comparisons between the present week on medication and past weeks before medication.

This questioning could naturally be followed by the creation of a clinical story or summary: "Okay, what I hear is that Andy is feeling overall less anxious this week about taking the bus, and you see that too, Mom, but the last 2 days were difficult, with almost as much anxiety as before medication." Then the doctor demonstrates flexibility and the ability to incorporate new information: "Wait a minute, Andy, it was very stormy outside these last 2 days. Does the weather impact how much you fear getting on the bus, as compared to how many kids are on it?" The doctor is considering a shift from thinking about the boy as having social anxiety (with fears that the other kids will look at him, make fun of him on the crowded bus) to thinking of him as having generalized worry (e.g., fears of the weather, of harm to self or loved ones).

A doctor with the capacity for flexibility shows that he can take in new information to fine-tune his understanding of your child. Of course, you can't predict exactly how consultations with a particular doctor will unfold over time, but as noted above, closed-mindedness that's evident during initial interviews might be a sign that you can't expect the appropriate flexibility down the road. As you work with a practitioner, you should have the sense that the doctor continues to fill in the gaps, circling closer and closer to a full sense of your child and her problems. Every visit should build on the last. In this respect it can be fine for the doctor to say, "As we've been talking about Emily's angry, sad mood I keep hearing a lot about impatience and quick temper and restlessness

... It sounds like impulsivity to me ... I think we need to talk more about possible ADHD symptoms. Poor impulse control might be fueling her moodiness and lack of response to the antidepressants."

On the other hand, be wary if every session or week or month brings a brand-new diagnosis and/or plan, without a sense that the doctor is developing a better understanding of your child or can back it up with a clear clinical story. Simplified, this would sound more like "Well, the antidepressant isn't working; it's time to try a mood stabilizer." Why? "Because the antidepressant isn't working, so there must be something else going on." This reasoning lacks detail and a clinical story to back up a shift in plan.

In addition, all treatments should be given a reasonable amount of time to demonstrate benefits before being replaced with something else. Generally speaking, medications require several weeks (e.g., stimulants for ADHD) to 2–3 months (e.g., antidepressants for depression) before a response can be determined. However, often within a month on a medication you have a sense that there is at least some positive change, and that's an indication that it's worth sticking with this medication trial. And, again, the doctor's ability to zero in on an accurate diagnosis and appropriate treatment, even if it takes a little time, is a sign that it's worth sticking with that doctor.

Should we expect the doctor to be able to follow through with treatment?

Once you have a good feel for the doctor's qualifications, philosophy, and way of thinking, you'll want to know if the doctor can follow up on the evaluation by treating your child. Ask:

- "Are you available to treat my child following this evaluation?"
- "If so, for how long, or, until what age?"

Whether the doctor can treat, not just diagnose, your child is a critical question to ask, perhaps even as your initial question. It's not unusual to wait several months for an appointment with a child psychiatrist. Therefore you want to be sure that you know whether the doctor is conducting only consultative evaluations or has room in her practice for ongoing care. This is a very appropriate question to ask at the time of initial scheduling. You don't have to wait until you see the doctor to know if this doctor has room in her practice to continue to treat your child following the evaluation.

If this practitioner is going to treat your child, you might want to ask about the doctor's hospital affiliations even though most children will not require psychiatric hospitalization. This affiliation may help in establishing trust in the inpatient team and greatly foster communication with your doctor should your child ever need hospitalization. Given the shortage of inpatient psychiatric beds, even with affiliations, children often are admitted to whatever unit has availability.

Our pediatrician's group now includes several nurse practitioners, and when we inquired about having our child evaluated for behavioral problems, we were advised to see one of them. Are these professionals qualified to perform an evaluation?

The nurse practitioner (NP) role originated during the 1950s and 1960s as one means of trying to address the shortage of physicians and address health care costs. The number of NPs in this country has risen steadily since the beginning of the 21st century, with numbers approaching 200,000 as of 2014. A nurse practitioner's training includes a college degree (bachelor's) in nursing, followed by a master's or doctoral degree program (Doctor of Nursing Practice; DNP) and additional specialized clinical training. The majority of NPs are training in primary-care programs, so it may become increasingly commonplace to have regular medical as well as behavioral health appointments with an NP. As noted in Chapter 1, nurse practitioners can prescribe medication, so they can follow through on your child's treatment after an evaluation.

NPs are also helping to fill the gap in available child psychiatry physicians. Your child may very well be referred to one. As with doctors, experience and competence vary, so ask similar questions to those listed above to determine whether a particular NP is the right professional to evaluate your child. Nurse practitioners may work independently or in collaboration with psychiatrists, prescribing all classes of medication; guidelines may vary by state. In Massachusetts, for example, Advanced Practice Registered Nursing (APRN) prescriptions for medications must contain the name of the NP's supervising psychiatrist, and it would be appropriate to ask for that doctor's name and to inquire about her experience as well.

Our doctor's office includes a lot of other staff. What can we expect them all to do?

In addition to the doctor—whether a pediatrician or a mental health specialist—it's useful to know what role is played by others in the prescriber's office, because in many cases these staff members will be valuable sources of information and even your primary contacts. In a growing number of medical practices, a psychologist, social worker, or nurse works with a prescribing practitioner. In these settings, the psychologist's role may include diagnostic assessments, treatment planning, and progress monitoring. A psychologist may serve as an important medication consultant with the physician. You might also end up working closely with a nurse during a medication trial. Nurses are often equipped to talk with you about what side effects to expect and what constitutes a response to the treatment. The nurse may also be checking the child's blood pressure as well as ordering or performing blood tests, depending on the medication. In this scenario, the nurse would be a good contact person if questions or problems arose during the treatment.

For ease in care delivery, whenever possible, try to consolidate your child's care in one setting, particularly if your child has multiple medical and psychiatric problems necessitating multiple treaters and medications. At the very least, try to use providers who have worked together in the past. It's very helpful when the treatment team shares the same philosophy and overall approach to treating psychiatric disorders in children and adolescents. When there are differences in perception between caregivers, stay focused on doing what's best for your child. Consensus among treaters is critical.

> **Knowing the "cast of characters" at any prospective evaluator's office is important since many of these staff members may play crucial roles in your child's care if this doctor will also be treating your child.**

What can I expect from a psychiatric evaluation?

Table 2 shows the different types of assessments that can be involved in a full psychiatric evaluation.

1. **The psychiatric history.** The basic psychiatric assessment involves a careful psychiatric history taken by the practitioner during a

Table 2. Elements of the Psychopharmacology Evaluation Process

Test	Reason
Family evaluation (with a social worker)	To determine what family dynamics, if any, may be contributing to the child's problem; may suggest having a family behavioral modification therapist involved in case
Psychosocial and school assessment (teacher or guidance counselor)	To assess child's peer functioning, determine academic and behavioral performance at school
Psychological testing (with a psychologist)	A broad group of tests that assess the child's emotional and cognitive (thinking) functioning; suggested if there are learning problems not attributable to a psychiatric disorder
Neuropsychological testing (with a psychologist)	Extensive and specific tests to evaluate a child's thinking or information-processing abilities
Structured interviews (varied)	Detailed questions about your child's history; available only at certain clinics
Medical assessment (pediatrician)	Physical examination, questions about medical health (e.g., heart, neurology), and laboratory studies; suggested prior to using medications and when there are concerns about a medical contribution to the disorder
Medication evaluation (medical personnel)	Thorough history of the child and his or her current and past emotional and behavioral problems; review of above

Note. This table presents potential assessments for children with behavioral and emotional disorders. The evaluation process varies greatly, depending on the region of the country, the type of practice, and the circumstances of the child.

1- to 2-hour face-to-face interview. The health care provider will elicit a thorough description of the current problems as well as information on any previous treatments your child has undergone for this problem. A thorough history will not, however, be limited to the primary concern—or "chief complaint" in doctorspeak—that brought you in. It will also include at least some basic "screening" questions about a range of other common psychiatric problems. For example, even though you may be convinced that your child has anxiety, the doctor should inquire about other areas too, such as depression and school or learning problems.

> **Asking questions about problems that don't seem to be affecting your child is an important part of the screening process by which the evaluator starts to rule out certain problems and zero in on an accurate diagnosis.**

Of particular interest are your child's prior psychiatric or psychological treatments, including successes and failures in therapy as well as medications prescribed. Details here are paramount. To prepare for this evaluation, think carefully about:

- Why you consulted the prior treater
- The diagnosis or impression given
- The recommendations made
- The specific form of treatment provided
- The skills or strategies developed during therapy
- How well your child connected with the therapist

When to Seek Help

Seek a professional evaluation when your child exhibits any of the following symptoms:

- Self-harm or suicidality
- Threats of serious harm to others
- Severe outbursts
- Social withdrawal or isolation
- Substance abuse (alcohol, marijuana)
- Bingeing (eating excessive amounts) and/or purging (vomiting)
- Weight loss with no medical cause
- Auditory or visual hallucinations (hearing or seeing things that are not there)

The bottom line: What worked and what didn't work? Sometimes, for instance, children connect better with a therapist who is young or one who is older, with either a female or a male. Therapists should be committed to success for your child, which might mean acknowledging that it's not a good fit. This thoughtfulness can turn a disappointment into a learning opportunity, providing you with perspective that can help you make the most of future doctor–patient relationships for your child.

2. **The medication history.** For medication history, details are similarly critical. Be prepared to be asked for:

- The name of each medication your child has been on
- The starting dose and maximum dose reached
- The duration of the treatment
- The changes in dosage and intervals
- Your child's response, including other factors that could have affected the response at the time—either positive or negative stressors
- Side effects, in detail, including their relation to the dose, timing during the day, and attempts made to address them

A child's medication history can be quite complex, particularly when multiple medications have been prescribed at the same time or when medications are changed at the same time. As discussed in Chapter 4, it's easier to keep track of all the details when you keep medication logs, which you can then copy and provide at the evaluation. Or, if you haven't done that in the past, the pharmacy where you fill prescriptions and/or your insurance plan can print out your child's prescription history, and you can add comments to that. These efforts will help the doctor reach the goal of figuring out what each individual medication contributed to the health of your child.

3. **A thorough medical, developmental, social, and school history** of your child from birth to the present may be taken before or after this discussion about psychiatric history. The doctor will want to know whether your child has had medical problems, including assessments by other physician specialists. For example, has your child had a head injury and seen a neurologist, or has your child passed out playing

sports and seen a cardiologist? The critical follow-up questions the doctor will likely ask you include "What was the diagnosis and what were the recommendations?" Ideally this information is easily accessible. If you have any records, including last visit summaries, you can certainly provide them.

4. **A developmental history** may follow, including questions dating back to pregnancy, delivery, and early patterns of sleeping, eating, social engagement, language, and physical skills. Think back to how easily your child slept, ate, and connected to you and the rest of the family.

- Was the child easily comforted?
- Did your child look for your attention, communicate his needs to you, by pointing and then through speech?
- How about walking and motor skills such as riding a bike or holding a crayon?
- Was the child's play imaginative, varied?

While not all psychiatric problems can be traced back to the early years, it is not uncommon to hear some reference to early observations. Parents of children with ADHD say, "he never walked—he ran!" Parents of children with anxiety might describe long-standing patterns of fear, avoidance, or hesitancy. Children with ASD may be described as never having quite connected with peers or reached out to parents for emotional connection as a sibling might have. Sometimes in the process of thinking about your child's social–emotional patterns, you begin to see more clearly that what seems to be a sudden change in your child actually has been developing for years. You should know that this is our expectation—that we will see patterns of moodiness, anxiety, and hyperactivity dating back years before you came to our office.

5. **A social and school history** includes important questions about the basics:

- Who is in the family or, more practically, who lives in the home?
- Are you and your child's other parent married, separated, divorced, remarried?
- Are you a guardian—a relative such as an aunt, uncle, grandparent?

- Or, if your child was adopted, when, and what information do you have about the child prior to adoption?
- Are there siblings?
- Any losses, stressors for the family?
- Anything you would consider traumatic for your child, or even simply changes in routines?

While getting a sense of your home is vital to the practitioner, your child does spend the bulk of the day in school, and therefore a school history is necessary. A school history can include academic skill development or struggles, as well as educational or neuropsychological testing that has been completed, with a summary and recommendations.

School is also an important setting for social–emotional challenges and growth. Doctors will benefit from forming a picture of your child in school: Is the child happy, sad, stressed, confident, social, isolated . . . ? You should be able to describe your child at school in that manner, based on conversations with teachers, administrators, perhaps even other parents or children.

6. **A family history** is often quite informative as well. Therefore, be prepared for questions about whether other family members have or might have psychiatric or substance abuse problems. Sometimes just your informal description of symptoms of a disorder, such as anxiety, in other family members will be sufficient for a psychiatrist to see a family history, which could predispose your child to a similar or even a different psychiatric disorder. For example:

- ADHD runs in families at a very high rate. In addition, studies of the incidence of ADHD have shown that families with ADHD may be at higher risk of tics and learning disabilities.
- It's also not uncommon to see Tourette's disorder in children of parents with obsessive–compulsive traits and vice versa.
- Sons of alcoholic fathers are at increased risk for a number of problems, including alcoholism, ADHD, and conduct disorder.
- Children of parents with anxiety, depression, or bipolar (manic-depressive) illness are at higher risk of developing those disorders.

Of course the severity of any of these symptoms or syndromes can vary widely, from, for example, a "little anxiety" to severe crippling panic disorder. Having a family history doesn't destine your child for the same problems. If, for example, your child's father and grandmother both have very disabling depression, your child may not have any such problems. Or, if he does, early intervention and treatment might greatly minimize or even prevent the development of diagnosable depression.

Your review of family history is also an important moment in the interview for your child. Your child will benefit from your poise here, as you talk openly, candidly, and comfortably about psychiatric problems that "run in the family." Some details may not be appropriate or necessary to share with children or teens present, but seize the moment to provide the message "I am okay talking about this" just as you would if the discussion were about a family history of headaches or diabetes or asthma.

7. **A mental status examination** includes direct questions to your child or teen. This component is considered the physical examination of mental health and is a crucial part of the basic interview. It is a standard part of all psychiatric/psychopharmacology evaluations. How exactly your child will be involved in the evaluation varies, though (see page 64). Generally the mental status exam involves questions asked directly of your child to find out how the child is feeling and to assess the child's thinking abilities. The doctor may ask the child if he is bothered by something in particular, if he is sad or mad, or more seemingly unusual questions such as whether he is hearing voices or seeing objects that others are not. Don't be offended by the types of questions covered. Some questions may not apply to your child, but it's valuable for an evaluator to stick with a standard template of questions.

Don't be alarmed if your child doesn't respond openly, as the evaluator may be collecting valuable information just by observing. While the evaluator is observing your child and interviewing both of you, she may be mentally answering a running list of questions such as these:

- Is he attentive to the examiner?
- Does he appear anxious or depressed?
- What is his pattern of speech?

- What is his sense of reality?
- How does he relate with the parent(s) or the examiner?

Do evaluations include any form of medical or physical testing?

Whether your child's evaluation includes a physical exam depends on whether she has had a complete checkup by the pediatrician that includes all the elements required for psychiatric diagnosis and psychopharmacological evaluation. Generally, children who are being considered for medications should have a thorough medical check, including a physical exam, by their pediatrician to ensure that (1) the child is well, (2) an underlying medical problem (such as low thyroid hormone) is not causing or exacerbating the child's psychiatric disorder, and (3) the child has no major medical problems (such as heart defects) complicating the use of medications.

All medical conditions need to be brought to the attention of the mental health practitioner who is evaluating your child. In particular, a clear history of neurological or other conditions that are closely related to psychiatric disturbances should be made available. Additionally, any previous or current medical problem that may put your child at risk with certain medications should be brought to the attention of the doctor.

If mental health problems are so firmly founded in biology, shouldn't we be able to do a brain scan or a blood test for my child's problem?

Our field still lacks objective methods of testing children and teenagers for psychiatric disorders. At present, no acceptable "biological test," including pictures of brain activity or blood tests, is recommended to diagnose any psychiatric disorder in children. However, remember that doctors in other fields still base much of their diagnoses upon the clinical story or narrative that patients provide. While we don't ever expect a blood test to replace your physician, it is reasonable to hope for a test that can provide additional support for a diagnostic impression and guide the selection of the best treatment for your child.

In considering the development and widespread use of tests one must take a public health perspective. A critical question must always be "What is the cost of this test?" in addition to "How good is it?" Cost can be thought of as actual cost in terms of dollars, but it can also be thought of as the time involved in taking the test and the risks of the test. One important risk not always considered is "What if the test comes out negative (e.g., my child does not have OCD) but it's wrong?" Or conversely, the test could conclude that your child does have OCD and be wrong. Finally the same test could be positive for OCD and for fear of heights. So a positive test could mean your child has one or the other condition, or perhaps both! These important test attributes are called test *sensitivity* and *specificity*. In other words, how good is the test at picking out one and only one condition? As psychiatric tests begin to appear on the market, remember to ask these critical questions and to think about the impact not only on your child, but on the thousands of children who may be exposed to the tests. A false positive or false negative result impacts many children if thousands or hundreds of thousands are using the test.

If there's something wrong with my child's brain, won't she need a neurological test?

Not necessarily. Whether your child needs a neurological test, or other medical test for that matter, will depend in large part on the types of concerns you take to the doctor and how quickly those concerns have surfaced. For example, if you provide a very typical description of inattention and hyperactivity and state that you've been seeing it in your child since he was quite young, the doctor who is now evaluating your 10-year-old will probably feel comfortable suspecting ADHD. In that case, there is no need for a brain scan or other neurological test. But if your previously healthy child suddenly, in a matter of days, started behaving angrily, having memory problems, and suffering headaches, the doctor would be concerned that he had a neurological/medical condition and would likely recommend a brain scan to look for a change in the brain itself, such as a brain tumor that would require medical treatment.

Two major types of scans are used to take pictures of the brain: a CT scan and an MRI. Although the scans are painless, children may feel claustrophobic in the scanning equipment or be bothered by the knocking noises. Talk with your child about the machine and what it is doing and also inform the scanner technicians as to how your

> **CT scan:** Computed tomography; a detailed, cross-sectional picture of structures in the body and brain made by using X-rays.

child is feeling or may react. Just as you asked your doctor about his experience working with children, it's wholly appropriate to ask about the imaging center's experience with children, particularly if it's a younger child, not an older child or teen. Technicians in children's hospitals are very savvy about children's needs and perspectives.

> **MRI**: Magnetic resonance imaging; an imaging technique that uses magnets and radio waves instead of X-rays to produce better resolution (sharper images) and more varied pictures of structures of the body and brain than CT scans.

Additionally, your doctor may be concerned about certain types of seizures, particularly if the child appears to be confused or unresponsive at times. In that case, the doctor may order a particular test called an electroencephalogram. This painless procedure may require your child (and you, the brave parent) to stay awake most of the night before the test. Abnormal brain wave activity is often brought out during phases of sleep, so it will help if your child sleeps during at least part of the test. This test includes attaching sensors all over your child's head to capture abnormal electrical activity.

> **electroencephalogram (EEG):** A "brain wave test" to detect electrical signals produced from brain cells. The test uses small discs (electrodes) attached to wires, briefly stuck to the scalp to collect information, not to stimulate the brain. An EEG is a diagnostic test for epilepsy and can help in diagnosing other brain problems.

What is the purpose of psychological testing, and how does it differ from the psychiatric evaluation we're already planning to get?

The evaluator may refer your child for psychological or neuropsychological tests for two main reasons: (1) learning disabilities are suspected and/or (2) the evaluator cannot reach a diagnosis based on the information gathered. These tests are not part of an evaluation done by a child psychiatrist or other practitioner performing a psychiatric evaluation.

The "psychological" part of testing includes questions and tests intended to give the practitioner a sense of the child's emotions and thinking. The psychologist may look for signs of anxiety, sadness, loss, and the like. Psychological testing could be helpful, for example, to answer the questions "Is this sadness or a loss of reality?" and "Is this depression or psychosis?" about a teen who is withdrawing socially and taking poor care of himself. The "neuro" part of this testing examines academic skills (e.g., reading, writing, math) as well as other cognitive capacities, such as memory, processing of information, attention, and organizational abilities.

Currently, psychological testing may cost in the thousands of dollars if paid for privately. Neuropsychological testing is, however, often done by the public school system, because that's where problems that affect learning are often noticed first. If the school has not already alerted you to the need for testing, you can request an educational assessment through the school system based on your child's academic difficulties or information gathered by your psychiatric/psychological evaluator. The school pays for testing completed by the school. If your child's evaluator recommends neuropsychological testing to clarify a diagnosis and you have to seek it privately, an individual psychologist or testing service may give you guidance on the likelihood that your medical insurance plan will cover all or part of the costs and how to get preapproval.

> **neuropsychological test:** A group or "battery" of performance-based assessments, including cognitive skills (memory, attention) and capacity (IQ), academic achievement (reading), and psychological functioning. Results are compared to the performance of others of similar age and gender.

Will the evaluation include blood tests?

As with medical/neurological tests, blood tests should be done only to gain specific information that will help the doctor figure out what may be wrong with your child and how to treat it. It's important that you understand every single test's purpose so that you can assure yourself and your child that all tests are justified—especially with a child who fears needles!

Children with behavioral difficulties may be asked to have a ceruloplasmin (copper-containing protein) or lead level test. Whereas lead exposure and elevated levels may cause behavioral and intellectual disturbances, elevated ceruloplasmin levels indicate a treatable metabolic disorder called Wilson's copper storage disease. Both high and low thyroid hormone levels may cause or worsen underlying behavioral or emotional problems in children. Similarly, genetic testing may unveil less common problems such as fragile X (a genetic syndrome causing learning disabilities, intellectual disability, hyperactivity), and metabolic testing may unveil metabolic diseases. However, despite our field's attempts and parents' wishes, no blood testing is available to diagnose any of the psychiatric disorders we treat in children and adolescents. Instead blood tests are done to rule out medical illnesses causing or contributing to psychiatric symptoms.

> Be sure you know the purpose of any test before approving it for your child.

Tests should not be ordered for liability protection, research without consent, or compensation to the institution or practitioner. For example, some clinics suggest expensive "biochemical analyses" of a child's brain or blood. These tests have yet to be validated scientifically and do not provide a foundation for treatment. Again, your best protection against unnecessary tests is to ask the purpose of each and every one.

We've read a lot about biochemical and genetic testing. What could those tests tell us that would help our child?

The two areas in which biochemical or genetic testing may be indicated would be (1) in looking for medical causes of psychiatric symptoms, such as abnormal thyroid as a cause of fatigue and low mood, and (2) for genetic disorders associated with intellectual deficits or autism. Besides this, such tests are not yet recommended for routine psychiatric practice. In the future, biochemical and/or genetic testing may help in making psychiatric diagnoses, in directing treatments, or in predicting how treatments (medication) may be tolerated.

Can we keep the school out of the evaluation for now, to protect my child's privacy?

Academic functioning and peer relationships are two major domains in a child's life that are important for a psychiatric history. The school (or day care center for younger children) is in a unique position to provide input in these areas, so the doctor will greatly benefit from having this information from the start. Parent/guardian signatures are necessary to release any information about a child *to* the school. However, you may provide this information to the evaluator without direct communication being necessary. That is your prerogative, to protect your child's privacy.

While schools are expected to keep diagnostic and treatment information confidential, you don't need to disclose information that is not relevant to the school's direct needs. One option after your child is diagnosed is to have the treating physician write a succinct letter with the major diagnosis and reason for the communication (such as special education needs or medication administration).

Privacy-related laws have restricted the flow of information between schools and parents. In some states school faculty and staff are not allowed to advise parents that their child seems to have problems that would warrant a mental health evaluation; nor are they permitted to report on their observations of how a child is doing during a medication trial. While your child's privacy may be better protected than it was in the past, collaboration between parents and schools in the interest of a child's improved mental health may be restricted significantly. One source of additional information regarding these laws is found at *www.hhs.gov/ocr/hipaa*.

> **Your signature is required for information about your child to be released *to* the school, but you can freely provide school records to your child's evaluator without notifying the school.**

Will my child be involved in the evaluation?

Providers may differ considerably in how they conduct the evaluation process, including how children are involved. Ordinarily time will be allowed for you and your child to be interviewed together, as well as you alone and/or your child alone. The order of interviews may vary, starting out all together or with parents alone or with a teenager alone. The composition and order of interviews may also reflect the setting of the evaluation. Expect that in a typical clinic setting, such as a hospital-based clinic, the evaluation will mirror a general pediatric visit, with much of the time spent together. In contrast, in a private practice setting, the evaluations may be more spread out and may include wholly separate appointments with parents and chil-

> **Ask *all* of your questions about what an evaluation will entail so both you and your child will feel comfortable right from the start.**

dren. As to other involvement, obviously if psychological, cognitive, neuropsychological, or other tests are called for, the child will participate. Never hesitate to ask the doctor or the doctor's clinic what to expect from the evaluation and/or these testing processes.

The doctor refers to my child's problem as a "disorder" and to something called the DSM. Our pediatrician never used these terms—what do they mean?

DSM stands for *Diagnostic and Statistical Manual of Mental Disorders,* a book published by the American Psychiatric Association that contains a standardized method of diagnosing mental illness. The DSM attempts to create a guide for clinicians so they can make valid and reliable diagnoses. The DSM includes descriptions of symptoms that form a given diagnosis, like depression, OCD, ADHD, or ASD. These symptoms are derived from the scientific literature and are considered valid, describing a "true" disorder. If the symptoms are well understood by all doctors, then separate doctors should come to the same, reliable conclusion in seeing the same patient. Thus OCD is a valid and reliably diagnosed disorder.

Furthermore, the DSM gives credence to emerging information on new treatments because it has defined exactly what constitutes a specific disorder. Clinicians reading a study on a successful new therapy for schizophrenia, for example, should feel confident that what the researchers called schizophrenia in their study is the same thing that the clinicians see and call schizophrenia in their practice.

The current DSM (fifth edition; DSM-5) had its origins in meetings with heads of the National Institute of Mental Health (NIMH) and the American Psychiatric Association (APA). A DSM-5 Research Planning Conference was convened in 1999, gathering experts in genetics, neuroscience, cognitive and behavioral science, development, and disability. Work groups met over 5 years, reviewing the current known science and clinical expertise. The current edition was published in 2013.

What should I take to the evaluation?

First and foremost, take along your calm, confident self. In addition to the best attitude that you can muster under what may be difficult circumstances, take whatever information you've collected about your child's problems, including any information requested specifically by the evaluator's office. Some clinics will want specific paperwork, tailor made for their clinic. Doctors are interested in summaries of prior therapies and medications, as discussed above. Educational or cognitive neuropsychiatric testing done in the past is valuable as well. Summaries of services provided in schools via individualized educational plans (IEPs) or Section 504 of the Rehabilitation Act of 1973, including recent descriptions of the child in action in school, may help the doctor in making a diagnosis as well as guiding educational recommendations. Revisions to Section 504 were made in 2008 to incorporate information about the Americans with Disabilities Act Amendments Act, to broaden the interpretation of disability.

> **Individuals with Disabilities Education Act (IDEA) and Rehabilitation Act of 1973 (Section 504):** Federal laws that guarantee a free and appropriate public education and provide services or accommodations for children with disabilities. A student is eligible for Section 504 if a physical or mental condition substantially limits learning; relatively simple accommodations or services are provided (e.g., tests in quiet settings; directions for homework). IDEA services are provided if there is a qualified disability that needs special education services; these are intensive, broader services given through an IEP.

Parents sometimes are wary that we might be overly influenced by a prior conclusion, and they choose not to bring in any previously collected information. While we understand this perspective, we would argue against this approach. A true professional would want to know past history, yet remain committed to forming his own impressions. Therefore, we feel that there is far more to be gained than lost by supplying any prior assessments and treatment records to build on past impressions and treatment efforts.

Don't assume that a more objective, open-minded evaluation will result if the evaluator does not see prior assessment or treatment records. Providing all the information you have will produce the most accurate diagnosis.

How should I prepare my child for the evaluation?

Preparation for your child depends greatly on the child's attitude toward being evaluated in the first place. Children and adolescents vary widely in their reaction to the news that their parents are going to take them in for a mental health evaluation. If your child expresses opposition, remember that you've made the decision to pursue an evaluation for all the right reasons. In this respect, there is no reason to apologize. Saying you're sorry seems empathic, but your child might interpret your apology as meaning that this appointment is a form of punishment. We suggest firmness, telling your child that the decision is nonnegotiable. The most important thing is to get the child in for the evaluation.

When you discuss your decision with your child, be honest (with explanations appropriate for the child's age) about why you think an evaluation is necessary. Don't hesitate to bring up the problems that you and the child have been experiencing, but try to avoid negative comments or blame. Say, for example, "I know it bothers you that you've been having trouble with your friends" rather than "You're causing so much trouble in the neighborhood that I don't have any choice."

Your child's willingness to be evaluated may depend on the type of problem the child has. Youngsters with "internalizing" mood and anxiety symptoms may be easier to get into a practitioner's office because they may more readily connect to the internal distress in their lives. These children may be more likely to want to talk about these feelings. On the other hand, children with "externalizing" disorders, such as oppositional defiant disorder, are by definition oriented externally toward other people, not inwardly toward feelings. Therefore, these children may be more likely to deny their problem or blame it on others. They may be more resistant to the evaluation.

The child's reaction to the evaluation may also depend on age. In general, young children tend to be more malleable but may be governed by typical fears of doctors. If you know your child is afraid of shots, for example, assure her ahead of time that she will be seeing a "talking doctor" who does not give shots. Adolescents can be more difficult and may even try to sabotage your efforts by oversleeping or not coming home from school on time for the appointment. Adolescents, however, may be more eager to go if they understand that this doctor is really theirs. The psychiatrist is ideally seen this way, as being an advocate for the child or teen, interested in all she has to say. Adolescents want to be listened to; they want to teach the doctor about "what it's like to be me." This can be a helpful approach.

Whatever the child's age, be prepared for the child to be closed-mouthed once you're in the practitioner's office. It may help if you assure your child (again, especially teens) that whatever is said in the doctor's office will be kept confidential. But don't be too concerned if your child refuses to talk to the doctor at all. Considerable information is gathered simply from observing the child. Yet, rest assured, the evaluator will be taking more than firsthand impressions of your child into account in making conclusions. All practitioners are aware that children often act differently in their office than at home, at school, or with peers, so they do not rely solely on what they see or hear face to face.

In the evaluation interview, the doctor asked many questions that scared me, such as whether my son ever felt suicidal. Won't these questions put dangerous ideas in his head?

Asking about sensitive mental health concerns such as suicidality (i.e., thinking about suicide) is a critical part of the evaluation. Asking questions about suicide does not place the idea in your child's head. In fact, young people are frequently relieved to be able to talk openly in a safe environment about these often hidden thoughts and feelings. When the evaluator asks direct questions such as "Have you ever felt hopeless and wanted to kill yourself?" the message is one of openness—that both the evaluator and the parents want to know what's really going on in the child or teen's mind so they can help.

Sixteen-year-old Sean, for example, was brought in for an evaluation because his pediatrician thought his low energy might have been related to depression. In addition to many depressive symptoms that he had not discussed with anyone, Sean said he had been suicidal for almost 3 months but had felt ashamed to tell his parents and scared of the feelings. The interview proved to be a catalyst for open communication by the parents about his depression and treatment. Fifteen-year-old Susan reported in front of her parents that she had copied the key to the gun cabinet and was planning to shoot herself the following week. Needless to say, the parents were both terrified to hear this news and relieved to know about it. Remember, discussions that may very well cause you great anxiety may save your child or teen's life.

Follow-up questions about details—any planning involved, intent to be dead, knowledge about whether rescue was likely—can bring out information of the type Susan revealed and are critical to distinguish children who are thinking about suicide without any plan to carry it out from those who are planning on killing themselves. Fortunately it is more common to be thinking about suicide than planning suicide.

We haven't had a final report from the doctor yet, and I'm worried that he's going to tell us nothing is wrong because Jenny acted perfectly normal in his office!

Many parents become alarmed when their children don't manifest the particular symptoms of concern during the actual meeting with the practitioner. Remember, the symptoms of the disorder occur as interactions between the environment and the child. Some problems, such as academic difficulties, may appear only at school. The practitioner evaluating your child is no more likely to base her conclusions only on your child's behavior in the office than a cardiologist would be to discount the chest pains you report having while walking upstairs simply because you don't have those pains in her office! Children may not be inattentive or hyperactive in the structure of a practitioner's office; however, in the school and home environment, they may have disabling ADHD. Likewise, depressed children may "hold it together" during the examination, only to fall apart at home. Traumatized children may have the bulk of their difficulties at night. In contrast, some children will act worse at the evaluation.

We've put our child through all of this testing, and now the doctor says she's not sure what's wrong. Why is it so difficult to diagnose my child's problem?

The goal of the evaluation process is to come up with a diagnostic hypothesis of your child's problem. However, confidence in a diagnosis may take time and may also change over time, as certain problems lessen and others emerge. Even though an evaluator may be unsure about the nature of the problem, he should share his thinking with you. What should emerge is a "differential diagnosis"—the top several diagnoses that the doctor thinks are likely for your child. For example, it may include "generalized anxiety" or "social phobia," the former being a general state of worry and the latter being anxiety in social situations.

Mood disorders, bipolar disorder in particular, may be difficult to diagnose. Thus, the differential diagnosis of a moody child might include depression, bipolar disorder, and possibly ADHD. Depressed children often can't express their feelings clearly and may display confusing symptoms such as anger or temper tantrums rather than sadness. Children with bipolar disorder may have explosive angry moods, followed by sadness, hopelessness, and even giddiness, near euphoria. On the other hand, if the moodiness consists of brief bursts of frustration, the diagnosis may be ADHD, with poor emotional regulation. A critical question in this differential diagnosis is "What is the child's day-to-day [or baseline] mood?" A disturbed, sad, or angry mood at baseline indicates a mood disorder, whereas emotional blow-ups in a "really sweet, happy boy" are more consistent with ADHD.

A 12-year-old boy with a family history of depression was brought to our clinic because he was somewhat anxious, isolating himself, and sometimes appeared sad to his parents. He thought something was awry but was unable to be more specific and denied frank depressive symptoms. We opted to follow him, and his parents observed him diligently. Over the ensuing 4 months, he withdrew further from his family and friends, had difficulties in school, and noted feeling sad. In follow-up visits it was more apparent that he was suffering from depression, and he was started in psychotherapy, along with an antidepressant.

> **differential diagnosis:** The process of figuring out which of several conditions that have similar symptoms is affecting the child being evaluated.

This is a typical example of the collaborative process that accurate diagnosis often requires: We describe concerns and speculations to a child's parents and ask for help in watching for certain symptoms. If you fear that you're reading something into your child's behavior that doesn't exist, discuss what you've observed with the doctor, who should be able to help highlight meaningful observations.

Unraveling children's psychiatric and psychological disorders poses many challenges to even the most astute diagnostician, including factoring in age and developmental level. Simply put, what is normal behavior for a 2-year-old could be signs of a disorder in an 8-year-old. Excessive activity in a preschooler may still be within the normal range, but by age 8 the child should be able to sit still for long enough to focus on schoolwork.

Similarly, some symptoms of psychiatric disorders overlap with the signs of a typical reaction to a stressful event. It's perfectly natural, for example, for a child to become depressed or anxious following the death of a loved one. But if the child's depression or anxiety is protracted, the child may be suffering clinical depression that has been triggered by the stressful event.

Differentiating inherent from external causes of a child's problems is even more difficult when major stressors exist within the family. For example, financial problems and parental separation, unfortunately common problems, often result in a certain type of response from the child, who is trying to adjust to the situation. When does that typical and expected reaction become a problem? It depends on the severity of the child's reaction, how long the symptoms last, and how seriously impaired the child becomes.

Studies show that the vast majority of children whose parents have separated or divorced have some type of reaction, such as sadness, anxiety, or more overt acting-out behavior such as oppositionality or rebelliousness. Usually this behavior is self-limited, and the parents can deal with it effectively by talking and maintaining a nurturing home environment. Yet a smaller group of these children may have prolonged, severe difficulties such as extreme reluctance to leave the remaining parent or caregiver, leading to a child's refusal to go to school or play with his friends. These children might benefit from individual or group therapy to discuss the parental separation and what it means to them, and/or medication treatment if anxiety is severe or persistent.

We've seen some instances in which too much emphasis is placed on the immediate cause, or trigger, of the child's problems. Although there are clear cases in which a stressor appears to be the major cause of a child's behavior (such as severe trauma), any event may not be directly related to the disorder. Many parents wonder, for example, if a fall out of a high chair caused their child to develop ADHD. It often emerges, however, that the child was overactive, perhaps resulting in a fall in the first place. Since we have no method of truly assessing what leads to what, it's useful to keep in mind that there is an important interaction between the environment and your child's biological constitution.

3

The Diagnosis and Treatment Plan

Laying Out a Strategy to Help Your Child

Now that the psychopharmacology evaluation has been completed and you have a better understanding of what's going on with your child, your next question, of course, is "What can we do about it?" At this point you should have a diagnostic hypothesis from the evaluator, along with an initial treatment recommendation. The phase you and your child are entering now may be the most difficult in the diagnosis and treatment process. Now you must deal with the full reality of your child's problem and its possible treatment, and many parents find that all their lingering doubts and fears come to the surface. "Is the doctor's diagnosis correct?" and "Does the proposed treatment seem reasonable?" are questions that every parent asks—and *should ask*.

As you move toward action—and toward treatment—you and the doctor must have a clear sense of direction, based on the doctor's diagnostic impressions, beginning with the evaluation. As we mentioned, sometimes doctors will tell you that they have confidence in a given diagnosis, and other times the clinical picture may be less clear. As long as the possible diagnoses are shared with you, are understandable, and seem consistent with your child's problems, moving toward treatment is reasonable. For example, a doctor may say, "The symptoms your child has are most consistent with depression . . . Bipolar disorder is an unlikely diagnosis but possible." Based on this impression, the treatment recommendation may include an antidepressant, with the expectation that the child's sadness will lessen. On the other hand, if the antidepressant causes serious worsening of mood with irritability, pressured speech, and insomnia, the medication will be stopped and a bipolar disorder diagnosis will be considered.

We have a diagnosis, but the doctor wants to come up with what he calls a "comprehensive" treatment plan. That sounds a little ominous to us. What should we expect?

Overall, a broad treatment plan should follow the evaluation. When a family comes to us for an evaluation of their child, we consider how the biological, psychological, and social aspects of treatment might be combined in the best possible comprehensive plan. Biological treatments include psychiatric medications. Psychological treatments include various forms of therapy, including individual therapy, family therapy, and group therapies. Social systems treatments or supports could include provision of basic family services in the community related to housing, employment, and food needs, as well as state services and educational interventions. You should always feel that your child's treatment takes into account psychological and social factors in his life and that the doctor is doing more than just writing a prescription. For example, following a psychiatric evaluation that resulted in a diagnosis of ADHD and depression, 13-year-old Anthony received a recommendation for a stimulant medication for ADHD, as well as therapy for mild depression and low self-esteem.

Sue, age 17, came to the office due to persistent depression, having had no response to several prior antidepressants. In a thorough diagnostic evaluation, it was determined that Sue had depression, as well as social anxiety and a learning disability. Her father had chronic untreated depression, and her school was not providing any supports despite her failing grades in math and science. A comprehensive treatment plan was developed over time to include biological treatment (an antidepressant), psychological treatment (individual therapy to work on her negative self-critical thinking style; family therapy to address Dad's depression), and an IEP for her math disability. Previous treatment, which had been limited in scope, had not been successful because factors exacerbating Sue's depression (i.e., learning disability, parental depression) were not being addressed.

This is not to say that biological, psychological, and social treatments will all be equally important to your child. For some kids, one form of treatment seems more critical than another. These differences may reflect the type of condition (e.g., ADHD vs. generalized anxiety), the severity of the condition (i.e., mild, moderate, severe), or the age of the child (e.g., preschooler vs. adolescent).

Always ask the doctor why specific treatments are being recommended or not recommended. The doctor's response could be something like "Well, it's my impression that your child has an anxiety disorder, but given that he is young [6 years old] and the anxiety is not keeping him from attending school right now [relatively mild symptoms], I am recommending therapy as a starting point." If you feel the need for additional assurance that the treatment makes sense, one way of determining this would be to ask "How do your recommendations line up with others, like those of national organizations like AACAP?"

> A plan should include only treatments recommended for specific reasons, with clear goals.

The different aspects of your child's situation and general practice in the field should govern treatment recommendations, and not the idiosyncratic practice of the mental health professional. The latter would sound more like "I use X medication for boys his age—I know it works best." That response could indicate that the doctor is guided solely by his experience and is not influenced by the advances in the field.

If our daughter ends up seeing three or four different practitioners, who's going to keep track of everything?

In the meetings following the initial evaluation, the comprehensive treatment plan that takes shape may involve several other professionals besides the doctor. Your child's team may include a psychiatrist, a therapist, a school counselor, and a family behaviorist or family therapist. While these practitioners are experts in their fields—and you should ask who will coordinate all the different aspects of your daughter's care and who is in essence the "captain" of the treatment team—don't minimize your role in a successful treatment plan. Communication is paramount, and you can help greatly in connecting these professionals together.

If you're seeing a psychiatrist in private practice, which typically means paying outside of insurance, that doctor may offer weekly therapy in addition to a medication prescription. But doctors in hospital or community clinics typically don't provide weekly therapy as well as prescribing medications. They should, however, refer you to a therapist and other professionals, and it's reasonable to expect that the prescribing doctor and other professionals you're referred to have some communication, at least at the onset of the treatment, to confirm that they are on the same page, with the same goals. Communication may become critical again if there are significant changes in your child's condition or situation, worsening of symptoms, or if there appear to be differences of opinion on the direction of treatment. This is where your involvement may help keep things on track. Do your best to help facilitate communication among team members in these ways:

- Have the contact information for each professional on hand to provide to each of the others.
- Encourage the members of your child's treatment team to connect, to discuss your child's treatment plans and progress.
- If you feel that one treater is acting without sufficient information from another, it is your right to ask that they confer prior to moving forward with the recommended plan.

For example, 7-year-old Tommy came in with his parents for a psychopharmacology evaluation because he had suddenly started to experience a very high degree of anxiety in the last couple of months. Tommy had been seeing a therapist the family was referred to by their pediatrician. Prior to recommending any treatment, we asked the parents about some stressors on Tommy that they had alluded to, and Tommy's parents suggested we call the therapist and provided the office number. The therapist told us about recent losses in the family and parental conflicts and said they were starting to be addressed in therapy. We determined it was most appropriate to defer medication and to monitor Tommy, as long as the therapy gains continued, which they did. This approach worked well due to excellent communication between treaters and the family. The family and therapist were appreciative that our opinion was consistent with their treatment plan and that we were available should Tommy's anxiety be less responsive to therapy over time.

We have doubts about the treatment plan. Should we agree to it anyway?

First of all, try to determine exactly what your doubts are about. Think carefully and share your concerns thoughtfully. Share doubts often and early. There is a common adage in medicine: "Don't worry alone." This can apply to those we treat as well. If you are uncertain and/or worried, let the doctor know. Most likely others have expressed your uncertainties before you. You can help resolve any doubts by being as clear as possible about them: do you question the diagnosis, or the treatment, or is it something else? Since the doctor's goal is to help your child and your family, most doctors will be more than willing to address whatever doubts you have. They may find that you've brought up something that has been overlooked inadvertently and would call for modifying the treatment recommendations. Or they'll be able to clear up your misgivings, which will make you a more effective collaborator in your child's care.

Don't worry alone.

Sometimes parents feel uncertain about a treatment plan because they lack a clear understanding of a psychiatric condition or treatment. Or uncertainty can reflect personal history with a poor outcome in treatment, or something heard or read in the news or online. While there are some excellent sources of information on the web, there is no shortage of dramatic stories of poor outcomes, which can be misrepresented as commonplace when in fact they may be quite rare and, importantly, not clearly caused by the treatment. One common theme you might encounter involves a healthy child who took a medication, such as an antidepressant or a stimulant, and immediately tried to harm himself or someone else. In actuality, by the time most children begin a medication they have been ill for a long time, typically years, and have had ideas of self-harm long before taking the medication. So take whatever concerns and stories you have heard to your doctor. She should be able to help you assess whether these are relevant to your child's condition and/or treatment.

Naturally you should beware of any website whose main purpose (or even a significant goal) is to sell you anything. With that caveat in mind, you should know that the pharmaceutical industry has developed excellent websites with updates, links, and other resources related to their medications (especially those with FDA approval in children). Such websites may also link to major parent support groups and the National Institutes of Health's related information.

> **FDA:** The Food and Drug Administration (FDA), an agency within the U.S. Department of Health and Human Services that is responsible for monitoring the safety, effectiveness, and quality of drugs.

Always balance proprietary (business) information with unbiased independent sources, but don't deny yourself the help you can get from these websites. The FDA website does provide clear information about what the medication is approved for—and, importantly, it must adhere to discussions only about those purposes. The FDA has directed pharmaceutical companies to create simple "Medication Guides," which are useful summaries about how to take the medication, what side effects to look for, and so forth. These medication-specific guides may be found as links within the website.

It's critical to ask the doctor about any doubts you have, because you don't want to put off help your child could get while indecision festers unproductively in your mind. On the other hand, don't allow the process to be rushed—unless the doctor can present convincing reasons to try to ease certain symptoms quickly,

> **medication guides:** Handouts that come with many prescription medicines, discuss specific issues for a given drug, and contain FDA-approved information to help patients understand serious side effects.

such as a child thinking of harming himself. If you have serious doubts, one option that should be shared with you is to wait and observe the symptoms of your child's disorder over time. Maintain contact with the treating practitioners regarding your plan. If your child gets better, your hesitancy in initiating medication treatment was well founded. If your child continues to have problems, or they worsen, you now have more data on which to make your decision. Either way, if you are carefully watching your child, along with mental health professionals, you win.

> **You want your child to get necessary help as soon as possible, but when you have serious doubts about a treatment plan, "waiting and watching" to see if the problem eases without treatment should always be an option if it poses no apparent risk to the child.**

You may never like placing your child on medicine, if that is the decision, but should you decide to take that route, you will have the satisfaction of knowing you've weighed all the pros and cons and engaged in informed decision making.

I'm inclined to go with my doctor's recommendation for medication, but my husband thinks our son just needs more discipline. How do we decide who's right?

It's not unusual for one parent to agree with a plan and the other to have doubts or even refuse to move forward with treatment. This common dilemma can be related to a number of factors. Considering them may help you and your husband determine how the disagreement originated, with the ultimate goal of coming to agreement. Being on the same page will get your child the help he needs, as well as your unified support so that he can make the most of that help. See the box on page 76.

One case immediately comes to mind as an illustration. Mrs. Jones brought 10-year-old Sam into our clinic because Sam was not listening to her parents or teacher, was hitting other children, being mean to her baby brother, and having bad temper tantrums. Mrs. Jones noted that her daughter did not respond to requests from either parent and said they had been "yelling at Sam a lot lately" and felt guilty about this. Now both parents were "at the end of our rope." Mrs. Jones's sister's kids were all doing well, and similarly, her friends' children did not seem to have any major behavioral problems. There was one younger son who was doing well. Mrs. Jones's marriage was described as "rocky," which in large part was related to their daughter's acting out. Mr. Jones, who was from a large family with a strict upbringing, thought that Mrs. Jones needed to be tougher and more consistent in disciplining Sam. A daughter of an alcoholic father, Mrs. Jones was conflicted, viewing Sam's acting out as being at times willful and "behavioral" and at other times out of her control, and her daughter as in need of her unconditional love.

As parents we can't prevent our parental perceptions from being influenced strongly by our individual upbringing and childhood experiences. If, like Mr. Jones, you were raised in a discipline-oriented family, you may naturally view your child's behavior as somewhat manipulative, requiring more discipline. If, like Mrs. Jones, your upbringing was less strict or you had a family member who suffered from mental illness, you might be more likely to blame the child's acting out on an underlying

> **What's behind your disagreement about the treatment plan with your child's other parent?**
>
> - "We have different perceptions of our child." (What are they?)
> - "Our separate observations of the child." (What do you each see?)
> - "We spend different amounts of time with our child, in different settings." (How might this affect what you see?)
> - "The different notions we bring to parenting from our own childhoods." (What do you each expect from your child and your role as parents?)
> - "We have different disciplinary styles." (Is one of you more permissive than the other? How could this be affecting your perceptions?)
> - "We each have a different relationship with our child." (Is there goodness of fit? Chemistry that makes you feel a natural bond—or the absence of one?)
> - "One (or both) of us has problems similar to our child." (Does this make the problem hard to recognize in your child?)

problem in the child or a system in which the child is participating (e.g., school, peers). Obviously conflict is going to result when one parent empathizes with the child, perceiving disturbing behaviors as ramifications of a problem, while the other parent or other family members see the disturbing behavior as calling for the child to be reined in. In most cases there's some truth to both perspectives. The trick is to ferret out the cause of the disagreement and come to some agreement on what's going on with the child and what to do about it.

One key is for both caregivers to feel involved in the process and mutually supported. Children need the adults to work at being unified and supportive of each other, no matter how difficult this may be. Your child's doctor should have your child's best interest at heart and should be able to articulate the necessity of coming together as parents around a psychiatric treatment plan. Instead of risking appearing to take sides with one parent or the other, a wise doctor will suggest counseling for parents who can't seem to come to a meeting of the minds. We well understand that seeing your child in pain can be quite painful and can cause a rational parent to get a bit (or a lot) irrational. Keep an eye on your emotions. Admitting how intensely worried you are about your child can be the best way of keeping communication lines open. Besides admitting to your emotions, stating that you have your child's best interest in mind is another key to success in these difficult situations.

> Expressing how worried you are about your child can keep communication open between you and your child's other parent by reminding you both that helping your child is your primary goal.

When all else fails, in rare cases the courts might need to be involved in resolving disputes about the psychiatric treatment of a child. More often, another professional opinion can help bring people together.

Should we get a second opinion?

"Second opinions" serve the purpose of having your child reevaluated from a different perspective. This can result in either reaffirming the first diagnosis or legitimizing your concerns about it. When there is no response to treatment, understand that it is quite reasonable to ask whether the diagnosis is the correct one. That does not mean, however, that everyone should seek a second (or third) opinion. If you're satisfied with your child's doctor's background, approach, and understanding of what is wrong, and the treatment is consistent with the diagnosis, don't feel obligated to seek an alternative opinion just to get a confirmation. However, also don't worry that there is only one time to seek a second opinion. Second opinions or consultations can be sought months or years into a child's treatment.

In today's medicine, most practitioners welcome the opinions of others. In fact they may recommend a second opinion themselves, particularly if the child is not responding to treatment or the child's case has been difficult. But even if the doctor is confident about her impressions and plan, she should be able to recognize when you are not and should want you to be comfortable with the plan before moving forward. If you're the one who wants to seek a second opinion, direct talk with your child's doctor is the best approach. It certainly helps all involved in the process to be frank, polite, and respectful. If you wish to continue with the original practitioner, it's wise to be supportive of the care that doctor has been providing. To reinforce your desire to be collaborative even if the practitioner doesn't feel the need for a second opinion, ask the practitioner what she would like to see from any outside evaluation you plan to seek. This would confirm that you still value her advice and intend to keep her involved.

As you will probably be seeking out a highly specialized doctor for the second opinion, you will have to endure the usual waiting time to be seen. In addition, remember, if the second consultative doctor has a full patient load, this doctor may not be available to follow your child through treatment. However, the second opinion may be quite valuable and may direct subsequent treatment. Consider the process a success if you gain useful insight into your child's condition or if you are reassured that the current diagnosis and treatment recommendation are correct.

On the other hand, you have to be prepared for the decisions a conflicting second opinion might force. How will you integrate a new opinion into the current treatment plan? Both providers may arrive at the same diagnosis but take different clinical approaches and use different judgment in establishing a treatment plan. Neither may, in fact, be "wrong." In that case you may have to make a subjective judgment on which provider to go with if neither agrees to a compromise plan. Are you prepared to switch providers if necessary (and if it's an option)?

Getting a second opinion will be productive only if you're certain of why you're seeking one.

If you get a completely different diagnosis the second time around, you may have to seek a third opinion to confirm one or the other. Therefore, before seeking another opinion, again, be sure you know what is moving you to seek it, the basic diagnosis or the prognosis and treatment recommendation. Do a little soul searching to make sure you're not just looking for reassurance that in fact nothing is wrong with your child at all. And, consistent with the response above, ensure that you're not seeking a second opinion to find someone who will be on your side of a disagreement between you and the child's other parent regarding treatment.

> **prognosis:** What is expected to happen to the disorder and the child over time.

How do we find the best possible practitioner to give us a second opinion?

Generally, a second opinion should come from a doctor with a more specific knowledge base than the first one had. To find one, you can try the same avenues that took you to the first doctor, including your insurance company, your child's pediatrician, friends, and family. It is not unreasonable to ask your current doctor for ideas about a second-opinion physician. The more specialized the request, the more your doctor may be the best person to provide that referral. If the initial evaluation was done by your pediatrician, for example, referral to a child psychiatrist, pediatric psychopharmacologist (a child psychiatrist specializing in diagnosis and medication management), developmental pediatrician, or pediatric neurologist is probably best. Although generally not familiar with the details of using medication, a child psychologist may be very helpful in diagnostic and systems consultation (e.g., review of school, community services, and involved professionals).

To save time, can we just ask another doctor to review the information gathered in the first evaluation and give us a conclusion?

This may seem like the most efficient and economical route, but to get an objective second opinion, you will need a reassessment of the clinical situation and previous treatments. If the primary physician has the facts incorrect or has some bias that the second doctor doesn't know about, it will be difficult to spot an error based on the data provided. One thing you're after with a second opinion is anything the original evaluator has missed, so it is much more fruitful to start with an in-person comprehensive consultation.

Won't our current doctor be offended—and uncooperative—if we seek another opinion?

You have the right to request a second opinion without the blessing, or even knowledge, of your child's doctor. *As a parent, you need to do what is in the best interest of your child.* If possible, it is generally advisable to discuss your wish for a second opinion with the original evaluator. As we discussed, most physicians welcome outside consultation.

We are concerned because the doctor says he's not sure what's wrong but says Ritalin has helped other kids with the hyperactivity he sees in our daughter. Should we agree to this without a diagnosis?

We can't emphasize enough how important it is to have a firm diagnostic hypothesis before any treatment. This doctor may have accurately put a name to one of your child's *symptoms* (e.g., restlessness) but has not fully identified the *syndrome* and therefore has not yet named the *disorder* (e.g., ADHD). It is crucial to distinguish among these three terms in any evaluation, diagnosis, and treatment recommendation. While certain medications do seem to have a specific effect on a particular symptom, the practitioner should always be treating the entire constellation of symptoms that makes up the disorder.

Exactly how does a doctor decide which medication to prescribe?

The doctor decides on a medication—and every other aspect of your child's treatment—on the basis of the risk–benefit ratio involved in using that treatment. The practitioner will compare all the benefits of the treatment—the improvements in symptoms that the medication should produce and the future damage that may be prevented by treating the child now—with the risks, or side effects, of taking the medication. If the benefits outweigh the risks, the doctor may decide to prescribe that medication for your child. How great the ratio must be in favor of the benefits depends to some extent on how severe the impairments are that your child and family are suffering because of the child's disorder.

Yet side effects don't always have to be seen as the enemy. At times a doctor may decide to use specific medications in part *because* of their side effects. For example, your doctor may choose to use a medication with more sedative properties to be given at night if your child is having prominent sleep problems. Conversely, children who are withdrawn or low in energy may benefit from a medication that stimulates the child's energy, often reducing sedation.

> **sedative:** Sleep-producing.

The specific medication choice will therefore reflect a balance of anticipated benefit and side effects characteristic of the chosen medication. Most of the major classes of medications used in child psychiatry have multiple agents in the class. For example, there are several SSRI-type medications (e.g., fluoxetine or Prozac; sertraline or Zoloft) and many methylphenidate medications (e.g., extended-release methylphenidates such as Concerta, Metadate, Focalin). These medications differ in some significant ways, including time to onset of effect and duration of effect. Yet their similarities are likely greater than their differences, meaning that your child's depression may be similarly responsive to any SSRI and your child's ADHD may respond to any of the stimulant-class medications.

Therefore, while your doctor's explanation for choosing a specific medication should reference unique aspects of the drug, there is little scientific literature to guide doctors in choosing a specific medication from among a group of medications. From a practical standpoint, if one medication ("D") in a group of similar medications ("A, B, C") works well, scientists have to decide collectively whether to spend limited research dollars and researcher time proving that medication D works as well or better in some way.

A reasonable discussion of medication choice can touch on details of the medication and presence of FDA approval for certain conditions (more on FDA approval appears on page 82). Be wary if the bulk of the conversation is centered on the doctor's experience with the medication or if the doctor describes the medication as working in "teen girls" or "moody boys" without any mention of the scientific literature or FDA approval.

The nurse practitioner doesn't seem to think FDA approval is that important. Is it really okay for our daughter to take a medication that hasn't been approved for use in children?

FDA approval means that the U.S. government has carefully reviewed studies on the effectiveness and tolerability of the medication and has deemed that the medication can be marketed and sold for a specific "indication"—a specific disorder in a specified age group. However, the lack of FDA approval does not preclude the use of any given psychoactive medication in children (or in any other group). The age limit on any FDA-approved medication generally means that the testers did not study the use of the medication in a younger group.

The use of medications in groups of individuals outside of the "indication" is not necessarily dangerous but simply has not been studied and therefore has not received the FDA "stamp of approval." It is important to note that in the practice of medicine clinicians frequently use medications for reasons not specifically addressed in FDA guidelines.

> The absence of FDA approval for use in children does not mean that a medication is dangerous or ineffective; it simply means not enough research has been done to give it the FDA stamp of approval.

For example, while all of the serotonin-specific antidepressants (SSRIs) appear clinically effective for treating obsessive–compulsive disorders in children, only sertraline (Zoloft) has been formally approved by the FDA and hence it is the only SSRI indicated for this condition in advertisements. Note, too, that although sertraline is commonly prescribed for children suffering from depression, sertraline is not FDA approved for that use. It is important to point out that the FDA monitors serious problems arising from medication use through voluntary physician reporting. Based on its review of such problems, the FDA sends physician alerts about the possibility of medication-related problems.

If these medications don't need FDA approval to be used in children like mine, how are they tested for safety and effectiveness?

As mentioned earlier, doctors know that the medications are effective for the use prescribed mainly from clinical evidence—information obtained from the actual practice of medicine. Clinical evidence may include experience derived from day-to-day practice as well as data from studies performed in human subjects. Studies may result in FDA approval or may not be used for that purpose, and instead remain as scientific inquiry.

There are two common types of clinical investigations: "open" studies and placebo-controlled studies. Both types of investigations are based on knowing what is wrong with the child (diagnosis) and carefully observing the child through the study to determine whether the medication works

> **placebo:** An inactive compound such as sugar pills, used in scientific studies to determine how much of a medication's positive effect comes from the medication and how much from other factors, such as seeing the doctor frequently.

(*efficacy*) and whether there are side effects. An *open study* is a trial in which the doctor prescribes a medication to the patient and both the patient/family and the doctor are aware of the study medication being used.

An example of an open trial would be having a child on a specific medication for a given disorder with weekly monitoring for 6 weeks. At each visit, the child and parents (and sometimes teachers) are asked questions and rated as to how the medication is working and asked about side effects. Open studies are often the first type of clinical trial done on a medication that doctors wish to study formally. However, these studies are clearly vulnerable to bias, in that even well-intentioned families and doctors might be hoping for benefit and rate the medication more favorably than is appropriate.

> **clinical trial:** A systematic and scientific evaluation of a new treatment for a disorder.

In the more relied-on and less potentially biased "controlled" trials, an inert substance referred to as a *placebo* is employed. In a placebo-controlled study, the placebo and active medication tablets or capsules appear identical.

To further eliminate bias from the study, the child, parent, or doctor may not know whether the child is taking a placebo or the active medication. This purposeful attempt to mask whether the child is receiving active medication is referred to as a *blind*. If both the child/parent and doctor are unaware whether the child is receiving the active medication or placebo, the trial is referred to as a *double-blind study*. You can see that by using this mechanism you can eliminate the bias of unconsciously having a response based on receiving the active medication. In some type of studies referred to as *parallel design,* a child will receive either the active medication or the placebo throughout the study. In contrast, in a *crossover* investigation, the child will receive both placebo and active medication at different points in the study.

The overall response is derived from comparing the response of the children receiving placebo and the response of those receiving the active medication being tested. An effective medication might work for 70% of children in a study, whereas only 30% of children receiving placebo register a similar response (e.g., reduction in a scale measuring depression after 8 weeks). Large placebo-controlled double-blind studies might enroll several hundred children across 10–20 centers across the country. As you can imagine, these controlled trials can cost millions of dollars to develop and conduct, are highly labor-intensive, and often take from 3 to 5 years to complete. Even if a medication has not received FDA approval for use in children for the specific disorder your child has, the prescribing doctor may have access to these types of research studies and clinical reports regarding safety and effectiveness.

I've heard various groups of medications referred to by different names—how are these names arrived at, and what do they mean?

The names of medications can indeed be quite confusing. One group of medications, for example, is the antidepressants, and within that group is the class of antidepressants called SSRIs. Then there are the generic names and brand names for specific formulations within a given class of medications. This doesn't, however, help you understand why your child who has anxiety, not depression, is prescribed one of these antidepressant medications. Just as with other medications, like antipsychotic medications, the name is based on the initial area of study or treatment. But once the medication is on the market, evidence may appear that the medication works for other conditions, like anxiety for an SSRI antidepressant. The initial name, antidepressant, sticks. Likewise, antipsychotics have been found to be effective for mood disorders, such as bipolar disorder, but they are still called antipsychotics, even when prescribed to someone without psychosis. In this edition of the book we have updated many of the medication class names to reflect their method of action rather than their original application, such as using *alpha agonists* rather than *antihypertensives* or "blood pressure medication." If you have any questions, always ask your doctor and/or pharmacist for clarification.

The doctor keeps talking about my child's treatment as a medication "trial." Not settling on one drug regimen is making me and my son really nervous. Is it typical to have to try medication after medication?

medication trial: A systematic test of a medication that usually takes 1–3 months.

It's not uncommon to have a child try several medications before settling on one medication that is both effective and well tolerated. That is the goal, effectiveness without adverse side effects: reduced anxiety without upset stomach or headaches; improved focus without low appetite and trouble sleeping; aggression control without weight gain.

All medications do have side effects, so you and your child should be prepared for them. Preparedness can be used to reinforce the overall vision that "we want you to feel less anxious, but in the first week or so you may have some feelings, like stomach upset, that you don't like . . . we will expect these to go away, leaving you feeling just less anxious." Monitor along with your child, aiming for an occasional, inquisitive "How are you feeling today?" To get accurate feedback from your child, beware of the power of suggestion (see the box on page 86).

In addition, when you do share concerns with the doctor, make sure not to miss the benefits that can occur at the same time as the problems. Try your best to document without judgment. Your best role in the process is to observe and take to the appointment evidence of possible side effects as well as possible response to the medication.

Together you may conclude that there is some clear benefit to the medication as well as some side effects, which have persisted over several weeks. In this situation it would be quite reasonable to switch to a similar type of medication for the same problem. For example, if your child has a favorable response to one form of stimulant for ADHD but trouble sleeping, the decision might be to switch to another form of stimulant that is shorter acting.

The big picture is that it is quite reasonable to go through a number of medication trials of a certain type of medication if benefit is seen, supporting the diagnosis, but the tolerability is not optimal. The general rule is to use a medication at a reasonable dose (if it is well tolerated) for at least 1 month. Always ensure that the medication is being taken properly (or at all). There is no upper limit on when to call it quits with medication for those disorders that are known to respond pharmacologically. On the other hand, if the medication trial results in side effects and no evidence of response, then you and the doctor should be flexible in thinking that the diagnosis may not be correct and/or that there are other problems warranting a different medication approach.

Why does my child have to take three medications instead of one?

It may be comforting to know that multiple agents are commonly used in both clinical practice and research for the treatment of child and ado-

> ### Eliciting Accurate Information from Your Child during a Medication Trial
>
> You can get valuable reports to share with your child's doctor if you aim to be curious and interested in how your child is doing. It's important not to appear hypervigilant ("Are you okay? . . . Are you sure you're okay?") or fearful of adverse effects. Hypervigilance and worried questioning offer a not-too-subtle suggestion that you don't expect that your child is okay.
>
> Collect information, but don't draw any conclusions without a discussion with the doctor. Strive for careful remarks such as "Maybe your trouble falling asleep has to do with medication. I'm not sure—it could be another reason—so let's call the doctor and see what he thinks." You're a powerful influence on your child, and your interpretation of what is going on will carry far more weight than the doctor's. If you rush to judgment, it may be difficult to backtrack later if the doctor reassures you that your child is tolerating the medication well.
>
> Henry, age 8, was highly anxious and rigid and focused constantly on certain ideas and fears. Unfortunately, his parents thought that his stomachaches the week before school started were due to the new anxiety medication started the prior month. Despite reassurance from Henry's doctor that the medication was not likely to be causing the problem, Henry was unable to shake their initial impressions and would repeat what they had initially concluded—it was disappointing that the medication was hurting Henry's stomach, since it was starting to work. Henry ended up becoming so distraught about this notion that the medication needed to be stopped and replaced with another. In this case another medication trial probably could have been avoided.

lescent psychiatric disorders. Doctors use combined pharmacotherapy (multiple medications) primarily to treat co-occurring or comorbid disorders (e.g., ADHD plus an anxiety disorder) or when there is inadequate response to a single agent (e.g., two mood stabilizers with children who have bipolar disorder). Your child's doctor will typically arrive at the decision to prescribe three medications based on information gathered during each individ-

comorbid: Occurring at the same time as another problem or disorder.

ual medication trial. It is not typical to start more than one medication at a time. However, if the first medication treats anxiety well, but the symptoms of ADHD persist, a second medication may then be added to treat ADHD.

While it's not your responsibility to make medication decisions, know that if your child does end up taking more than one medication and the prescriber wants to make changes to improve response or address side effects, it is quite reasonable to ask if medications can be changed one at a time. As noted in Chapter 2, when you keep a medication history for your child, an important goal is to separate out benefits and side effects of each and every medication prescribed for your child, something that would be difficult if more than one medication were changed at the same time.

Although not the preferred initial approach, there are other situations in which a second medication is added to the first to address side effects. For example, a medication that can help with sleep onset or weight gain could be added to a stimulant for a child with ADHD who has responded to stimulant medications only with associated, persistent side effects. When we say it's not the preferred initial approach, we mean that for such a child, several stimulant medications as well as nonstimulant medications can be tried first, before the prescriber is convinced that the stimulant, with its side effects, is the clearly superior medication in terms of effectiveness. If that is the case, it may be reasonable for the doctor to suggest a period of time with a second medication added to the stimulant, primarily to address the side effects.

> More than one medication may be needed to treat more than one disorder or to address side effects, but as with a single medication, the goal of each prescription should be clear.

Despite the common practice of prescribing combination medications, there is generally a lack of scientific evidence demonstrating the effectiveness and safety of using two or more agents simultaneously. There are two new exceptions to this fact, with two medications for ADHD approved by the FDA for combination prescription. Two new longer-acting forms of medications that have been used "off-label" for years (clonidine and guanfacine) are now approved for ADHD as treatment alone and as adjunctive medications: the nonstimulants Kapvay and Intuniv.

When combining medications, you should ask again about potential medication-to-medication interactions that may arise between the agents to be used. Don't forget to consider over-the-counter (OTC) medications as well, including herbal supplements. Finally, cost may be a factor, since two or more medications may cost more than a single agent, especially if you have to copay $10 to $50 per month, per prescription.

> **off-label:** Use of a medication different from that described in the FDA-approved drug label, such as for a different condition (anxiety instead of depression) or at a different dose (40 mg when the label recommends a maximum of 20 mg).

How will the medication affect my child's school life?

The medication trial itself does not necessarily have to affect your child's school life. The school does not have to be involved in the administration of medication for many disorders, including the extended-release preparations of commonplace stimulant medications for ADHD. At present only a minority of children require dosing of psychiatric medication during the school day (e.g., midday dosing of short-acting stimulants for ADHD).

> **extended-release preparation:** a form of a medication released slowly over time, such as over 6–12 hours, typically aiming for once-a-day dosing.

What should we tell the school about the upcoming medication trial?

You should decide at your discretion how much you wish to inform the school regarding your child's medication. First, consider asking your doctor to write a brief letter documenting the diagnosis, treatment (including specific medications), and educational or behavioral needs of your child. Based on your individual school's policy on mental health, and your comfort, you can then collect useful information as to your child's response to medication, particularly during the initiation of different pharmacological trials. Some parents disclose all of the specifics of the medication, including dose, expected action, and side effects. Others choose only to ask for a report of their child's behavior with a more limited, if any, acknowledgment of a medication trial.

If you choose to communicate openly with the school about the medication, it's helpful to identify an advocate or point person within the school, such as a guidance counselor or teacher, to serve as a vital link among you, your child, and the school. Both you and your child should feel comfortable talking to this person. Your child should have regular contact with him or her, and you should be in close contact with this advocate to get feedback about your child's response to treatment, particularly medications.

> **Disclosure about medication trials should be based on balancing the child's right to privacy with the benefits of greater understanding and collaboration from school personnel.**

There are pros and cons to speaking directly to the school about your child's medication. Keeping the school fully informed makes personnel feel more involved in the process, which can foster greater collaboration and understanding. It also means you can expect more direct relevant feedback. However, you will have to keep an eye out for teacher and school personnel biases, just as exist in the community at large. Be wary about others sharing family experiences or personal viewpoints on medication. Be wary if you hear more emotion than reason.

If your child is to receive medications during the school day, the school's nurse will likely become an important contact as well. School nurses are generally responsible for holding and dispensing any medication to be given at school and will play an important role in your child's care. The nurse can be of great assistance in monitoring your child, giving you feedback on problem side effects and the effectiveness of the medication during the school day. The nurse may also be quite knowledgeable about your child's medication and therefore can be a great source of information. How much communication and assistance you can expect, however, depends on the scope of the nursing staff at the school. Some schools have a staff of full-time nurses, some have only a part-time nurse, and some have no medical personnel at all.

Most schools have a well-worked-out procedure for dispensing medication. Generally state laws dictate that children are not allowed to carry and take their own medications in school. Therefore, schools are usually required to have forms filled out by both your child's physician and you regarding your child's diagnosis and the specifics of dispensing the medication. Many schools will not start giving medications, or change the type or dose of the medications, until these forms are completed, and at times a caregiver is required to bring in a labeled prescription bottle as well. It is a good idea to ask for a couple of extra forms and take them with you to your child's follow-up medication visits in case the medication dose is changed.

Has the doctor made a mistake? The dosage recommended for my 11-year-old daughter is the same amount prescribed to her adult cousin.

First of all, if you have any doubts at all about medication dosage, ask the doctor. It is reasonable to ask your doctor about the level of evidence in support of not only a medication but also a given dose of medication. You can also double-check with your pharmacist or review typical dosing guidelines online. The FDA can be a primary trusted source of this level of detail. The FDA has helped to ensure that pharmaceutical companies create clear, readable medication guides, which provide approved dosing ranges.

Understand that at times doctors may prescribe dosing that is greater than approved by the FDA. Consider two paths of specific research on dosing: one path is taken by a drug company for drug approval when it is seeking a minimally effective, well-tolerated dose; the other path is taken by doctor researchers searching for the maximally effective dose. So you can pose a very savvy question to the doctor: what's the dose range approved by the FDA and what's the literature to support a higher dose?

In addition, children may require relatively more medication compared to adults because they are more efficient in breaking down and eliminating medications. The younger you are, the more quickly your body breaks down medications, making them inactive and/or ready for elimination. The two major body organs involved in the breakdown (metabolism or catabolism) of medications are the liver (hepatic system) and kidneys (renal system). Many psychoactive medications are broken down by the liver and are passed out of the body in the stool.

How do prescribers determine an appropriate dosage for my child?

Doctors determine doses of medication based on safety, effectiveness, and strength of the compound. How well a medication works or, more technically, the amount of change the medication causes in the symptoms of a disorder is called its *efficacy,* or *effectiveness.* The amount of medication it takes to get a response indicates how strong the medication is and is referred to as *potency.*

It is common for two medications to be roughly equal in how they will work (efficacy). However, it may take different amounts of the medications to get a similar response (potency). Your child will require lower doses of a more potent medication and higher doses of a lower-potency agent to obtain the same effectiveness. The antidepressant agents offer a good illustration of this point. Whereas your child with depression may require 20 mg of fluoxetine, she may need approximately 100 mg of sertraline to get the same effect. In each of these cases, the medications have about the *same* ability to treat the problem (efficacy); however, different amounts are necessary due to their chemical composition.

Because children and adolescents vary so widely in body size, doctors may determine dosing of certain medications by the child's body weight, usually expressed via the metric system: milligrams of medication per kilogram of body weight (mg per kg). When considering this dosing approach, remember that 1 kg = 2.2 pounds. A 110-pound adolescent, for example, weighs about 50 kg, and for that child a 1 mg per kg per day dose of a medication would be 50 mg daily. Dosing of stimulant-class medications for ADHD might be determined based on weight, although this is not how the FDA approves medications. In other words, the FDA will recommend a dose of X mg for children and y mg for adults, without reference to body weight.

How will the doctor determine whether the dosage is correct once my child starts taking the medication?

As you will learn in more detail in Chapter 4, there are various ways to monitor the effects of your child's medication. To state it simply, the best way to determine whether the dosage is too high or too low is to observe the child. If your child's condition has improved as expected but side effects are bothersome, you and the doctor may want to consider a slightly lower dose. If there are no side effects but improvement is also minimal, you may want to try increasing the dose.

Of course to determine whether there really has been improvement, we have to know what the medication was intended to do. Having clear "targets" for the medication is paramount to assessing and getting

Table 3. Typical Pediatric Dosages of Psychotropic Medications

Medication	Daily dose (rough approximate)	Daily dosage schedule
Stimulants		
Dextroamphetamine/amphetamine compounds	5–70 mg	Two or three times (once for extended-release forms)
Methylphenidate	5–90 mg	Two or three times (once for extended-release and patch forms)
D-Methylphenidate	2.5–45 mg	Two or three times (once for extended-release forms)
Nonstimulants		
Atomoxetine	18–100 mg	One or two times
Antidepressants		
Tricyclics (TCAs)	10–300 mg	One or two times
Imipramine		
Desipramine		
Amitriptyline		
Nortriptyline		
Clomipramine		
Selective serotonin reuptake inhibitors (SSRIs)		
Fluoxetine	5–40 mg	One or two times
Sertraline	25–200 mg	One or two times
Paroxetine	10–30 mg	One or two times
Fluvoxamine	50–300 mg	One or two times
Citalopram	5–20 mg	One or two times
Escitalopram	10–40 mg	One or two times
Atypical		
Bupropion	37.5–400 mg	One to three times

Medication	Daily dose (rough approximate)	Daily dosage schedule
Serotonin–norepinephrine reuptake inhibitors (SNRIs)		
Venlafaxine	25–150 mg	One or two times
Duloxetine	20–120 mg	One or two times
Antipsychotics		
Phenothiazines		
Low potency (e.g., Seroquel, Mellaril, Thorazine, Clozaril)	25–400 mg	One or two times generally
Medium potency (e.g., Zyprexa, Geodon, Abilify, Saphris Trilafon)	5–60 mg	One or two times generally
High potency (e.g., Risperdal, Invega, Prolixin, Haldol, Orap)	0.5–20 mg	One or two times generally
Medications		
Lithium carbonate	300–2,100 mg	One or two times
Valproate	250–1,500 mg	Two times
Carbamazepine	200–1,000 mg	Two times with meals
Gabapentin	300–1,200 mg	Three times
Lamotrigine	50–200 mg	Two times
Topamax	50–400 mg	Two times
Trileptal	300–1,200 mg	Two times
Antianxiety medications		
Buspirone	5–45 mg	Three times
High-potency benzodiazepines		
Klonopin (long-acting)	0.5–3 mg	One or two times
Xanax (short-acting)	0.5–3 mg	Three times
Ativan (short-acting)	0.5–3 mg	Three times

(*cont.*)

Table 3 (*cont.*)

Medication	Daily dose (rough approximate)	Daily dosage schedule
Lower-potency benzodiazepines		
Valium, Tranxene	3.75–30 mg	Three times
Antihypertensives		
Clonidine	0.025–0.6 mg	Two to four times; at bedtime
Clonidine XR	1–6 mg	One or two times
Guanfacine	0.25–4 mg	One to three times
Extended release	1–4 mg	One or two times
Miscellaneous medications		
Naltrexone	25–75 mg	Two or three times
Desmopressin (ddAVP)	One to two times nightly	Intranasal; one or two times
	0.2–0.6 mg	One to three tablets at bedtime

the most out of treatment. For example, we hoped that the anxiety medication given to 13-year-old Timmy would reduce his social and separation anxiety enough for him to be able to order food in a restaurant and to tolerate being alone on the first floor of his home with others upstairs. And we aimed for 20 minutes of sustained focus for 7-year-old Ruth with the initiation of a stimulant for ADHD. In each case, we identified clear, relatively objective markers of treatment response. Compare this to "we wanted Timmy to feel better" or Ruth to "get good grades."

> Exactly what is a medication prescribed for your child intended to do? Knowing that is the only way to measure the effectiveness of the treatment.

The other, less common method for monitoring dosage is blood tests. Tests of the blood

> **blood level:** The amount or concentration of medication in the blood. Also called serum or plasma concentration.

levels of a medication can reveal whether your child is taking the medication in the first place (*adherence*), as well as whether the dose is high enough to begin causing toxicity in the form of side effects or too low to be effective. Blood tests can also identify children—about 1 in 10—who are particularly slow at breaking down medications. Because these slow metabolizers will end up with high concentrations of the compound in their blood, prescribers may order blood tests for some medications when starting treatment.

Only a minority of psychiatric medications require blood tests, and when utilized, they are typically for monitoring safety—to prevent drug levels from becoming elevated to the point of causing greater side effects or to watch for damage to body systems, such as damage to the liver, kidney, or blood cells. Another adage in medicine is "don't treat the level," meaning don't adjust the medication simply based on the drug level in the blood, without considering the response of the given child. While there is some literature informing us of what an effective level of medication may be for a certain medication (e.g., lithium, Depakote), this may not apply to an individual child. Therefore, it's appropriate to question the doctor should he suggest an increase in medication dose because the drug level is low, not because of ongoing symptoms of concern, such as mood instability. Some may have beliefs about the importance of a given blood level, but that is not supported by the pediatric scientific literature.

Similarly, blood tests are important when children are taking more than one medication because some medications interact and slow each other's metabolism. *Always discuss possible medication interactions with all of your child's doctors.* Mental health providers need to know about all medications your child is taking, because psychotropic medications can even interact with OTC medications, including herbal supplements. Your child's other doctors need to know about psychotropic prescriptions, especially if they

> **medication interaction:** A change in the concentration and effectiveness of a medication when administered along with another medication. One medication can increase or decrease the usefulness of another.

want to start your child on a medicine. Common relevant examples include Accutane for acne or an antibiotic for an infection.

Overall, no simple blood or other test will reveal the exact dosage that is appropriate for your child. Be prepared for an adjustment period, be observant, and stay in communication with the doctor.

Having our child evaluated and diagnosed has taken a lot of time, and now it might take a few months to figure out the best medication for him. How can we be sure he's really going to feel better after all this?

Parents often have ups and downs during medication trials because they're so eager to see improvements in their child's symptoms and overall well-being. To stay focused on what your child and you stand to gain from this entire process, keep in mind that you're going to gain a lot besides alleviation of symptoms for your child. You also stand to gain:

- A better understanding of your child's strengths and weaknesses
- Easing of your child's specific struggles, whether the diagnosis involves anxiety, depression, substance abuse, or hyperactivity
- Stabilizing of the environments in which your child lives, from home to school
- The comfort of knowing you are no longer alone in trying to help your child feel better and function at her highest possible level.

When asked about why they seek treatment, parents tend to express poignant desires: "I just want him to be happy." "I want my daughter to lead a good life." "We wish he would enjoy his friends . . . recognize his talents . . . work to better himself." Toward this end, biological, psychological, and social treatments should be considered individually and together. We understand the powerfully positive impact a healthy parent or a supportive school system can have on the gains a child makes in mental health treatment. That's why teams of treaters should collaborate to work on the whole child, for gains at home, school, and socially.

> **Remember, in child psychiatry, you and your child's treatment team have development on your side.**

Communication and collaboration are critical in what can be a complex and often painfully slow process of healing.

However, in child psychiatry we have development on our side. Thanks to emotional, behavioral, and cognitive development, many children have a greater ability to handle stressors and to work effectively in treatment as they age. So, while keeping an eye on long-term goals, do not miss short-term victories!

4

Treatment and Beyond

Collaborating in Your Child's Ongoing Care

The planning stages are over; now your child is embarking on treatment. Many of the questions we hear about this phase of the psychopharmacological treatment of children concern the definition of roles: "What can I do to make sure my child continues to do well?" "How much responsibility should my child take for his own care?" "When should I call the doctor?" Everyone who has an interest in your child's continued well-being plays an important part in the proactive measures described in the following pages.

In addition, there are questions related to countless practical details. Do you need to change the child's diet or lifestyle to optimize the treatment effect? Can you use generics as well as brand-name drugs? How do you time administration of the medication for the best effect and the fewest side effects? What do you need to know about other prescription medications and OTC medications? In this chapter we will address questions regarding roles as well as these practical details to help you get the most out of your child's treatment.

As a parent, what should I be doing now that my son's medication trial has begun?

By learning everything you can about the disorder(s) your child has, the accepted treatments, and specifically the medications used, you can be an active collaborator in your child's treatment rather than a passive bystander. Additional information on the medications can be obtained not only from this book and your child's doctor but also from a range of quality private and public Internet sites, good old-fashioned libraries, and the many parent-run support groups on the different child disorders.

There is much to be said for organization in this effort. We recommend that you develop a detailed record of your child's treatment history that includes copies of tests and evaluations. We also advocate creating a medication log, containing information on each medication tried: when, at what dose, and what happened—whether it worked as expected and whether it produced any side effects. An example of a filled-out medication log appears in Figure 3, and another example, plus a blank log to photocopy and use as needed (or download and print), appears in Appendix B.

Parents who keep medication logs are not at the mercy of a clinic's medical records when they need information on their child's treatment history. This is particularly important today, when your child may end up transitioning from one doctor to another. This may be necessary due to ever-changing group health insurance plans or to frequent turnover in staff at your doctor's office. Parents who have their child's treatment histories at their fingertips simply have an edge.

> Having an up-to-date medication log at your fingertips can smooth the inevitable transitions between doctors or insurance plans.

Keep in mind that throughout your child's care you'll be handling multiple tasks, beyond keeping a medication log. Your involvement will be critical in the process of advocating for educational accommodations and/or services that your child needs from the school, as well as working with your insurance company or the state's insurance program for children to ensure that your child is eligible for a broad variety of treatment programs.

The challenge lies in keeping an eye on the big picture about overall treatment goals as well as the day-to-day details—that medications are ordered and filled at the pharmacy, that the child takes them at the correct times, and so forth. The most important job you have is to monitor your child's progress. You are the indispensable eyes and ears of the professional caregivers.

Medication Log

Start/end date	Medication	Daily dose	Response	Side effect(s)	Comments
Jan–Mar 2014	Methylphenidate, extended release	40 mg	More focused, still impulsive in classroom and baseball	Low appetite, weight loss ~ 5 pounds	Good school performance
April–Aug 2014	Mixed amphetamine, extended release	20 mg	Focused and less impulsive in school and sports too	Seemed more nervous after dose. Picking at skin but maybe due to hot summer, insect bites.	Good school performance
Oct 2014	Clonidine	0.1 mg twice a day	Less impulsive, not focused	Sleepy	Good school performance
Nov 2014–Feb 2015	Atomoxetine	60 mg	Good—focused and less impulsive	Stomach upset at first, then none	Good behavior, attention problems
Mar–Sept 2015	Atomoxetine + methylphenidate, after school	60 mg 10 mg	Most even response through the day, after school stimulant really helps with homework	Mild low appetite at dinner	Good school performance and behavior Improved mood

Figure 3. Example of a completed medication log for a child treated for ADHD.

Do I have to change anything in my daughter's daily routine to make sure she gets the full effect of her medication?

In many ways, the answer is no. The doctor's challenge is to determine whether the medication is helping and/or causing problems. To do this, it's best to have little to no other significant changes in your child's environment, such as different routines or interactions with family members. Such changes only complicate the assessment of the medication. A good example is anxiously questioning your child about how she's feeling, which we cautioned against in Chapter 3. Your child may pick up on your anxiety and feed off it, reporting more anxiety or physical complaints, which have nothing to do with the new medication but might be seen as a side effect.

So, as we discussed before, remain composed as much as possible. Monitor your child. Think about patterns of moods and behaviors over periods of days and weeks and report these to the doctor. Look for changes, positive or negative, over time. Maintain your perspective. If you start analyzing your child's progress on a minute-by-minute basis, you'll stop seeing the forest for the trees and make a premature decision about the medication's lack of effect or side effects based on limited data.

> **Consistency in taking the medication is the most important way you can help your child get the most out of the treatment.**

The one measure that is important to take is to make a plan to ensure that your child does take the medication consistently. Whether you tie in the administration of a dose with an event (mealtime) or the time on the clock, make sure it's easy for your child to make it part of her daily routine.

Will my son need to change his diet due to this medication?

The vast majority of psychotropic medications don't require any specific diet. The rare exception is the monoamine oxidase inhibitors (MAOIs), which require a strict diet but are not commonly prescribed for children. With the arrival of SSRI medications, MAOIs, given their dietary complexity, are rarely recommended for childhood mood or anxiety disorders.

However, many medications do have an impact on appetite, either reducing it (e.g., stimulant medications for ADHD) or increasing appetite (e.g., mood stabilizer medications for bipolar disorder or other conditions). Therefore, it's important to know about these possible changes in your child's interest in food, either to help encourage a high-protein or high-calorie diet on a medication that suppresses appetite or to discourage a doubling of your child's meals due to an increase in appetite.

Is it okay to use OTC medications at the same time as the prescription?

Most OTC medications can be used safely with the medications described in this book. However, it's always prudent to discuss this with your pharmacist and/or doctor.

> **over-the-counter (OTC) medications:** Medications you can buy (at a pharmacy counter, for example) without a prescription.

The majority of potential interactions are more minor and include the child being overly sedated, as is the case for the standard antihistamines, or mildly agitated, as with the decongestants.

> **antihistamines:** A class of medications that block histamine receptors or histamine release. Used primarily to treat allergies, they are used commonly in psychiatry to treat drug reactions and for their sedative properties.

Some OTC medications may have a more significant impact on a psychiatric medication by changing the blood concentrations of the medication (see information on blood tests on page 59). Be aware that it may be just as risky to have an OTC medication raise the level of a prescribed medication in your child's blood as lower it. Children receiving an MAOI, which is rare, need to adhere closely to their special diet as noted earlier, but there are also prohibitions against taking OTC medications without consulting their pharmacist and doctor.

What about other prescriptions?

Since you've undoubtedly stayed up all night with a sick child at some time in the past, it would be frivolous to remind you that children occasionally have medical problems necessitating other prescription medications. When that happens, it's important to notify the person examining your child of the current agent your child is taking. While it's important to discuss all medications with your providers, the majority of psychiatric medications can be taken safely with other prescription medications.

Can I substitute generics for brand names?

As you probably know, the brand name—Ritalin, for example—is the name chosen by the pharmaceutical company that developed that medication. The generic name—such as methylphenidate—is the medication's chemical name. Brand names are typically capitalized, whereas generics are not. Brand-name medication is generally more expensive than the generic, whether you pay directly or you have a copay insurance policy.

> **generic medication:**
> Refers to the chemical makeup of a medication, not the advertised (sold) brand name.

It is the brand-name product that has been studied extensively by the pharmaceutical company under guidelines and monitoring by the FDA. Both the pharmacological properties of the medication and the "vehicle" (specific capsule, pill, or tablet) that the medication is put in to keep it stable and palatable for humans have been evaluated. There is also a quality control from batch to batch of medication, which generally ensures that each tablet of the medication from month to month is virtually identical in the amount of medication and filler it contains.

Most generic medications' pharmacological properties make them acceptable, less expensive alternatives to the brand-name medication. On an individual basis, some parents report no difference between the brand and generic preparations, whereas others observe less effectiveness, allergic reactions, or increased or different side effects with generic versions.

There are no absolute guidelines for deciding between generics and brand names, and many parents have taken the approach of beginning with a generic for cost savings and continuing with it if it proves to be well tolerated and effective.

Be sure to discuss your concerns about different producers of the generic forms of the medication with the phar-

> **One common course of action is to start out with the less expensive generic version of a medication and continue with it as long as it's effective and doesn't cause intolerable side effects.**

macist. Knowing which pharmaceutical company is making the generic your child is taking can facilitate consistency in the way your child's body interacts with the medication. If your child has been on a stable regimen and doing relatively well and develops a drug reaction, or loses the response to the medication, first check to see if the recent batch of medication was a different version of the medication or if the pharmacist received other reports of problems with the medicine. Although infrequent, we have a number of parents who have noted loss of effectiveness related to a particular "batch" of medicine.

Don't interactions among medications make dosage timing important? What if we don't stick perfectly to the schedule?

Whether your child is taking one medication or several, timing of doses is not nearly as important as being sure that your child is actually taking the medication. The administration time of many medications can be adjusted to optimize response, improve compliance (giving once-daily medication instead of three times a day), and reduce side effects. In general, few medicines outside of the stimulant-class medications for ADHD and certain antidepressants need to be given at precise times.

However, your child will be more compliant using a routine or a schedule. Medications given once a day are certainly easier to remember—think of your own difficulties in remembering to take multiple-times-per-day antibiotics—but if your child has to take medicine more often, spread it out according to your family's schedule. Three-times-a-day medication does not have to be taken at exact 8-hour intervals; giving the medication at breakfast, lunch, and dinner is often quite acceptable. Most of the medications used for behavioral and emotional disorders can be given with meals, which not only makes it easier to remember but may result in fewer side effects. Agents that may cause tiredness are often given at night, before your child's bedtime.

Inevitably your child will miss a dose of medication. Generally a missed dose is not a problem. If you plan to give a missed nighttime dose the next day, be aware that your child may be tired during school. More problematic is giving your child the medication twice. Inadvertent double dosing is generally not dangerous, but it may create a problem and should be discussed with the pharmacist or your doctor. Most pharmacies provide a printout on the medication that includes contingencies for missed or double doses. You should also be aware of what medications can be held (not given) if your child is ill. Children who are nauseated or vomiting may not tolerate certain agents, and it may be advisable to hold single doses of the medication.

How do we tell whether the medication is working?

First, be open-minded and objective while you watch for positive effects (as well as side effects). Ask the doctor for precise signs of response in target symptoms (the major problems being treated) as well as a time frame in which they should appear. Determining effectiveness of an agent is easier if your child's problematic behavior or disturbed mood occurs all the time, as with hyperactivity or anxiety, and thus may respond more dramatically. Behaviors such as intermittent outbursts or infrequent panic attacks are more difficult to assess and are best described by how often they occur and how severe they are when they do.

> **positive effect**: A beneficial outcome of a treatment—the anticipated effect for which a medication is prescribed.

> **side effect**: An adverse reaction to a treatment that accompanies the effect for which a medication is prescribed. Side effects can either be predictable, such as tiredness, or idiosyncratic, such as liver problems.

The signs that a medication is working may include improvement in mood, as well as in sleep, interest, and socialization for depressed children. Anxious children, in addition to feeling less nervous, might have fewer stomachaches or less of the other common anxiety-related physical complaints. Obsessional children will not spend as much time with rituals or obsessions and/or find the intensity of the urge to do a compulsion to be less. Youth with bipolar disorder may have less mood volatility, including reduced aggression/irritability as well as less sadness. Children with ADHD may have improved attention and greater impulse control with fewer risky or reckless behaviors.

These are all very general examples. If you and your child's practitioner have developed a solid understanding of your child's problem, together you will be able to come up with signs of improvement to watch for in your particular child: If Tommy usually retreats to his room after school when depressed, talking to you or going out to play when he gets home may be a sign that his medication is working. If Tanya's biggest

> **If the medication is working . . .**
>
> - A **depressed** child may sleep better, be more interested in activities and other aspects of life, and become more sociable, in addition to experiencing better mood.
>
> - An **anxious** child might have fewer stomachaches or other physical complaints, in addition to feeling less nervous.
>
> - A child with **OCD** might spend less time on obsessions and rituals and feel less intense urges to respond to a compulsion.
>
> - A child with **bipolar disorder** may feel less irritable and behave less aggressively, in addition to having less volatile moods.
>
> - A child with **ADHD** may be less hyperactive, less impulsive, and behave less recklessly.

ADHD challenge is concentrating on homework, finishing a 30-minute assignment on her own may be a major milestone.

Very roughly, it typically takes 1 month or more to determine whether a medication is working, leading many physicians to request a routine follow-up visit in 2–4 weeks. Monthly to bimonthly visits are typical during the first few months of treatment. During these visits your doctor will be assessing the effectiveness of the medication and inquiring about side effects. Once the regimen is working and your child's condition is improving or stable, the interval between visits may be widened to every 3, 4, or, 6 months. Children with greater complexity of illness (e.g., ADHD, bipolar disorder, OCD all together in one child) will likely require frequent visits for a prolonged period of time. Sometimes what begins as an apparently straightforward treatment of one problem can change as a child worsens, and as other conditions emerge. Then the treatment course must adapt and appointment frequency must increase.

> When watching for improvements during a medication trial, keep in mind that it usually takes 1 month to tell whether a medication is working.

As a parent, you should be satisfied that your child is benefiting from a medication. You should see proof of efficacy in your dealings with the child and get information from other sources too, commonly the school. Don't be surprised if your view or the school's view differs from your child's view. Some children are poor reporters of their own illness and response to medications. It's not uncommon to have a child or adolescent report no difference in behavior while the school and family state that the medication is working very well.

How do I monitor a medication trial without hovering?

Monitoring doesn't have to mean hovering. You'll probably find, in fact, that once you settle into a routine, you no longer feel the nervous need to check on your child constantly. Still, because adherence is crucial to the effectiveness of your child's treatment, you'll have to plan to talk to and observe your child to ensure he's actually taking the medication.

adherence: Following the guidelines agreed on by you and the provider, including taking medication as prescribed.

Watching for side effects is also important, not only for safety purposes but also to ensure adherence. Subtle side effects like indigestion can deter your child from taking the medication and should be reported to the doctor.

> One of the major reasons for medication failure in adolescents is simply nonadherence.

Collaboration Equals Safety

If your child is experiencing severe psychiatric symptoms or is abusing substances, you'll have to ensure vigilance and diligence in communications with your child's treatment team. Any of your child's physical (e.g., pediatrician) or mental health professionals (e.g., therapist, psychiatrist) should alert you if your child develops active suicidality (i.e., talks about a specific plan to kill himself) or psychotic symptoms (e.g., hallucinations), or becomes a danger to himself (e.g., high-risk substance abuse) or to others (e.g., threat to harm someone else). Should your child require psychiatric hospitalization, your child's treatment team should be in communication with the inpatient team for shared treatment planning.

How can I monitor a medication trial when my child spends most of his day at school?

With the use of extended-release medications (for ADHD), parents can observe the child's behavior long after the school day ends. In addition, you can monitor medication effectiveness during the weekends, afternoons, evenings, and mornings. The school should be able to give you frequent updates on your child's progress if the state's privacy laws allow, possibly using behavior rating scales. The child's school performance itself, in fact, is a way of measuring the effectiveness of the medication. Follow the suggestions in Chapter 3 for communicating with your child's school.

What types of side effects should I watch for?

Parents and children should expect side effects; no medication comes without them. Without a doubt, side effects remain among the most problematic aspects of using medicines in anybody, particularly children. During clinical research, it's not uncommon to see side effects reported before the administration of the study medication, as well as for those children who are receiving a placebo (an inactive substance used for comparison with the medication). So, yes, many common complaints (e.g., insomnia, stomachache, headache) do occur, but they are not always due to the medication.

In general doctors view common mild side effects, which may fade over time, as typically of less concern, and they are not necessarily a reason to change treatment. These could include stomachache in the morning, slight difficulty falling asleep, and occasional headaches. Then there are common but moderate side effects, which occur less often than the mild versions but may warrant changing the dose—or at least avoiding an increase. Such moderate side effects could include a reduction in appetite, to the point of not eating lunch every day, or the opposite, a 5- to 10-pound (2 1/4- to 4 1/2-kg) weight gain. These problems might lead to a reduction in dose or a change of medication.

Then there are the rare but typically more serious side effects. These could be grouped into emotional/behavioral changes and physical/general health changes. Such side effects would include suicidal thinking, a very serious medication rash, and a sudden dramatic increase in aggression. It's important to note that any of these "side effects" may be caused by the medication or just related (by timing) to the medication but not caused by it. Figuring out causality can be quite tricky at times.

For example, a teen was started on an antidepressant and within 3 days had a rash across his chest and back. The medication was thought to be the cause of the rash until the family realized that the teen had borrowed a shirt from a friend. The friend's family cleaned their clothes with a detergent known to cause this teen a rash. Or, in another case, a young child was started on a stimulant and the next day became unusually angry at school, fighting with a peer. Again this was thought to be caused by the medication. Fortunately it was soon realized that the fight was started by a boy known to bully, who had just moved to town and to that classroom that day.

Because anyone can make a mistake at times, including the child herself, the doctor should also describe the signs that your child has received an unintentional overdose of medication. Fortunately in this day and age, psychiatric medications for children are generally quite safe, with a large "safety window," meaning that even in overdose it's unlikely the child will become seriously ill or die. This was not true of medications commonly used in the past, such as the tricyclic antidepressants. The following are several types of side effects you should know about.

Side Effects

- **Mild side effects**: Low in intensity and infrequent (morning stomachaches, occasional headaches, slight difficulty sleeping, etc.), for example, once-a-week mild headache or upset stomach in the morning after the medication, taking another 30 minutes to fall asleep.
- **Moderate side effects**: More bothersome and more frequent (daily)—for example, significant change in appetite and body weight; weight loss of more than 5 pounds (21/4 kg) in a young child; taking an hour or more to fall asleep at night.
- **Severe side effects**: Intense, even life threatening (suicidal thoughts, serious rash, radical behavior change, etc.), for example, ideas about killing oneself, violent aggression toward family members, body rash, and difficulty breathing.

1. **Sedation.** Sedation (sleepiness) is a frequent side effect that often gets less severe with time. Sedation can occur 1–3 hours after the agent is given, or it can be present throughout the day. Commonly prescribed medications that cause sedation include clonidine, the antipsychotic medications, and the benzodiazepines. If a medicine causes your child to become tired, consider giving the medication before sleep. In that way, the sedation caused by the agent occurs during sleep. Sometimes doctors prescribe sedating agents with the intention of helping the child who is having difficulty with sleep.

> The appropriate response to noticing a side effect in your child generally depends on whether it is mild, moderate, or severe, but you and your child's doctor should form a specific plan for reporting adverse effects to any medication.

Sedation occurring many hours after the medication is given may be related to a wear-off or "crash" from the medication. This, however, more typically feels like physical fatigue or weariness than pure sleepiness. It's not uncommon for stimulant medications to cause this phenomenon. Often, changing to an extended-release preparation of the agent or giving an additional low dose of short-acting medication may eliminate this effect.

2. **Rashes.** Generally, rashes associated with psychotropics are more a discomfort than a life-threatening side effect. Typical rashes are generally fine red dots or bumps, occurring mainly on the trunk of the child and spreading to arms and legs. The presence of this type of rash may not mean that your child will have to be taken off the medication and may also be viral instead of medication related. Consult the doctor if your child develops this type of rash and decide together how serious the reaction is, including whether it should keep your child from resuming the medication or similar medications.

A severe rash may include blistering or peeling of the skin, hives (e.g., swollen itchy or burning bumps), or painful sores of the mouth or eyes. This may represent an infrequent but very dangerous reaction reported in those receiving certain psychiatric medications, including lamotrigine (Lamictal). It's important to be aware of the risk of this type of rash, because in some cases it can be life threatening. *If your child develops a rash that fits this description at all, contact your child's practitioner immediately.*

3. **The opposite reaction.** A disconcerting side effect of psychiatric medications and some other medications as well (e.g., Benadryl) is the worsening of the problem for which the child is being treated (*paradoxical response*). A small group of children may become more hyperactive with an ADHD medication intended to reduce hyperactivity, or more anxious or moody with a medication intended to treat anxiety. Similarly, some children become "wired," or energized, with Benadryl, whereas the majority of children become sleepy.

Does my child need blood tests or other tests once the medication starts?

Some effects of the medication may not be observable by you or your child but occur within the body. For this reason, your child may require medical monitoring. The most commonly employed tests for the psychotropics are the electrocardiogram (ECG) and blood tests. The ECG produces a display of the electrical activity of the heart. This test may be completed before starting your child on certain medications and again during treatment. The less commonly used older tricyclic antidepressants (i.e., imipramine and desipramine) may impact the electrical system of the heart; therefore an ECG is used to ensure that these changes are not significant. This use of the ECG is different from conducting an ECG to look for signs of a heart defect or prior injury.

Other medications may influence blood cell production. However, these medications are also less commonly used than other newer or safer medications. Examples include Tegretol and Clozaril. Blood tests may also be necessary to ensure that your child's kidneys or liver can process/excrete certain medications. Kidney functioning is monitored with lithium and liver functioning with Depakote.

What should I do if I do notice a side effect in my child?

It's always important to step back and ask yourself whether what seems like a change in your child is not, but rather is due to heightened attention to your child since he started taking medication. But this doesn't mean you should shrug off any concerns. If you believe your child has developed a problematic side effect, what's most important is to have a plan for communicating with the child's practitioner.

1. **For the majority of concerns,** routine messages left with the office receptionist or on the doctor's voice mail are likely adequate. Leave the times and numbers where you can be reached and be clear about your concerns and specific questions.

2. **For emergency situations,** you'll need to know how to contact the practitioner. Doctors are quite aware that you may need to page them in case of an emergency. An emergency would include concerns that your child is going to harm himself, such as talking about suicide, or others, such as threatening someone with a weapon. If you are requesting an immediate callback, try to keep the phone line clear and provide the doctor with basic information on your child. If you should reach another physician covering for your doctor, give a very brief history of your child: "Dr. Smith treats my son, who is a 14-year-old with depression who has become very aggressive in the last several days, which is quite unusual for him. Dr. Smith started him on fluoxetine 2 weeks ago because he was depressed and was concerned that he might get agitated and asked me to call him immediately if this occurred. This is the first antidepressant that he has been on, he hasn't had a similar reaction before, and has never been so out of control as to need a hospitalization."

3. **It is also a good idea to have a contingency plan** for when you cannot get in touch with the doctor, including calling the child's primary-care physician or accessing your local emergency room or acute care medical clinic.

It took us a year and four different drugs to find something that worked, and now my son's symptoms are returning even though he's still taking the medication. Why?

We don't know why this phenomenon occurs, perhaps most notably and frequently with sicker children. Although there are no clear-cut reasons that children stop responding to their medication, there are several speculations about what may be occurring: (1) the condition is fluctuating; (2) another disorder is emerging; (3) the amount of medication actually reaching the brain is changing; or (4) the brain is adapting to the medication.

However, two initial questions must always be answered: (1) Is the child taking the medication? (2) Has the environment changed in any way? It's always important to review compliance with medications (and

> **Emergencies**
>
> *Any severe side effects such as shortness of breath, chest discomfort, severe agitation, fainting, or disorientation call for immediate contact with your child's doctor, even if they are occurring infrequently.*

therapies) when the child's symptoms are worsening. In addition, teasing out the influence of environmental change versus "biology," meaning the natural course of the disorder, is quite challenging but must be done when the child's condition worsens.

Figuring out when worsening means a medication needs to be changed and when something in the environment needs to be changed is one of the biggest challenges for doctors and parents during the course of a child's treatment. Even if the environment seems to be causing some problems, it's not always realistic to modify it. Not every child who is struggling with attention in a class of 25 children, for example, can be moved to a class of 10 children. Nor can we predict that that will be the answer for all children!

In these situations, patience and doctor–parent collaboration become paramount. Together you can have perspective and consider patterns of response, or lack of response, over time. Taking a long view can help you realize that your child has responded best to the environment (e.g., having an experienced teacher) versus a medication, or vice versa. Taking notes as you go will help you with this eventual review; for example, your notes may say "on anxiety medication for the past 2 months, clearly less anxious every day and no other changes at home or school to explain this" versus "on anxiety medication for the past 2 months, clearly less anxious every day, but it is summer and we have been home, with no social demands on him."

I don't think this medication is working, but my doctor wants us to stick with it. How do I know if he's right?

It helps to limit your expectations of medication trials and to anticipate "bumps" along the way. Your child's doctor does not have a crystal ball and will not be able to foretell which medicine will be most effective and tolerable for your child. Therefore, you and your child need to be ready to try different agents with the understanding that there will most probably be successes and failures along the medication journey. The keys are persistence and systematic trials of different agents within and between classes of medication.

In the case of Gene, an 11-year-old treated for anxiety and ADHD, an initial stimulant medication had little effect on the ADHD and increased his anxiety. Two separate SSRI anxiety medications made him feel moody and upset his stomach. Alternate anxiety medications were then attempted as his anxiety continued to worsen, with minimal positive impact. Then a shift back to a nonstimulant ADHD medication began to show success in his attentional control, which in turn started to lessen his anxiety. "I know what's happening in class now," Gene said. "I'm not just spacing out all day!" Both Gene and his mother were patient through this protracted series of trials, which spanned 6 months, and now Gene is doing much better because of their perseverance.

Even in the face of a medication trial failure, you need to have the attitude that it's worth hanging in there to continue finding out what may be helpful for your child. It's also important to be sure you have a doctor with the same philosophy.

We've already tried three medications, and they've had awful side effects and little positive result. Isn't it time to try something besides medication?

If after multiple trials there is still no response, a careful review of the situation is warranted. First, make sure you and the doctor still agree with the original diagnostic hypothesis. If the child's symptoms seem to have changed, or new ones have appeared, you may want to reevaluate the child. Next, go over possible contributing stressors, your child's adherence to the medication regime, and any medical conditions that may be interfering with treatment.

A thorough review of past trials and outcomes is also in order. By keeping a log of medication trials, including maximum doses, outcome, and major side effects, you can work with your child's doctor in determining classes (such as stimulants) and specific agents that have not been considered. Don't be shy about suggesting different agents that may not have been tried.

Sometimes, on the other hand, a break from a medication trial is advised. If the child has had to suffer debilitating side effects such as a painful rash or disturbing panic attacks on medication, both the child and the parents may be understandably hesitant to keep trying. Unfortunately, we still rely on trial and error in finding the correct psychotropic medication for young people.

In terms of other options, as has been stressed before, medication is one part of a comprehensive treatment plan. So in the absence of medication response, revisit the overall treatment plan, including therapy and school supports. A lack of medication response is not necessarily a "failure" of overall treatment. This can be an important time for doctor and therapist to communicate, including considering the options for school services.

We've gotten along fine with this doctor so far, but now that we can't seem to find the right medications, everyone is getting very testy. Should we start looking for a new doctor?

The relationship between you and your child's doctor is often tested during both a crisis and ongoing unsuccessful medication trials. Obviously it's important to have good communication with your child's treater through this process. As with most of life, keeping your sense of humor while sharing your frustration over the situation can be useful to maintaining your own mental health and keeping communication lines open.

Although you may feel angry, exasperated, and helpless about the situation, try not to blame the doctor or the medication if your child is not responding to treatment—as long as the doctor has been working with you and has been systematically trying reasonable agents for your child.

Doctors are vulnerable to the same emotions and disappointments as patients and their families. We try to see children who are not responding to treatment as a challenge and to maintain our intellectual objectivity. Sometimes without realizing what is occurring, however, doctors may blame patients or families for the child's condition, becoming less responsive to the needs of a patient or simply unavailable.

Eight-year-old Robert's treating pediatrician had a "frank" discussion with Robert's parents in which he told them they were responsible for his poor response to the traditional ADHD medication because they were not taking the situation seriously. Apparently they were in the habit of joking about his impulsivity and talking openly about his spaciness:

"Just like his Aunt May." He in turn would joke that he really was quite smart but that knowing everybody's business in class would make him a better principal when he grew up. In fact, everyone in this family was very committed to treatment but was exercising the healthy defense of humor. They were well aware of the ongoing ADHD problems, but rather than damaging Robert's self-esteem (or letting him berate himself), they brought up the problematic symptoms in a less direct manner. In this case, the more pressing problem was with the doctor, who felt frustrated, angry, and injured because the young man did not respond to treatment.

If you notice this type of attitude in your child's doctor, discuss it if at all possible. Voicing your commitment to working with your child's doctor as a team, toward whatever treatment will help the child, may give your collaboration the boost it needs. You can also do your part as a team player by being sure to keep appointments and acknowledge the frustration and hopelessness that both of you feel during these medication trials.

You must also take an honest look at yourself, and at the home environment, to consider whether there are additional changes you, your spouse, or any siblings can make. Although you might not think of it this way, your child is working hard by going to appointments and taking medications. Therefore you should be working hard as well!

If, despite your best effort, you remain dissatisfied with the level of care provided by your child's practitioner, seek alternate care. You want to be receiving care from a doctor who is thoughtful, positive, and confident and who exudes hope.

Hope from your child's doctor is essential.

Offering hope is critical. One of the true joys of working in child psychiatry is appreciating the awesome potential even the most ill child has for change, growth, and healing. Hope must be present at every appointment, whether that means every week, month, or year. Any doctor can tell you hope-filled stories of children who in the span of 6 months or a year had a major turnaround. Maybe the child started to see the importance of homework, of being kind in the home, of challenging himself to try something despite feeling anxious. Children who show newfound maturity, independence, thoughtfulness, and emotional control bring parents back to hope.

Besides actually taking the medication, what should my child's role be in the course of medication treatment?

Children should be encouraged to be involved in their treatment from the diagnostic evaluation through adherence with the prescribed regimen and monitoring of the drugs' effects on them. They should also be taught to recognize and report side effects.

Despite the use of medication, children need to be encouraged to work hard at mastering their academic, social, interpersonal, and behavioral skills. It's very important not to attribute improvements in symptoms solely to the medication. Help family members and school staff avoid statements such as "You've been doing so well this week—you must be taking your medication!" Rather, emphasize that medicine is one part of the overall treatment plan and that you know your child is trying hard to do her best.

> **It's important to empower the child, not the medication.**

We work hard to emphasize that the medicine is there to help but (with younger children) that they are "the boss of their body." We want to encourage children to have a strong sense of self-agency, not to suggest that the power to "make it all better" resides entirely in the medication. We may say that we are glad the medication is helping the child focus better or feel less sad or less anxious, but your child should be proud of his efforts to overcome these struggles himself. Say "The medication helps, but you are the one with the smarts!" or "The medication is helping, but good for you for raising your hand in class even though you still felt a little nervous."

What can we expect from our 15-year-old now that he's about to start on medication?

Teenagers are a special breed. Depending on your point of view, or your degree of optimism, you can see teenagers as remarkably challenging or remarkably resilient. From a parental standpoint, the teenage years bring great risk, with social complexity (cars, drugs, dating . . .) and greater autonomy. Therefore it's natural to be concerned about how your teenager will handle prescription medication.

As children become adolescents, they will (and should) have more say in their medications. To enhance adherence, be sure your adolescent is talking with the prescriber about his condition and the positive and negative effects of the medication. We want to raise well-informed medical care "consumers." It is truly important to start taking a longer-term view of the teen, with the goal of education and self-awareness versus simply taking the medication every day.

Given their desire for independence, adolescents will often request a trial off medication to see if in fact the medicine is needed. In general, this can be managed by agreeing to taper the medication but to restart it if symptoms reappear. When carefully executed, this may be invaluable to engage the teenager in the responsible care of his own condition.

> Reductions or cessation of medication is better done while your teen is still living at home than at college.

Particularly for seniors in high school, we would prefer that teens reduce the dose and even stop the medication before leaving for college instead of stopping it by themselves in college. We have to admit that once they are in college they are the ones deciding whether or not to take the medication every day. In that setting there is little observation of the teen, as compared to what has occurred in the home. So if the teen is determined to stop and saying, "The second I get to college I am done with this medication," instead of getting into a power struggle that you can't win, consider starting a taper before he leaves, to at least allow for some observation and attempts at self-observation of how he does without the medication. This strategy, of course, does not apply to all teens, but it is one to consider.

Everyone can see that our daughter's condition has improved with this new treatment, but for some reason she takes every opportunity to skip a dose. Why?

For a variety of reasons, children and adolescents will refuse to take medications. One common cause of children missing or skipping doses is the presence of side effects. Typically, young children will not alert their parents to their headaches or stomachaches but instead refuse to take the medicine at times. Children may not like the taste of the medicine or may complain that the medicine is getting caught in their throat—a very uncomfortable feeling! In that case, you can have your child practice swallowing with small candies. Speaking to the pharmacist about different formulations (sprinkles or chewable formulations) and methods of taking the medication (such as opening capsules) may help eliminate many of these problems.

New forms of medications make it easier for children to take their medicine; you'll find more information on these in Parts II and III. If getting your child the medication she needs means mixing it with applesauce, and the pharmacist says that's okay, just do it—insisting on her swallowing a pill is not worth the battle. Be careful that you talk with someone knowledgeable prior to changing how your child takes her medication, though. Children should not, for example, chew long-acting, extended-release tablets (commonly how stimulants for ADHD are given).

> **If your child resists taking medication, make sure simply swallowing the pills is not uncomfortable— there are other ways to take medicine in almost all cases.**

My teenager avoids taking her medicine because she says it just keeps reminding her that she's not "normal." How can I help her with this?

Just like adults, children and adolescents worry about whether their bodies and minds are okay. It's important for them to understand that they have treatable problems that they did not bring on by themselves, and that these problems are not products of moral weakness, do not indicate intellectual deficits, and are simply not their fault. Often fears and fragile self-esteem are what underlie a child or teen's resistance to taking a medication. Your daughter may simply say, "No, I won't take it" or declare that medication is a "stupid idea—I'm fine, I'm normal . . . it's you." The actual fears may not be voiced explicitly.

Avoid the power struggle, particularly with adolescents. As the saying goes, you may win the battle (getting her to take the pill tonight) but lose the war (she hides the medication instead of taking it for the remainder of the school year). Try instead the approach of saying (1) "I hear you" and (2) "Help me understand more what you mean." If your immediate response is closer to "Teach me; help me understand" than "Do it because I'm the adult," you're likely to have more success. Adolescents love to explain their lot in life, to discuss all that it means to be them. Explore what it means to be normal, and you're bound to gain some ground on the topic.

If the problem is that your son feels ashamed of having a disorder, you can help by pointing out examples of the many others who have the same problems—either friends and relatives that you know about or, even better sometimes, famous adults who are leading successful lives with the same disorder. Websites dedicated to your child's disorder as well as books on the disorder aimed at parents often contain these names.

More and more public figures, whether athletes, business moguls, or actors, are opening up about mental health conditions that affect them or their families. In addition, fictional characters in books and movies are increasingly portrayed openly as having depression, OCD, ADHD, and learning disabilities—sometimes fascinating, accurate portrayals, sometimes weaker stereotypes. Regardless, mental health is becoming a more natural part of public conversations and daily experiences.

> A thoughtful discussion of what "normal" means can help you sidestep power struggles with a treatment-resistant teen.

If you can get your child to talk about what taking the medication means for him, terrific. But you may need help, and you shouldn't be afraid to ask for it. Take these conversations back to the doctor. Resistance to taking medication should be considered a therapeutic issue—it has some meaning that should be understood. Do not engage in a solitary power struggle over a medication.

Should my teenager be responsible for her medication?

As your child's parent or guardian, generally you will need to assume responsibility for the medication until your child is 18 years old. You are responsible for her well-being as well as the safety of the home. Because many of the medicines can be fatal in overdose, you should keep them safely away from siblings who may inadvertently mistake the colorful pills and tablets for candy. Unfortunately, many overdoses and deaths on medications occur not in the patient but in a sibling—who has taken the medication either accidentally or in a suicide attempt.

You are the keeper of the medicine and should dispense daily doses to your child. That is not to say that you can't share some of this responsibility with your child as she gets older. A gradual transition to her having primary responsibility makes sense. And this transition can occur beginning 6–12 months before the teen leaves home, not just weeks before.

> ## Discontinuing Medication by Tapering
>
> Rather than stopping a medication abruptly, your doctor will likely choose to taper the medication slowly, instructing you to observe your child's behavior closely during that time. Tapering medication may reduce the chance of withdrawal symptoms caused by the sudden removal of certain medications and allow you to hold or resume the dose if psychiatric symptoms start reemerging. In addition, remember that timing is everything. Choose when to taper medication carefully. The goal is to change one variable at a time, the medication being only one variable in your child's life. Other variables with great impact can be major events, such as the last week of school, a move to a new town, or loss of a good friend. If you stop a medication while other significant events are occurring, you'll have trouble determining whether any symptoms are the result of being off the medication or of whatever else is going on in the child's life. In fact, it's during significant events that your child may depend most on the medication. These precautions should not deter you from discussing this important question with your child's doctor: "Does she still need this medication?"

For teens at risk of misusing their agents, such as substance abusers, the medication needs to be stowed and inventoried carefully. Medications with abuse potential such as the benzodiazepines or stimulants should be kept in a safe place (avoid medicine cabinets). Some parents have a locking drawer or cabinet in which they store their children's medication. Of interest, it's generally not the adolescent for whom the medication is prescribed who abuses the compounds but the child's friends or friends of a friend.

My son has been on medication for a year now, and I'm beginning to wonder if he needs his pills anymore.

It's not a good idea to stop giving a child his medication without talking to the doctor first. Some medications need to be tapered slowly (see the box above), but it's also possible that your child's doctor will disagree with trying to wean him from the medication right now. While psychotropic drugs do not cure psychiatric or psychological disorders, some conditions do improve in some children over time, which is one reason to reassess the need for pharmacotherapy by tapering and discontinuing the medications periodically. This taper should be considered if your child is free of symptoms for a significant period of time, typically considered to be 6–12 months.

After 14-year-old Maria had been treated successfully for depression with an antidepressant for 1½ years, we decided to try tapering her medication. First we reduced her dosage from 20 mg to 10 mg daily for about 2 months. Then we administered 5 mg every day for another month. When her symptoms did not reappear over this 3-month time period, we discontinued the medication altogether.

Additional considerations are whether there is evidence of change and growth in the child since the medication was begun. The ideal situation is one like 13-year-old Tanya's experience. We started her on a medication for severe anxiety that had kept her from attending school, and not only did the medication clearly reduce the anxiety but she also developed new skills. Tanya became quite skilled at talking about her emotions and quite brave at challenging herself to try new situations, which had been difficult in the past. In this situation, following 10 months of successes in school, we felt confident that she was doing well, due to a combination of a medication effect and the development of new coping strategies, leaving her far less vulnerable to stress than in the past. Given this change, we felt confident that the timing was right to taper and discontinue the medication.

What is a medication holiday, and why would we choose to do that?

A medication holiday is a period of time (weeks to months) during which the child's medication is discontinued, principally to address concern about longer-term side effects. Medication holidays are commonly used over the summer months, such as for children with ADHD whose symptoms predominantly affect academic performance when you are concerned about the medication's impact on the child's health. For example, a medication holiday may be used for a child on an appetite-suppressing medication to enhance his appetite and help him catch up on his weight over the summer. Medication holidays are not appropriate for children and adolescents who suffer from illness that is more serious and pervasive.

When Children Need to Be Hospitalized

Despite efforts at treating children with therapy and/or medications, some may still need a structured-day treatment or psychiatric hospitalization, whether partial or full. Although necessary at times, typically due to threats to harm themselves or unsafe aggression in the home, a higher level of care such as hospitalization can understandably cause anxiety in parents. Because children are being released from hospitals much faster now (the typical length of stay is 1 week), parents and families may feel they are facing the care of sick children without sufficient outpatient resources (counselors, psychiatrists) or school supports to manage youth while they are still quite unstable.

Commensurate with reduced hospitalization, there has been an increase in the utilization of day treatment facilities (caring for the child during the day in a semistructured setting). These facilities may accept a child to avoid a psychiatric hospitalization, or a child may be placed there following a psychiatric hospitalization, as a "step-down" transition to being back home full time.

Regardless, more intensive care for your child can involve time in commuting for visitations and for meetings. If your child is coming out of the hospital, you may want to plan to have ancillary assistance as well as more time available to supervise her at home. Parents can seek out reasonable agreements with their workplace under the Family and Medical Leave Act (FMLA; details are available from the U.S. Department of Labor at its website, *www.dol.gov/whd/fmla*).

What are the reasons for hospitalizing a child?

Practitioners decide on hospitalization based on a number of variables. As stated above, hospitalization is typically considered when children are acting in a way that is dangerous either to themselves (such as being suicidal) or to others (including the threat to harm a sibling, parent, or peer). Other reasons for hospitalizing children include a rapidly deteriorating condition, inadequate resources to manage them safely at home or in the community, severe behavioral medication reaction, or unstable eating disorders.

If I thought my child needed this type of care, what would I do?

The method of getting your child hospitalized varies among regions. In most cases, if you are concerned about your child's condition, contact the treating practitioner. If your child suddenly becomes out of control or dangerous to himself or to others, you may be in the position of having to take him to the nearest emergency room or local mental health crisis center. If your child refuses to comply, you may contact the local police and ambulance to transport the child to the nearest evaluation site.

What happens when we get to the hospital?

In the crisis center or emergency room, your child will be assessed for hospitalization. If your child is deemed dangerous to herself or others, the practitioner may "commit" the child to a psychiatric hospital or psychiatric wing of the medical center. This commitment will last for an initial 3 days, during which the hospital, in collaboration with the child's caregivers, will determine the necessity of continuing hospital care. However, most commonly, during the admitting process, you will be asked to voluntarily sign your child in to the psychiatric facility. This is typically what is done: all agree the child needs to be in the hospital for safety. You will be able to stay with your child throughout the evaluation process and transfer to the psychiatric hospital. You can be very helpful in aiding your child in the transition to the hospital as well as providing invaluable information to the admitting team. Unfortunately, due to limited capacity in the mental health system, it is not unusual for a child to wait in an emergency room for hours, even days, for a psychiatric bed to be available. Or a child may "board" on a pediatric medical inpatient floor, waiting for transfer to a psychiatric hospital. In addition, when found, psychiatric hospital beds may be available in communities far from a child's home, making visitation and treatment planning difficult.

Does insurance cover psychiatric hospitalization of children?

Depending on your insurance, the decision to pay for hospitalization may need to be reviewed with the evaluation team prior to transfer to a hospital.

Likewise, the specific hospital to which your child will be admitted may also be determined by your insurance and bed availability. Some families choose to pay privately for psychiatric hospitalization in specialized centers. The hospital will need to provide ongoing evidence of the need for hospitalization during the course of your child's stay. You and the treatment team can appeal decisions made by insurers regarding approval of length of stay. Of course, insurance for mental health care can vary widely, and it's best to contact your insurance company to know what is covered, and for how long, as some insurers may have total yearly limits.

How long will my child remain in the hospital?

It depends on the child's condition, the hospital, and outpatient resources. In the past, children (and adults) were often hospitalized for months. At present, hospitalizations average 1–2 weeks. Your child may be transferred from intensive inpatient status to day treatment or a step-down program, as discussed earlier. Day treatment encompasses having your child spend nights and weekends at home while going to the hospital during the day. Many of the specifics of the approach to your child's care are based on the resources available in your community.

Will the hospital be able to figure out why my child's condition worsened?

Having your child in the hospital affords the opportunity, while in a safe environment, to get an initial or fresh comprehensive view of the situation. Medication trials can move along more rapidly while the child is in this safe environment and can be monitored carefully for behavioral and medical complications. This is not to suggest that faster dose increases are always indicated or lead to greater effect.

How can I make this process productive for my child?

To facilitate your child's treatment, be sure the hospital team is in contact with your child's outpatient team. Make yourselves available for individual and family meetings. Provide information on your child upon request. Also be sure to familiarize yourself with the hospital policy on bringing in toys or food, visitation, and phone calls.

How can I stop feeling so awful about this?

Be ready for a flood of emotions. Hospitalizing your child may be one of the hardest experiences you will ever undergo. First and foremost, know that if your child is threatening suicide, you are doing the right thing to take that threat seriously and take action to protect your child. Some parents, probably out of fear of the reality of the situation, believe their children are only trying to get attention and may even try to talk their children out of feeling suicidal. This situation demands expert advice and may be urgent, in which case a hospital is a good source of help.

Added to the angst of the precipitating event leading to hospitalization, parents often experience guilt, separation anxiety, and helplessness due to their lack of control. Don't be surprised if you feel angry, sad, anxious, or detached while your child is hospitalized. Seek out understanding friends and family during this time. Parents also report that seeing their own or their child's therapist or talking with the hospital social worker can be very educational, comforting, and supportive. There may be the additional stress of providing for siblings who remain home.

Do your best to use your energy constructively in learning from the hospitalization and building the best treatment plan and team possible. For those whose children may end up needing multiple hospitalizations, often at different hospitals, work hard to create a narrative that builds on itself. Consider maintaining a simple one- to two-page summary of your child's key problems (e.g., social anxiety, sadness, poor body image), diagnoses (e.g., depression, social anxiety), treatments (e.g., CBT with Dr. *X* for the past 6 months), medications (see the sample medication logs in Figure 3 and Appendix B), and hospitalizations that you can bring to the hospital. It may be quite appropriate to demand that the inpatient team contact the outpatient team prior to any decisions regarding treatment. Communication within the field, from inpatient to outpatient and vice versa, remains poor but will be responsive to your direction.

Part II

Common Childhood Psychiatric Disorders

This section describes the most common emotional, behavioral, cognitive, and developmental disorders seen in children and adolescents. Because every child is unique and so many have more than one disorder, your child is unlikely to fit squarely into any one of these molds. You may, however, find it helpful to consult these summaries of symptoms and behavioral patterns during the diagnostic evaluation. Does the picture of the disorder in this book mesh with what you see in your child and what the practitioner is reporting to you? If not, what you read here may help you formulate questions that will push the evaluation process toward an accurate hypothesis. It's very important that you know and agree with what is going on with your child before you agree to treatment.

You may also wish to come back to this section if you notice a change in your child's behavior or other symptoms:

- Could a new problem be developing?
- Are these signs typical of the child's disorder at the older age your child has reached?
- What is the disorder's expected course?

The fundamental information in the following chapters should serve as a springboard for the ongoing dialogue between you and the doctor that will ensure continued good care for your child. In addition to a description of symptoms and some examples of how the various disorders look in real children, each chapter tells you what we know to date about neurological and other biological causes. Following the description of each disorder, you will find information on how we currently treat it—including methods for resolving the side effects of some treatments—and why. Full descriptions of the pharmacological agents used in treatment are given in Part III.

5
Attentional and Disruptive Behavioral Disorders

Attention-Deficit/Hyperactivity Disorder

ADHD is the most common psychiatric disorder that pediatricians, family physicians, neurologists, and psychiatrists treat in children. It affects from 6 to 9% of school-age children, at least 70% of whom will continue to have the disorder into adolescence. About half of all children with ADHD will still have the disorder as adults. With age, the hyperactivity and impulsivity tend to diminish; however, the attentional problems often persist.

The Disorder

In the past you may have heard basically the same syndrome called attention deficit disorder (ADD), ADDH, or ADD with or without hyperactivity. Today the disorder is known collectively as ADHD, as defined in DSM-5 (see page 62). The symptoms that characterize ADHD are inattentiveness, distractibility, impulsivity, and often hyperactivity, all to a degree considered inappropriate for the developmental stage of the child. That is, a 4-year-old who "can't sit still" would not necessarily be suspected of having ADHD. A 12-year-old with the same problem, however, would be suspect. Typically, children with ADHD also get frustrated easily, shift what they are working on frequently, get bored easily, are disorganized, and daydream a lot. Because ADHD reveals itself in atypical ways of feeling, thinking, and acting, it is known as an emotional, cognitive, and behavioral disorder.

The symptoms of ADHD are usually present in many areas—they show up in a multitude of situations—but they may not all occur in all settings. Children whose main problem is inattention, for example, may have difficulties in school and in completing homework but few troubles with peers or family. Children with more hyperactive or impulsive symptoms may do relatively well in school academically but have difficulties at home or in situations offering less guidance and structure. The symptoms of ADHD may impair the child's academic performance, overall behavior, and social/interpersonal relationships. But because the symptoms vary among children and in different environments, the disorder is not always easy to diagnose, especially when inattention is the predominant symptom.

Fifteen-year-old Steve, for instance, was doing worse and worse in school, taking an inordinate amount of time to complete homework, and becoming more and more frustrated and depressed. But cognitive (thinking ability) tests showed his intelligence was above average, and he had no major learning disabilities. It took a complete evaluation to reveal that Steve was highly inattentive and distractible, was unable to finish tasks, and was daydreaming a great deal of the time. After treatment with Metadate CD 20 mg in the morning, his inattention improved, and so did his school performance. In turn, his self-esteem rose, and his frustration dropped over the next few months.

It can take some digging to unveil ADHD when the more noticeable symptoms of hyperactivity don't appear, but it is crucial that parents and other adults in the child's life not ignore symptoms like Steve's. Many children with untreated ADHD not only become dejected and discouraged by the problems their disorder imposes but begin to have other secondary problems as well.

Research shows that ADHD commonly occurs with oppositional defiant disorder (40–60% of cases), anxiety disorders (35%), and conduct disorder (10–20%). More recent studies show that ADHD also occurs along with mood disorders—depression and bipolar disorder (10–20%). Increased rates of cigarette smoking and substance abuse also are associated with ADHD; however, treatment reduces or delays those problems. Learning disorders appear to co-occur with ADHD in up to one-third of children, so they should be considered in all kids with ADHD. If your child has specific learning problems in distinct academic areas such as reading, writing, or math, or has severe organizational issues, be sure to seek further evaluation—your child's school or pediatrician should be able to provide a referral.

We like to refer to ADHD as a neurobehavioral disorder. The *neuro-*part of the disorder relates to basic science investigations indicating that individuals with ADHD manifest disturbances in the neurotransmitters dopamine and norepinephrine (but not in serotonin, another neurotransmitter you may have read a lot about). These chemicals appear to be deficient in specific regions of the brain. The *-behavioral* part of the description refers to the behaviors that occur as a manifestation of having ADHD, such as impulsivity, hyperactivity, and the like.

Brain imaging used in research has shown that certain parts of the brain are usually different in individuals with ADHD: the frontal lobes; the striatum, which is rich in dopamine; the cingulate, involved in attention, emotions, and memory; the corpus callosum, which is the major connection among the lobes of the brain; and the cerebellum, which is involved in motor activities and diverse functions such as "keeping track of time." Brain scanning has in fact confirmed what neuropsychology has discovered: that these are the areas related to attention, vigilance, and distractibility. Research over the years since this book was first published is beginning to reveal a lot about the genetic basis of ADHD. For instance, children with ADHD have been found to have a few different types of variations in their genes that are linked to subtle, but important, problems in nerve-to-nerve communication.

Despite the neurological causes of ADHD, brain activity and brain imaging tests such as EEGs; brain electrical activity mapping, or BEAMs (fancy EEGs); and single-photon-emission space tomography, or SPECT (blood flow) studies are *not* considered reliable or valid in diagnosing ADHD; nor are blood tests. Some recent work on EEGs may prove to be useful for identification of ADHD and related conditions, however, so stay tuned. To date, a comprehensive history of the problem remains the best way to identify the disorder. The neuropsychological tests used in research studies—the CPT (Continuous Performance Test), Wisconsin Card Sort, Stroop Test, and TOVA—are also *not* part of the standard clinical evaluation for ADHD. There simply are not enough scientific data to support their effectiveness alone in diagnosing ADHD or directing medication management in day-to-day clinical practice. If an evaluator suggests such tests, therefore, you would be wise to ask why.

If your child was diagnosed with ADHD since the publication of the most recent revision of the DSM (DSM-5), he or she should have been diagnosed as having either the predominantly hyperactive subtype, the predominantly inattentive subtype, or the combined subtype. But diagnostic classification and criteria for ADHD seem to be in an ongoing state of flux as we learn more about the course of this disorder and its different manifestations. Approximately one-half of pediatric (and one-quarter of psychiatric) referrals have predominantly inattentive ADHD. But controversy exists over whether it is really intimately related to the combined subtype or whether the combined subtype, because of having more symptoms of ADHD, really just represents a more serious form of the disorder. For example, children with the inattentive subtype have fewer co-occurring difficulties, perhaps a different cognitive style (sluggish), and less overall impairment. Do kids who shed the predominant hyperactivity/impulsivity as they grow up really have the inattentive subtype, or are they really grown-ups with combined subtype ADHD? In general, the medication response for stimulants and nonstimulants is similar between the subtypes. In other words, kids with the inattentive subtype respond as well to the stimulants and nonstimulants as those who have the more classic "combined" subtype.

Also, it used to be thought that girls were overrepresented in the inattentive subtype, but that no longer appears to be true. Recent information on girls with ADHD indicate that they often internalize much of the stigma yet share many of the same characteristics and co-occurring problems that boys with the disorder have. For example, medications work equally well in girls and boys with ADHD.

The Treatment

Medication is considered one of the most important treatments for ADHD; the medications currently in use are listed in Table 4. In fact, its use with this disorder has been studied more extensively than any other application of psychopharmacology in children. One recent large study of children with ADHD and without other disorders completed in New York and Montreal demonstrated that, compared to intensive multimodal treatment including medications and psychotherapy, properly prescribed stimulants alone had the greatest positive effect after 2 years. Another very important study, funded by the National Institute of Mental Health, produced similar results, showing that medications were superior to behavioral treatments alone for the core symptoms of ADHD. The study also found that behavioral treatment along with

multimodal treatment:
The use of two or more different distinct types of therapy (such as medications and psychotherapy).

medication management was the most effective treatment to address some of the noncore symptoms (self-esteem, peer relationships, family functioning, and social skills).

The best-studied class of drugs for ADHD, and in most cases the treatment of choice, is stimulant medications—notably Ritalin (methylphenidate), Ritalin LA (extended-release methylphenidate), Daytrana (methylphenidate transdermal system [patch]), Metadate CD (extended-release methylphenidate), Focalin (Focalin XR—extended-release D-methylphenidate), Concerta and Quillivant XR (extended-release methylphenidate), Adderall (amphetamine), Adderall XR (extended-release amphetamine), Dexedrine (dextroamphetamine), Vyvanse (an extended-release dextroamphetamine prodrug, and Aptensio or Aptenso—the new methylphenidate drug; see more on this type of agent in Chapter 12). Stimulants generally work immediately when the correct dose is achieved. Although it is unusual for children to develop a tolerance to these drugs, they may need increasing doses as they grow.

Practitioners have found that if one stimulant is unsuccessful, it is worth trying another, but if your child cannot tolerate the stimulants or has prominent anxiety, mood symptoms, or tics, Strattera (atomoxetine) should be tried. Strattera is the first FDA-approved nonstimulant noradrenergic medication that is useful for ADHD. Strattera usually takes a few weeks to see its full benefit and is sometimes used with stimulants.

For children as young as 3–5 years, in aggressive or especially overactive kids, the alpha agonist (antihypertensive) medications Kapvay/Catapres (clonidine) and Intuniv/Tenex (guanfacine) may be useful. Alpha agonists are named based on their effects on a select group of receptors (molecules that "catch" the chemical messengers on nerve cells). Alpha agonists stimulate (activate) norepinephrine receptors. Norepinephrine is related to ADHD. These medications also have been found to be useful for inattentive symptoms. The alpha agonists may help with the sleep problems that sometimes plague children with ADHD or that result from its treatment with stimulants. Extended-release forms of guanfacine (Intuniv) and clonidine (Kapvay) offer the benefit of a once- or twice-daily, well-tested form of this class of medications for ADHD and have been approved by the FDA for use with children. For kids who respond partially to stimulants, alpha agonists are also FDA approved to be used along with the stimulant.

Second-line treatments include the antidepressants, both the tricyclics (desipramine, imipramine, nortriptyline) and Wellbutrin. Although you may see an effect immediately, antidepressants may take up to 4 weeks to reach full effectiveness. As with the stimulants, if one antidepressant is not effective, your child's doctor would be wise to try another.

Another nonstimulant medication that has been tested and shown effective for ADHD, though not FDA approved, is Provigil (modafinil). Provigil has had mixed results in trials for ADHD: positive in kids but not in adults. At a dose of approximately 200 mg in the morning and 100 mg in the afternoon, it has a moderate response in reducing ADHD symptoms with the most common side effects being headaches, stomachaches, edginess, and insomnia, and a rare side effect being a serious skin rash.

There was initial excitement about a newer group of medications that stop the breakdown of a neurotransmitter related to memory called cholinesterase. These medications, which have been successfully used in adults with Alzheimer's disease and are called cholinesterase inhibitors (Aricept [donepezil], Reminyl [galantamine], and Exelon [rivastigmine]), have had generally negative results for ADHD. One unique medication used in Alzheimer's disease, called memantine, is still being studied, however, and may help a select group of individuals with ADHD who also suffer from executive functioning issues ("the secretary in your brain"). Stay tuned.

Don't be surprised if your child's doctor ends up prescribing a combination of medications, such as Focalin XR with Intuniv, Concerta with Strattera, Wellbutrin and stimulants, or stimulants with clonidine. That is the way we often get the best possible improvement in ADHD symptoms. More than one drug may also be necessary if your child, like about half of the children who have ADHD, has other psychiatric disorders as well. Naturally comorbidity (see pages 16–17) complicates treatment. Atomoxetine (Strattera) may be particularly useful as monotherapy (single medication) in comorbid ADHD with tics, anxiety, or depression.

In children with ADHD and anxiety disorders, the stimulants may worsen the anxiety, in which case atomoxetine, an alpha agonist (Intuniv or Kapvay), a tricyclic antidepressant such as nortriptyline, or another antidepressant (including Zoloft, Effexor) may be helpful. Your child's doctor may need to combine agents, such as a medication for ADHD plus one for anxiety such as Buspar or a Valium-like agent.

For children with ADHD and depression, the use of an antidepressant such as Wellbutrin, a tricyclic antidepressant (imipramine, desipramine, etc.), or Effexor may be effective on its own. Or, as documented by the experience of many clinicians and research, the Prozac-like medications (SSRIs) along with the stimulants could work. Fifteen-year-old Sara, already taking Metadate CD (extended-release methylphenidate) for ADHD, did very well with 20 mg of Prozac daily and 20 mg daily of Metadate CD after the depression she had developed failed to respond to changing medications and psychotherapy. (There are, however, concerns about treating children and adolescents suffering from depression with the SSRIs; see Chapter 13.)

Treatment of children with bipolar disorder and ADHD is complicated. These children should be treated with an antipsychotic or a mood stabilizer for the bipolar disorder and then cautiously with a stimulant, alpha agonist, or Wellbutrin for the ADHD. Data for adults suggest Wellbutrin alone may be a good choice for less severe moodiness plus ADHD.

The sizable group of children and adolescents with intellectual disability or developmental disorders who show prominent ADHD symptoms may also benefit from pharmacological treatment of the ADHD. Although untested scientifically, the use of Strattera for kids with ADHD and learning disabilities and/or ASD has elicited some interest. Clinicians have reported improved ADHD symptoms, improved socialization and interaction, and less anxiety.

It is important to realize, however, that the care of specific developmental disorders, including learning disabilities, is largely remedial and supportive. That is, medications don't treat the intellectual or learning disabilities but may help remedial treatment work better.

Children with ADHD who have prominent organizational and time-management issues ("secretary in the brain" executive function problems) may benefit from a medicine for their ADHD plus atomoxetine (Strattera), and sometimes an Alzheimer's medication (e.g., memantine), although the effectiveness of these has not been demonstrated in controlled clinical trials.

Whatever medications end up being prescribed, when you should give them to your child depends on the severity and pervasiveness of the child's problems, and you need to rely largely on your judgment. Most children should remain on their medication all the time. However, your child may need the medication only during school, with weekend and vacation holidays off the medication, or around the clock and on vacations. If, for example, your child has made lasting friendships only since being placed on a stimulant, you probably won't want to limit the medication to school hours. But for a child whose main problem is inattention at school, weekend and vacation holidays may be fine. Also, some kids on stimulants have significant loss of appetite and weight loss and will need times off their stimulant to "catch up." Whereas the stimulants can be discontinued on weekends, it is advisable not to change the dosing of Strattera (atomoxetine), the alpha agonists clonidine (Kapvay) or guanfacine (Tenex, Intuniv), or the antidepressants.

Oppositional Defiant Disorder

Eleven-year-old Tim snaps at his mother when limits are set, argues incessantly, and frequently uses foul language. He instigates trouble among his siblings but is quick to blame them for problems for which he is clearly responsible. Tim is typical of children with oppositional defiant disorder. He creates problems for his family and others, although he doesn't inflict major harm or damage property, or steal.

The Disorder

Like Tim, children with oppositional defiant disorder are extremely difficult to care for or be around because their ongoing behavior falls at the extreme end of normal on a continuum. Parents and other adults often bear the brunt of the child's behavior since the child's oppositionality is usually directed at authority figures. These children often appear inflexible and have a quick temper in response to limit setting. The degree of inflexibility, however, is often key to understanding why your child may react to situations the way he does. While children who have oppositional defiant disorder will not necessarily be depressed, they will appear to have a pretty consistently negative attitude, taking the opposite side against you, teachers, or other authority figures; being quick to blame others for their behavior; frequently swearing and acting like "tough guys"; and being annoying to or being annoyed easily by others. The good news is that a large group of these children grow out of the disorder as they become young adults. The bad news is that a small group will progress to conduct disorder, generally by a young age (see page 137).

No specific brain region has been implicated in oppositional defiant disorder, although a disruption in serotonin may be involved in those who are oppositional and aggressive.

The Treatment

If your child also has ADHD or a mood disorder, as is common with oppositional defiant disorder, the medications for the former typically reduce the intensity of the oppositionality as well. The alpha agonists clonidine/Kapvay and guanfacine/Tenex or Intuniv, the stimulant drugs, Strattera, the tricyclics, or Wellbutrin also may reduce some of the symptoms and impairment associated with the disorder. Risperdal and Abilify (and presumably the other atypical antipsychotics) have been shown to be effective in more severe cases typically associated with conduct disorder (see below). Fortunately, medication is not your only option—behavioral modification and other conflict-resolution-based therapies such as collaborative problem solving appear to help both parents and children develop strategies for managing and reducing the impact of the symptoms.

Conduct Disorder

The Disorder

What mental health professionals of today call *conduct disorder* has often been viewed informally as juvenile delinquency—behavior that consistently violates the basic rights of others and disregards societal norms and rules. Bullying of younger children, cruelty to animals, fights (sometimes with weapons), and purposeful destruction of property are common among children with conduct disorder. The stealing, truancy, and lying that occasionally appear in normal development are rampant and persistent in the child with conduct disorder. A hallmark of conduct disorder is lack of remorse for these problematic behaviors or refusal to take responsibility for them.

Children with conduct disorder are usually very aggressive. Some have uncontrolled outbursts and may be described as having a bad temper; their outbursts may be triggered by individual external events or related to having some psychiatric disturbance such as a mood problem like depression or bipolar disorder. We have found that these children often have excessive "mood reactivity"—that is, they overreact greatly to minor provocations that result in negative outcomes and consequences. Others behave in a more predatory fashion, and their behavior may come across as cold, callous, and premeditated.

The Treatment

In some cases, conduct disorder appears to be passed on from parent to child, especially to the sons of alcoholic and antisocial fathers. Despite the fact that serotonin levels have been found to be lower and EEG activity may be different in children with conduct disorder and aggressive adults, pharmacotherapy has not proved to be a very satisfactory sole treatment. It is imperative to examine what seems to be the root of the problem and determine whether co-occurring difficulties such as a mood disorder are evident in the child. Children with the outburst type of aggression may respond more favorably to pharmacological intervention such as a mood stabilizer (e.g., Tegretol or Depakote) or an antipsychotic (Abilify) than those who perform calculated aggressive acts. But medication seems most likely to help when it is used to treat a co-occurring problem, such as depression or bipolar disorder. One study found that children with conduct disorder and depression who took imipramine had a substantial reduction in both their conduct symptoms and their depression. Similar findings were reported in youth with ADHD and conduct disorder who were treated with methylphenidate. Aggressiveness shared by youth with conduct disorder and bipolar disorder is reduced significantly with the atypical antipsychotics (e.g., Risperdal, Zyprexa). Research also shows that medications like Abilify, Geodon, and Risperdal are effective in managing the core symptoms of conduct disorder (e.g., aggressivity) in children and adolescents.

If you suspect that your child has conduct disorder, be sure to ask your doctor to look for other conditions: not only depression and bipolar disorder but also ADHD, posttraumatic stress, or anxiety. These disorders respond not only to pharmacological intervention but also to psychotherapy.

In the final analysis, intermittent treatment with behavioral and family therapy may be necessary for both the child and the family. Studies indicate that most children will continue to have the disorder, or aggressivity, for a long time. Long-term information indicates that an intact family may be one of the most important factors in an eventual positive outcome for the grown-up child with conduct disorder.

Table 4. Pharmacotherapy of ADHD and the Disruptive Behavioral Disorders

Disorder	Pharmacotherapy
Attention-deficit/ hyperactivity disorder (ADHD)	Stimulants—Ritalin, Ritalin SR, Ritalin LA, Metadate CD, Vyvanse, Dexedrine, Adderall XR, Concerta, Focalin XR, Quillivant, Daytrana
	First-line drugs of choice (FDA-approved)
	Extended-release preparations preferred (Concerta, Ritalin LA, Focalin XR, Metadate CD, Daytrana [methylphenidate patch], Quillivant [suspension]; Adderall XR, Vyvanse)
	Caution in patients with tics, marked height/weight problems or cardiac concerns
	Strattera (atomoxetine)
	First-line agent (FDA-approved)
	May be particularly useful in comorbid cases (tics, anxiety, substance abuse)
	Caution with bipolar disorder
	Catapres, Kapvay (extended-release clonidine), Tenex (guanfacine), Intuniv (extended-release guanfacine)—alpha agonists
	First-line agents (FDA-approved alone and in combination with stimulants)
	Effective for hyperactivity and impulsivity as well as inattention, preschoolers
	First line for patients with ADHD + tics
	Tricyclic antidepressants—desipramine, nortriptyline, imipramine
	Second line after stimulants/Strattera/alpha agonists
	May be effective for co-occurring depression, anxiety, or tics
	Caution if cardiac problems

(*cont.*)

Table 4 (*cont.*)

Disorder	Pharmacotherapy

Attention-deficit/ hyperactivity disorder (ADHD) (*cont.*)	Wellbutrin (bupropion)
	    Second line after stimulants/Strattera/alpha agonists
	    Caution if tics or seizures
	    May be effective for comorbid depression or bipolar disorder
	
	Modafinil (Provigil)
	    May be effective for ADHD, low motivation, low arousal states
	
	Combined pharmacotherapy for resistant cases

Conduct disorder, oppositional defiant disorder (ODD)	No specific pharmacotherapy available for core disorders
	
	Look for and treat other disorders (e.g., ADHD, bipolar disorder, depression)
	
	Consider stimulants, alpha agonists, Strattera, antidepressants (tricyclics or Wellbutrin)
	
	For serious agitation, aggression, and self-abuse consider
	    Antipsychotics (e.g., Seroquel, Risperdal, Abilify)
	    Beta blockers (e.g., propranolol)
	    Clonidine, guanfacine
	    Benzodiazepines (e.g., Ativan, Klonopin)
	    Lithium, anticonvulsants (e.g., Tegretol, Valproate, Trileptal, Neurontin)
	    Naltrexone

6
Anxiety-Related Disorders

Anxiety Disorders of Childhood

These disorders vary widely in how they arise and how they affect children, but they all have one thing in common: ongoing excessive anxiety, worrying, or nervousness. Children with these disorders are not just "worry warts." Their anxiety is exaggerated, inappropriate for their age or developmental level, pervasive, and out of proportion to the situation at hand. It can make the child's daily life a misery. The child not only feels the agony of mental and physical distress but may engineer his entire life to avoid anxiety-provoking situations—all without really understanding what is happening. Needless to say, such machinations can have far-reaching social ramifications. For instance, these children will avoid playing with other kids, be uncomfortable meeting new kids, be unable to speak in front of even a small group of children, and in more severe form refuse to go to school or extracurricular activities.

Childhood anxiety disorders are relatively common, with an estimated 4% of 11-year-olds having separation anxiety disorder and 2% having simple phobia. In 14- to 16-year-olds, 5% have phobias. A phobia is a fear that leads to avoidance of situations in which the fear might be triggered, such as not going outside because of a fear of snakes. A simple phobia is a specific fear (and generally avoidance of the thing feared), such as of spiders, heights, or animals.

Research tells us that shyness can be identified in very young children and that it may continue into adolescence and in some cases turn into an anxiety disorder. In many cases, anxiety disorders apparently continue into adulthood. Of interest, a majority of adults being treated for anxiety problems say their disorder began in adolescence.

It is interesting that the parts of the brain related to emotion and fear (e.g., the amygdala and others) are thought to develop quite early in a child's life. It is thought that these systems are important to help children develop the fight-or-flight mechanism necessary to protect them from potential harm. When children develop abnormal anxiety, their brain prematurely and too frequently triggers the intrinsic fight-or-flight response—leaving children feeling scared, unnerved, and causing them to avoid certain situations (phobic). Compounding these issues, the child's cognitive/executive/frontal brain areas develop later than the emotional centers, so the child may have little insight as to what is occurring and/or control over her anxiety symptoms without formal cognitive training (cognitive and/or behavioral therapy).

By their very nature, anxiety symptoms are often turned inward. If we consider the shame many children feel over their "weakness" and "fear," it should be no surprise that they often don't report these problems to their parents or others. If your observations lead you to suspect your child may have anxiety problems, ask her directly if she worries, feels nervous, or sometimes just feels bad for unknown reasons. Observe whether your child has many physical ailments without a cause (called *somatization*). Here's what to look for—the most common ways that anxiety disorders appear in children and adolescents.

The Disorders

Separation Anxiety

Among the common disorders of childhood, separation anxiety is characterized by excessive worry and fear over being away from a caretaker or familiar surroundings. Although some separation anxiety is normal in younger children, when this problem continues, say, into the school years, it may prove to be an anxiety disorder. Toddlers, for example, are notorious for forcing their parents to go through absurd gyrations to "sneak out" when leaving the child with a sitter; however, similar behavior in an 8-year-old is problematic.

Obviously the problem can be debilitating to an older child, who may refuse to go to school or develop stomachaches or headaches at school that force the child to return home. These children will often comment that they are afraid something "bad" will happen to their parents or siblings when they are away from home.

Generalized Anxiety Disorder

Michael, age 7, worries incessantly about performing well in school, particularly before a quiz. When I saw him, he had been evaluated by his pediatrician for multiple stomach problems, none of which were found on more extensive testing. He appeared anxious and reported feeling "funny inside." He noted "worrying all the time" but said he'd never experienced panic attacks. Michael is typical of children who have generalized anxiety disorder.

Children who worry excessively about minor matters or schoolwork, are overly concerned about what others think of them, and are perfectionists may have generalized anxiety disorder. These kids often complain about feeling on edge or restless inside. They commonly obsess over upcoming tests or projects. They also usually have multiple physical complaints, such as stomachaches, diarrhea, headaches, and muscle tightness, and have been seen multiple times in the pediatrician's or school nurse's office for minor medical complaints.

Panic Disorder

Children with panic disorder have discrete attacks of excessive fear for no particular reason. They may feel that something terrible is wrong but not be able to name it. The racing heart and rapid breathing that accompany these attacks often land the child in the pediatrician's or pediatric neurologist's office. When put in a situation that makes them feel trapped, these kids may also have "anger attacks," lashing out at someone who is handy or is instrumental in putting them in the "threatening" situation—often you, the parent.

Agoraphobia, the fear of going where escape is limited, is another frequent companion of panic disorder. This fear may greatly restrict the child's travel away from home and thus cause other problems for the child and the rest of the family. Children with agoraphobia might fear being in a car (or bus or train), going to school, going over bridges, driving through tunnels, or riding in elevators. Being unable to get into a car to be driven to a friend's house to play after school puts obvious crimps in a child's social life. Kids with agoraphobia may need a companion to help them stay calm when traveling somewhere or when in any place other than home. In some cases, though, the behavior is mystifying and difficult to recognize as agoraphobia. Seven-year-old Zoe, generally soft-spoken and described as "very sweet," would whine and then suddenly lash out at her mother in anger right before they left home to go shopping. It wasn't until her parents found out the same behavior was occurring to a lesser extent on the school bus that they began to suspect something was wrong.

Social Phobia

Among the most common anxiety-based problems to affect children, adolescents, and adults is social phobia, a fear of humiliation in social situations. Kids with social phobia have marked difficulty talking or making a presentation in front of other kids and adults because they are nervous about saying something embarrassing. Although more minor social phobia is generally not treated, the condition can be debilitating when the child has prominent symptoms such as stomachaches or panic attacks and begins to avoid talking in front of his peers even in informal groups. It can result in kids missing school on days with scheduled oral presentations or group discussions. Certainly, if your child has developed severe anxiety and/or panic attacks or is demonstrating substantial avoidance of activities, he should be considered for treatment of social phobia. In evaluating your child for an anxiety disorder, it is very important that the doctor look for the possibility of coexisting emotional problems such as depression as well as behavioral problems such as ADHD. Interestingly, children with shyness seem to be at reduced risk for later substance problems, whereas adolescents with active anxiety such as generalized anxiety are at increased risk for a substance use problem. It may be that some of these children are self-medicating their distressing anxiety symptoms.

The Treatment

Both psychotherapy and medication have been shown to be effective for anxiety problems. Cognitive-behavioral therapy, behavioral modification, and mindfulness/ relaxation techniques can reduce anxiety and the resulting avoidance in children and are considered first-line treatments for these kids. Seven-year-old Michael, for example, gained much improvement in his generalized anxiety disorder with behavioral modification focused on relaxation imagery. It's important to remind your children to practice the skills learned in therapy many times *while not experiencing anxiety*, so that when they are in an anxiety-provoking situation, they will be able to access the learned skills successfully.

The psychotropic medications used for anxiety in children are listed in Table 5. Although there are not a large number of studies in this area, children and adolescents with anxiety disorders appear to respond to the same pharmacological approaches as adult patients. We have some solid data on SSRIs (e.g., fluvoxamine) and serotonin–norepinephrine reuptake inhibitors (SNRIs) such as duloxetine for anxiety disorders; hence SSRIs and SNRIs are first-line medications for generalized anxiety, separation anxiety, and panic disorder. (See page 231 for information on the SSRIs.) Some children will respond favorably in the short term to the sedative, over-the-counter older antihistamines (such as Benadryl or Atarax). Unfortunately, these agents often are overly sedating and work for only a few days. Therefore, the pharmacotherapy of anxiety relies on the antidepressants, Buspar (buspirone), and benzodiazepines (Valium-like medications), often used along with behavioral modification. Seven-year-old Zoe, introduced on page 143, got much relief from the agoraphobia stemming from her panic disorder with behavioral modification plus the brief use of Ativan.

The antidepressants have been used increasingly for anxiety disorders in children, particularly when the anxiety appears chronic (long-standing). The newer antidepressants—Cymbalta (duloxetine), Prozac (fluoxetine), Luvox (fluvoxamine), Paxil (paroxetine), Lexapro (escitalopram), Celexa (citalopram), Effexor (venlafaxine), and Zoloft (sertraline)—probably are not quite as effective as the benzodiazepines, but they may be an excellent choice if your child has co-occurring depression or OCD. Duloxetine recently received FDA approval for the treatment of children with anxiety disorders. One drawback is that these medications generally need to be used at full antidepressant dosing. To avoid the risk of initial worsening of anxiety or panic, we usually start children on these medications at a very low dose (e.g., Zoloft at 25 mg) and increase them slowly until the parents and we see improvement in the child's anxiety.

If anxiety co-occurs with ADHD, Strattera (atomoxetine) is a good choice. The role of Strattera for anxiety disorders alone is unstudied. The older antidepressants, called the tricyclics, including nortriptyline, imipramine, and others, are considered second- or third-line drugs of choice for anxiety. These agents may, however, be a very good choice if your child has anxiety plus ADHD.

For your child, one of the benzodiazepines—Ativan (lorazepam),

Klonopin (clonazepam), Valium (diazepam), Serax (oxazepam), Xanax (alprazolam), and Tranxene (clorazepate), to name a few—may be the practitioner's first or second medication choice. Almost any of the anxiety-breaking medications will be useful for a typical anxiety problem. For children with panic disorder in particular, the stronger medications in this class, such as Klonopin, Xanax, or Ativan, are usually prescribed.

The benzodiazepines have been used for many years for a host of problems, including seizures and muscle spasms. Because of their effectiveness, excellent margin of safety, and minimal interactions with other drugs, benzodiazepines, along with antihistamines, are also used to treat agitation and insomnia. As a parent you should be aware, though, that these anxiety-breaking agents may produce an opposite reaction in children called *disinhibition* (see page 258). While not dangerous to the child, this paradoxical effect results in restlessness, anxiety, panic, giddiness, and more disturbed behavior, which often starts within 20 minutes of taking the medication. If this reaction should occur, just carefully observe your child and wait it out; the behavior generally subsides within a couple of hours.

The benzodiazepines can be abused and hence should be supervised closely. While we are not so concerned about your child's developing an addiction to these medications, other kids may approach your child about using the medication. These medications generally should be avoided in adolescents with a substance problem. By the way, if you are taking these medications, keep them safely stored as they are the second most common prescription medication "misused" by adolescents (the first being narcotic/opioid painkillers).

Of the nonbenzodiazepines, a novel drug called Buspar (buspirone) is also useful for children with anxiety. See page 259 for more details on the drug. If you have reason to seek a medication with little or no abuse potential that is typically less strong than a benzodiazepine, you may want to read about and discuss Buspar with your child's doctor.

When kids do have anxiety and another disorder, they often need a combination of agents. I (T. E. W.) treat an 11-year-old boy with generalized anxiety and OCD who is doing very well on Ativan 0.5 mg twice daily as needed and 40 mg of Prozac. I also treat a 12-year-old boy with panic disorder, ADHD, and depression who, after many failed pharmacological trials, is now stable on 50 mg of nortriptyline at night, 1 mg daily of Xanax as needed, and 50 mg of Zoloft with breakfast. Strattera is an extremely useful and demonstrated addition for youngsters with ADHD and prominent anxiety. I treated Kyle, an 11-year-old boy with ADHD and generalized anxiety disorder, successfully with 60 mg daily of Strattera. He reported much less anxiety, better attention, and improved quality of life.

Since anxiety disorders are known to wax and wane, periodic tapers to evaluate the continued need for medications are recommended. In some cases children require the medications (or higher doses) only around the beginning (August to November) or end (May to June) of the school year.

Posttraumatic Stress Disorder

The Disorder

Posttraumatic stress disorder (PTSD) is just what its name implies: a combination of ongoing symptoms caused by the stress of having suffered a trauma. A trauma is considered a severe stressor that falls outside the sphere of normal human existence. It may include emotional, physical, or sexual abuse or the witnessing of a calamitous event and may consist of a single incident or repeated exposure to a stressor. Remember, however, that although many children are exposed to trauma, only a small group develop PTSD. PTSD is often accompanied by other psychiatric disorders, including depression and anxiety. The symptoms of the disorder may last less than a month, in which case they are referred to as *acute*, or continue for a long time (*chronic*). The most common symptoms are a physically overaroused state (*hyperarousal*), emotional numbing or callousness, *dissociation* (feeling as if the child is outside of her body), avoidance of situations reminiscent of the event(s), nervousness and excessive startle, and recollections of the event that intrude on the child's thoughts.

There is a growing consensus in the field that, given the ability of the brain to change during development, severe or repeated trauma in children may result in persistent subtle structural and biochemical changes in the brain. The extent of this process and the specific changes have yet to be fully understood, however.

The Treatment

When the trauma suffered is some type of ongoing abuse, the first step in treatment of PTSD is to ensure that the child is in a safe environment.

Whatever the trauma, over time, stability in the environment and the child's communication with parents or caregivers are often very helpful in reducing the impairment caused by the PTSD symptoms. Various psychotherapies can be invaluable in helping children disentangle what occurred and why and in working through many of the issues associated with the trauma, particularly if it continued over a period of time. Specific therapies directed at diminishing the manifestations and emotions derived from the trauma and reliving the trauma are effective and considered first-line treatment for these youth.

No particular medication regimen has been found effective for PTSD, so your child's doctor is likely to target the child's most impairing and persistent symptoms for pharmacological treatment. For example, I (T. E. W.) found clonidine (0.1 mg) very helpful in reducing not only the sleep disturbance but also the nighttime anxiety of a 7-year-old girl who had been sexually abused and was unable to sleep despite months of counseling. Prazosin, a blood pressure medication (antihypertensive/alpha agonist), has been reported helpful when given at night to relieve nightmares associated with PTSD. For physically overaroused children who tend to startle easily, antihypertensive agents or a beta blocker such as propranolol can be useful. The antidepressants or the Valium-like medications (benzodiazepines) such as Ativan can help children whose functioning is disrupted by severe avoidance or nervousness.

For those who are plagued by repeated breaks with reality or "out-of-body" experiences (called *dissociative episodes*), techniques such as grounding can reconnect the child to the current environment. Grounding entails, for example, reminding the child where she is and what is going on around her. If these dissociative episodes are prominent, impairing, or scary to your child, the doctor may also try antipsychotic agents such as Abilify or Risperdal at low doses.

Children suffering from posttraumatic stress often have depression and anxiety disorders at the same time. If an evaluation produces such a diagnosis for your child, the practitioner may try an antidepressant such as one of the SSRIs (Prozac, Lexapro, Zoloft, Luvox, Paxil, Celexa), an SNRI (Effexor, Cymbalta), tricyclic antidepressant (nortriptyline, imipramine, and others), Serzone, trazodone, Remeron, or other medications. Emotional numbing, however, responds less well to pharmacological treatment. If your child has several problems related to posttraumatic stress, a combination of agents may be needed. We have used very low doses of Prozac (5 mg per day by suspension) and Catapres (half a tablet twice a day) or Intuniv (guanfacine, once daily) with excellent response in children with agitation, overarousal, irritability, depression, and sleep disturbances. It is important to remember, however, that many children with multiple PTSD symptoms will overcome them with time, environmental change, and therapy. If your child is among these kids, think of any medication prescribed mostly as temporary treatment, and make sure the child's doctor closely monitors your son or daughter to assess the continued need for it.

Obsessive–Compulsive Disorder

The Disorder

Obsessive–compulsive disorder (OCD) has been estimated to affect 1–2% of the population and is believed to begin most often in childhood or adolescence. Children with OCD are subject to persistent ideas or impulses (*obsessions*) that may lead to repetitive, purposeful behaviors (*compulsions*) that they feel they must complete. Their obsessions are intrusive and senseless and may center on their having caused violence, on sexual perversion, on the need for symmetry, on the danger of becoming contaminated, or on severe self-doubts. Children with OCD may at times appear so severely mentally ill that they have been confused with schizophrenic children.

One less common problem related to OCD is hair pulling (*trichotillomania*). A child who has trichotillomania may pull out his hair, eyebrows, or the hair of pets or stuffed animals, to the point of suffering complete hair loss (*alopecia*) that requires a hat to cover. Like OCD symptoms, this hair pulling seems to occur more often when the child is not involved in activities.

Most children report being aware of their obsessions and/or compulsions and not liking them. However, when they are prevented from completing the rituals intended to neutralize the obsessive worries, whether these rituals involve hand washing, counting, checking, or touching something, the children become very anxious.

Recent research indicates this syndrome is related to a disturbance in the neurotransmitter serotonin, particularly in the front areas of the brain above the eyes. Rarely, OCD (and tics) can be connected to recurrent streptococcal infections—called pediatric autoimmune neuropsychiatric disorders (PANDAS) or pediatric acute-onset neuropsychiatric syndrome (PANS). PANDAS/PANS is thought to be related to an individual's autoimmune reaction to a strep infection—specifically to antibodies that continue to interfere with an area of the brain called the basal ganglia, causing and/or worsening the symptoms. PANDAS/PANS can be difficult to diagnose, often relying on the abrupt or sudden onset of obsessive–compulsive and/or limb or motor movements and tics after (or severely exacerbated by) a streptococcus infection (such as a sore throat caused by strep).

The Treatment

Cognitive-behavioral treatment (especially a form called "exposure plus response prevention") is an effective form of psychotherapy for OCD and is often used initially or along with medications. Within the pharmacological domain, antidepressants that make more serotonin available seem to be the most effective in reducing many of the disabling symptoms of the disorder. The SSRI class of medications (Zoloft, Paxil, and others) is well studied in pediatric patients with obsessive–compulsive disorder, as is Anafranil. Studies indicate that relatively higher doses of these medications—300 mg of Luvox in the case of 16-year-old Peter—may be necessary for adequate treatment of juvenile OCD. In more severe or poorly responding cases of OCD, the doctor may need to use Anafranil with an SSRI such as Zoloft, an SSRI with a benzodiazepine (like Klonopin), or an SSRI with a low-dose atypical antipsychotic. (See Chapter 13 for a discussion of the black-box warning currently on the labels of SSRIs.)

If your child has trichotillomania, the practitioner will probably recommend similar therapy and medication treatment. Don't expect too much, though. Anecdotal information suggests that the disorder responds only partially to treatment, particularly when the child's trichotillomania begins before puberty.

Treatment for children suspected of having PANDAS/PANS is generally the same as for those with movement disorders, tics, and OCD; however, some researchers believe the disorder is more difficult to treat than regular OCD. The current treatments include cognitive-behavioral therapy and medications used to treat OCD, such as the SSRIs. There are also a number of less studied treatments including the use of intermittent antibiotics, intravenous immunoglobulins, clearing of antibodies in the blood (plasmapheresis), and prophylactic continuous antibiotic treatment to avoid strep infections.

Table 5. Pharmacotherapy of Anxiety-Related Disorders

Disorder	Pharmacotherapy
Generalized anxiety disorder	Antidepressants SSRIs: Zoloft, Lexapro, Celexa, Prozac, Luvox, Paxil SNRIs: Cymbalta (duloxetine) and Effexor XR (venlafaxine) Other antidepressants: Remeron, Effexor XR, Cymbalta, Viibryd (vilazodone) Anxiety-breaking agents (benzodiazepines): Ativan, Klonopin, others Buspar (buspirone) Strattera (atomoxetine)
Panic disorder, separation anxiety	Higher-potency agents: Ativan, Klonopin, Xanax Antidepressants SSRIs: Zoloft, Lexapro, Celexa, Prozac, Luvox, Paxil SNRIs: Cymbalta (duloxetine) and Effexor XR (venlafaxine) Other antidepressants: Remeron, Effexor XR, Cymbalta Combined pharmacotherapy for nonresponders or children with other disorders (e.g., Tranxene + Cymbalta, imipramine + Klonopin)
Posttraumatic stress disorder (PTSD)	Treat target symptoms (e.g., anxiety, psychosis) Antidepressants: SSRIs, SNRIs, atypical antidepressants, tricyclic antidepressants Alpha agonists/blood pressure medications: clonidine, guanfacine, propranolol Anxiety-breaking medications: Tranxene, Klonopin, Ativan, others If problems with depersonalization or psychosis, consider antipsychotics

(cont.)

Table 5 (*cont.*)

Disorder	Pharmacotherapy
Obsessive–compulsive disorder (OCD)	SSRIs: Zoloft, Prozac, Lexapro, Celexa, Paxil, Luvox May need higher doses Anafranil Combined pharmacotherapy for nonresponders (e.g., Zoloft + Anafranil or SSRI + atypical antipsychotic [Abilify] or + benzodiazepine) or for children with other co-occurring disorders

7
Mood Disorders

Many parents who bring children to our clinic because of "emotional problems" end up describing what mental health professionals term *mood disorders*. Mood is generally considered your child's ongoing emotional state, and any disturbance in that state that lasts continually for more than 2 weeks or occurs for most of the day over a substantial period of time should be evaluated as a possible mood disorder. Typically, children experience mood as sadness, crying spells, nihilism/negativism and/or irritability, anger, agitation, temper outbursts, and aggression. Mood disorders run the spectrum from just being down to cycling between feeling down and feeling up or giddy/euphoric. Previous and recent longitudinal studies (studies conducted over time) indicate that mood disorders tend to be chronic—that is, many of the children who are diagnosed with a mood disorder will tend to have that mood disorder 2, 5, and even 10 years later. We also know that mood disorders on their own will typically wax and wane—that is, children improve and then relapse, sometimes related to stressors and sometimes for no apparent reason at all. The good news is that treatment can help reduce the fluctuations and also reduce active symptoms and improve a child's functioning.

Mood disorders can be difficult to diagnose. It's not always easy to see that a child has been "down" for an extended period of time. Maybe your son isn't very forthcoming about how he's feeling; perhaps your daughter is too young to articulate her moods clearly. Consider, too, that children often seem moody, sometimes due to normal passing external pressures such as losing a sporting event or peer difficulties and sometimes due to transitions in their maturation. We've all known preteens and teens who seem pretty constantly crabby or glum, and it's difficult to determine when they're just "going through a phase" and when they're suffering from clinical depression and need help. Younger children may be giddy or goofy naturally—or the giddiness, if excessive, may be an "up" swing in a mood. Finally, we tend to view "real" mood disorders as an adult disease and don't often make the connection between less obvious symptoms—fatigue and listlessness, irritability, lack of concentration—and a mood disorder in a child. Fourteen-year-old Donny was referred to us by his pediatrician because the doctor could find no medical illness to account for his low energy level. It took a psychiatric evaluation to reveal that Donny could not report the last time he had been happy, that he felt blue and cynical "all the time," and that he was quiet and withdrawn. When we do evaluate children for mood disorders, we often find—as we did in Donny's case—that the child's problems began as long as a year or two ago.

As a parent, you can be guided to some extent by the fact that the rate of mood disorders increases with age. For instance, major depression is estimated to affect 0.3% of preschoolers, 1–2% of elementary-age children, and 5% of adolescents. Bipolar disorder is estimated to affect fewer than 0.5% of preschoolers but up to 3% of adolescents. In other words, the younger your child is, the less likely she is to be suffering from a mood disorder. For depression, until adolescence, roughly the same number of boys and girls suffer from the disorder. Then the more typical adult pattern starts, with approximately two-thirds of cases affecting females. Depressive disorders commonly occur together with anxiety, ADHD, conduct, and substance use disorders in older children and adolescents.

Depression versus Bipolar Disorder

Mood disorders in children are classified most commonly as depression alone or bipolar disorder (also called manic–depression). They can also be considered episodic (the child's mood is okay for a while and then gets worse) or continuous (the mood is problematic most of the time with some minor variation). The more typical symptoms of depression in children are sadness, anger, gloominess, nihilism, withdrawal, and loss of interest and enjoyment in life. When a child's "moodiness" falls generally into those categories, the child is likely to be diagnosed with a depressive disorder. But when emotional symptoms that seem the opposite of depression also appear—euphoria or severe and prolonged irritability or rage attacks, explosive energy, racing thoughts, marked insomnia, and driven behavior—bipolar disorder may be suspected. These "high" or "severely agitated" symptoms are called *mania,* and their contrast with "lows," or depression, results in the term *bipolar* (meaning two poles of mood). Complicating the distinction between depression and bipolar disorder, however, is the fact that depression may manifest itself in children as irritability or anger instead of sadness—and, depending on the frequency and intensity of the anger, may be a symptom of either disorder.

Other Mood Disorders

A less severe form of depression called *dysthymia,* commonly mistaken for a personality or character flaw, should be taken quite seriously because it can significantly damage a child's quality of life. Dysthymia is very long-standing, requiring at least 1 year's duration for diagnosis but often lasting more than 2 years. It does not involve full-blown depression, but the child may have a long-term negative and somewhat irritable mood, appearing somewhat unhappy, low in energy, and uninterested in activity. Not surprisingly, the child may have problems with friends and classmates and with parents and siblings. Often the disorder is a precursor to more severe depression that begins later in adolescence or adulthood. Disruptive mood dysregulation disorder (DMDD) is characterized by severe and frequent temper tantrums without many other continuous mood symptoms. This disorder is newly described, but what we do know about it appears at the end of the chapter.

Depression

The Disorder

As already mentioned, depression in a child may appear as a sad and/or irritable mood or a continued loss of interest or pleasure in favorite activities. Understand, though, that children have difficulty distinguishing sad from mad, so if asked how they feel they may confuse the two or report feeling sad and mad at the same time. Your observations may be more informative to the practitioner than the child's reporting. We frequently talk with kids about sadness and irritability being like a railroad track—one track is sadness and the other irritability.

What Does Depression Look Like?

Be alert for irritability, school difficulties, refusal to attend school, withdrawal, isolation, physical complaints, persistent negative or nihilistic attitude, frequent crying spells, and/or aggressive, antisocial behavior—all indications of possible depression in a child. The physical symptoms that many depressed adults have may also occur in a child: fatigue, changes in appetite and weight, abnormal sleep patterns (either too much or poor quality), physical slowing or agitation, and trouble thinking. Depressed kids and teens may report feeling worthless, hopeless, trapped, guilty, or preoccupied with suicidal thoughts. Many are unable to think positively of the future or see no future at all. Severe depression may even include disturbances in reality (psychosis), most typically hearing voices (*auditory hallucinations*).

You can see why depression may be hard for parents to identify with any certainty. Both overconcern and underconcern can lead you astray. Unless you look carefully at the context of your child's moods, you may have trouble differentiating depression from temperament (such as a tendency toward negativism) or passing emotions such as unhappiness or disappointment that commonly occur during childhood, particularly during high stress. A good distinguishing rule of thumb is that if the mood continues after the stressor that caused frustration or sadness has ended, the child *may* have a depressive disorder. Even if the symptoms do eventually end, a prolonged and exaggerated response, including many symptoms of depression, to a common stressor such as doing poorly on a test may indicate that the child is clinically depressed. As we discussed in Part I, some children inherit the tendency toward depression, which is triggered by certain stressors.

A child who has a full repertoire of depressive symptoms for at least 2 weeks is said to have a major depression. These symptoms may include irritability mixed with sadness, low energy and interest, physical problems (stomachaches, headaches), crying spells, withdrawal, a sad expression, problems with concentrating, and thoughts about harming himself. Adolescents with major depression have more adult-like features, including irritability, cynicism, sadness, low energy and interest, crying spells, social isolation and withdrawal, concentration difficulties, and suicidality.

No blood tests are used to diagnose any of the mood disorders. Psychological tests may help practitioners further understand depressive themes and any discrepancies in the child's thinking, but essentially mood disorders are diagnosed on the basis of the child's history of problems—symptoms, timing, and functioning.

What Causes Depression?

Clearly there is a component that is passed on through families and thought to be genetic—30 to 50% of children with depression have a family member with depression. But the environment and excessive life stressors can also cause depression. Most likely depressed children have a genetic vulnerability that becomes activated with stressors—a typical scenario in which genes and the environment interact. Medical causes can include injuries to certain areas of the brain (some types of seizures may mimic or cause depression), high or low levels of thyroid hormone, and drug abuse (such as cocaine and marijuana).

The Treatment

In general, juvenile-onset depression does not respond as well to treatment as adult depression. Psychotherapy continues to be the first line of treatment for mild to moderate depression, with medications used for moderate to severe depression. Both medication and psychotherapy should probably be considered for all kids with moderate or severe depression, because the combination has had the greatest overall short- and longer-term effect. Although traditional interpersonal and insight-oriented therapies can be helpful, more recently proactive, cognitive-based approaches that work on changing the child's perceptions and belief systems are gaining favor and have been shown effective in large studies. Be patient; these psychotherapies may take 2–3 months to start working. If your child refuses or is unable to engage in psychotherapy, medications should be considered. Likewise, if your child continues to have mood problems despite a reasonable course (8–12 weeks) of psychotherapy, you should consider a medication consultation. *Medication should be considered immediately in kids with previous recurring depression, suicidality, or severe depressive features with a lot of impairment.*

Medications for depression, which are mainly the antidepressants, are summed up in Table 6. The most effective and commonly used antidepressants are the SSRIs, including Prozac, Zoloft, Luvox, Lexapro, and Celexa. Studies of Prozac and Lexapro suggest their effectiveness for depression in kids. Prozac and Lexapro are the only FDA-approved antidepressants for adolescents and are usually among the first selected. (See more on recent studies of these medications in Chapter 13.)

The SSRI class of medications also appears particularly effective for dysthymia compared to the other antidepressants—20 mg of Prozac was the prescription that helped 14-year-old Donny, introduced earlier. Note, however, that we often use lower doses of these medications for younger children. For instance, we often start with 5 mg of Prozac or Lexapro in children and monitor their response to treatment for 1 month before increasing the dose. While we don't have similar studies of all the other SSRIs, it seems prudent to start younger children on one-quarter to one-half of an adult starting dose.

We increase the dosage of these medications as tolerated and necessary to control symptoms: Prozac or Celexa from 5 to 40 mg daily; Lexapro from 2.5 to 20 mg daily; Zoloft from 25 to 200 mg; Luvox from 50 to 300 mg. It's not uncommon to see improvement in the first week, but it may take up to 12 weeks to know if the medication is going to work. Two years of psychotherapy had helped identify the triggers of 12-year-old Jeff's more severe depression, but the low energy and low interest, the sadness and sense of isolation that went along with his dysthymia persisted. Prozac resulted in Jeff's having a panic attack, so we tried Lexapro. At 10 mg daily, the Lexapro proved instrumental in reducing Jeff's depressive symptoms.

Other antidepressants used less commonly for depression in children include Wellbutrin, Effexor XR, Cymbalta, Remeron, trazodone, and the tricyclic antidepressants (desipramine, imipramine, amitriptyline, and others). Very new medications like vortioxetine remain untested in children.

Less commonly, the mood stabilizers (see the next page) are used for depression that features prominent mood swings, or lability. Lamictal appears to help greatly with depression alone or with bipolar disorder. Another medication, the second generation antipsychotic Abilify, may also be used with an antidepressant for hard-to-treat depression. When using any of the antidepressants, monitor your child for the emergence of worsened mood or suicidal thoughts, as a small percentage of youths receiving antidepressants actually get worse and benefit from stopping the medication if this occurs.

lability: Rapid mood swings or moodiness.

When children exhibit depression and another disorder, the choice of a broader-spectrum agent that treats both disorders may be preferable. For children who have prominent ADHD and depression, Wellbutrin may be the initial drug of choice. Children with anxiety and depression may be tried initially on an SSRI (a Prozac-like medication), an SNRI (Effexor XR), a tricyclic antidepressant, or trazodone. When none of the antidepressants seems to work, the doctor may try a higher dose of an antidepressant as long as the child is having no adverse effects from the antidepressants. Or a different class of medication may be prescribed. A third approach might be to combine two antidepressants of different classes (e.g., Lexapro and Lamictal) or an antidepressant with another medication, such as lithium, stimulants, buspirone, or other anxiety-breaking medications. Some parents have treated their child's depression with natural substances such as omega-3 fatty acids ("fish oils") or St. John's wort, but results have been mixed. Research on these agents remains relatively scarce, and dosing and duration of treatment necessary for a positive outcome remain under study. If you're considering using natural compounds, speak with your practitioner to ensure there are no warnings about any particular type of compound or any drug interactions. Also be sure to get a well-regarded brand of the natural agents, since they are not regulated for purity in the same manner as standard medications.

Finding the right medication for your child leaves you and the doctor with the question of how long to treat the child, and unfortunately there is currently little information available to answer it. Often doctors are left relying on guidelines meant for adults with depression. Because most adults' mood will improve naturally in 6 months to 1 year, for example, doctors tend to prescribe medication for 6–12 months. In children, however, depression frequently lasts longer and is less likely to remit spontaneously. The solution in our clinic is to continue medication for 6 months or longer, until the child's mood is stable for at least 3 months, and then consider very gradually tapering the medication. If any symptoms of depression reemerge, we know we need to consider restarting the medication or boosting the dosage to the previous level that seemed to be helpful. Often, though, we find we can reduce the maintenance dose of the medication.

We feel strongly that parents and children should *not* feel any pressure to stop the medication if they are concerned about a recurrence of the depression and will continue prescribing it upon request. In the earlier case of Jeff, who had been on Lexapro for 8 months, we and Jeff's parents agreed to continue the medication for another 4 months before reviewing discontinuance. In that case, the theoretical risks of long-term treatment were outweighed by the real risk of depression and associated problems. This seems particularly pertinent in light of research showing that about half of adolescents with depression still have problems with their mood or anxiety as adults and that long-term treatment of depression continues to lead to improved outcomes.

Bipolar (Manic–Depressive) Disorder

The Disorder

Imagine feeling very depressed but at the same time very agitated and out of control. That, in a nutshell, is the "miserable feeling" that most children with bipolar or manic–depressive disorder and their parents describe. This intertwining of symptoms distinguishes childhood manic depression from its adult counterpart. Where adults are more likely to have broad mood swings, children with this problem typically experience manic and depressive features at the same time, and the symptoms stay with the child for long periods.

In children, mania commonly takes the form of an extremely irritable, rageful, and/or explosive mood, sometimes psychosis, with poor social interactions or functioning that is often devastating to the child and family. On top of the severe mood swings that make everyone's life difficult, the manic child may overflow with excess energy that makes it hard to sleep (without being tired the next day), propels the boy or girl into obsessively goal-directed activity, subjects the child to unrelenting racing thoughts, and turns the child into an overtalkative and loud individual. Many of these children exhibit markedly poor judgment, pursuing thrill-seeking, reckless, substance-abusing, or sex-based activities. Up to half of children with bipolar disorder have a relative with bipolar illness. Although mania in children should be differentiated from ADHD, conduct disorder, depression, and disturbances in reality (psychosis), these disorders commonly occur along with juvenile bipolar disorder. In fact, the younger the child with bipolar disorder, the more likely she is to have other psychiatric disorders.

Controversy continues to simmer over juvenile bipolar disorder. Does the disorder really occur in children? Is it overdiagnosed? The incidence in children and adolescents is reported to be anywhere from

1 to 5%. Also, does bipolar come with many related symptoms, or are these other symptoms an indication of co-occurring disorders (such as anxiety/panic disorder, ADHD)? And how many kids with depression actually go on to be bipolar? One paper says half, a significant figure: is it accurate? More research needs to be done, but we do have longer-term longitudinal studies that indicated a high rate of improvement and relapse with low rates of true remission or "cure" from the disorder 5–10 years later.

The Treatment

For bipolar disorder, it's essential to treat the child with a second-generation antipsychotic or mood stabilizer. As of 2016 a number of second-generation antipsychotics (SGAs) have been approved for treating bipolar disorder in adolescents (and adults), including Saphris (asenapine). Traditional mood stabilizers include lithium and the older anticonvulsants Tegretol and Depakote. More recently, the less-tested anticonvulsants Neurontin (gabapentin), Lamictal (lamotrigine), Topamax (topiramate), Gabitril (tiagabine), and Trileptal (oxcarbazepine) have been used in children with bipolar disorder, generally with mixed or negative results. There have also been positive reports on the use of omega-3 fatty acids ("fish oils") in both adults and children, used alone or in combination with other treatments. Typically, at least 1,000 mg daily of a high-dose EPA/omega-3 is recommended in children with unstable mood disorders.

High doses of these medications may be necessary, which means your child's blood levels should be checked, and she should be watched closely for side effects. While many of the SGAs (such as olanzapine) work within 2 weeks, you may not see the drug's full effect on the child's mood instability and associated problems until 3 months have passed. If, at that point, the child hasn't responded or hasn't been able to tolerate the drug, the doctor should consider other agents. In some cases—such as when the child does not respond to lithium or an anticonvulsant individually—your child may require two mood-stabilizing agents. I (T. E. W.) will combine Depakote or Trileptal with lithium, as I did with 12-year-old Jay, who is now doing well with 600 mg of Trileptal twice a day and 300 mg of lithium twice a day. In my practice it is common to use a full dose of one medication and a lower dose of the second mood-stabilizing agent.

Over the past decade, with the results of multiple trials and FDA approvals, clinicians tend to employ the SGAs as first-line agents for the treatment of children and adolescents who have severe disruptive disorders, self-injurious behavior, and bipolar disorder. The SGAs have been of invaluable assistance in controlling not only the manic symptoms (e.g., explosiveness, grandiosity) but also the depressive symptoms of the disorder. The use of SGAs for a whole host of disorders in children and adolescents (including tic disorders) is predicated on a number of studies demonstrating their efficacy for mania and depression in youth with bipolar disorder, tic disorders, explosive disorders, and disruptive disorders. In addition, these agents appear to work very quickly, with some trials showing vast changes in behavior after only 2 weeks.

We have continued to amass more information on the SGAs—risperidone (and its derivative, Invega [paliperidone]), Zyprexa (olanzapine), Seroquel (quetiapine), Geodon (ziprasidone), and Abilify (aripiprazole)—since this book was first published.

Antipsychotics should be considered immediately for children with prominent mixed symptoms, severe agitation, acute mania, or nonresponse to mood stabilizers, and/or hallucinations. Because the traditional antipsychotics such as Thorazine have longer-term side effects of concern (e.g., tardive dyskinesia), the second-generation ("atypical") class of antipsychotics is being used in the evening to assist with sleep and reduce the moodiness of the disorder; and in the morning for moodiness during the day, with very good success. Some clinicians will shift from Risperdal to paliperidone, an extended-release form of a breakdown product of risperidone, for kids who are having breakthrough symptoms of bipolar disorder or irritability in the afternoon as it may last longer. Others use Invega if risperidone has been helpful but weight gain has been problematic, since weight gain seems to be a bit less common with Invega. We have found that Abilify or Geodon can be effective for bipolar symptoms and are associated with much less weight gain and increases in blood sugar and blood lipids (fats), which potentially cause metabolic issues.

When prominent symptoms of depression (negativism, isolation, looking sad) are part of your child's bipolar disorder, the doctor may prescribe a medication for the bipolar/manic symptoms such as an antipsychotic and an additional medication such as an antidepressant. If an antidepressant is added, it is recommended that it should be short-acting to reduce the risk of severe activation or worsening of mania. The SSRIs

(Prozac, Zoloft, Paxil, Luvox, Celexa, Lexapro) are noted for making mania worse (activating mania) in individuals with bipolar disorder, but Lamictal or Wellbutrin can be introduced gently with less concern about activation. Other agents such as Effexor XR appear to be relatively well tolerated at low doses in youth with bipolar disorder. Other options include the use of Lamictal (lamotrigine), which seems particularly helpful for the depression commonly experienced as part of the "mixed" picture of bipolar disorder in kids.

> **activation:** The stimulation of emotional, cognitive, or behavioral processes.

What are you to do if your child has bipolar disorder and ADHD? Data show that ADHD responds to treatment *only* if the mood (mania or depression) is being treated. Data also show that you can safely and effectively treat the bipolar disorder and the ADHD at the same time. The key: the bipolar symptoms need to be treated completely *first.* Your child's practitioner may try an SGA and/or a mood stabilizer for the bipolar disorder and a stimulant, clonidine, guanfacine, Wellbutrin, atomoxetine, or a tricyclic antidepressant for the ADHD.

Many young people with bipolar disorder have multiple other problems and do not respond to a single antipsychotic. It is unfortunately not uncommon for these children to receive a few different classes of medication. After multiple hospitalizations and medication trials, one 12-year-old boy with bipolar disorder, ADHD, and anxiety whom I (T. E. W.) treat has finally stabilized on Risperdal, Lamictal, and Concerta. As a parent, you must be sure you are aware of what each agent is targeting and the potential drug interactions among all of them. The Risperdal and Lamictal are for the mood and anxiety, and the Concerta for the ADHD.

Usually, SGAs and/or mood stabilizers will need to be continued indefinitely until there is little evidence of mood swings over a period of time. Children and their parents often mistake the long-term effects of these medications for a "cure" and understandably, when the child has been doing so well for a few months, question the need to continue the medication. I strongly recommend that you discuss the matter thoroughly with your child's doctor. Prematurely discontinuing treatment imposes the risk of major relapse and perhaps psychiatric hospitalization (see Chapter 4). If you are leaning in the direction of a trial off the medication, talk to the doctor about trying a very slow taper off one medication at a time so you can observe your child's behavior as he safely comes off the medication. Data in adults suggest that rapid discontinuation (less than 1 week) compared to slow discontinuation (1 month) may lead to recurrence of the bipolar disorder and more difficulty treating the disorder in the future. Close communication with your child's school and frequent contact with your child's doctor are paramount during discontinuation phases on mood stabilizers or SGAs.

Disruptive Mood Dysregulation Disorder

The Disorder

Severe temper tantrums without many other symptoms appear to be the hallmark of this newly described disorder. Children with DMDD have severe and frequent temper tantrums that interfere with their ability to function at home, in school, or with their friends. These kids appear likely to develop problems with depression or anxiety over time. While occasional temper tantrums are a normal part of growing up, children who have very intense and persistent temper tantrums at least a few times a week over a year may have DMDD. Some children with DMDD also have other issues, such as oppositional defiant disorder, anxiety, and/or ADHD. Some professionals believe that DMDD is really just a manifestation of co-occurring oppositional and mood disorders. Others feel as if children diagnosed with DMDD have a complicated personality disorder referred to as borderline personality disorder, characterized by features including black-and-white thinking, difficulty with mood regulation/irritability, and outbursts at perceived injustices.

The Treatment

The treatment for DMDD is not well established, and clinicians who believe it is not a separate disorder but a manifestation of co-occurring oppositional and mood disorders think it should be treated that way. It is anticipated that psychotherapies directed at stress and anger management will be utilized initially. Medications used for the symptoms suggested for DMDD include the alpha agonists (Intuniv [guanfacine], Kapvay [clonidine]), low-dose atypical antipsychotics (Abilify and others), mood stabilizers, and SSRIs (Lexapro and others). Given that there is no set medication treatment for DMDD, psychotherapies and medication will need to be customized for the needs of the particular child and based on an understanding of co-occurring issues and the objective of reducing potential triggers of the disorder.

Table 6. Pharmacotherapy of Juvenile Mood Disorders

Disorder	Pharmacotherapy

Depression
  Major depression
  Dysthymia
	SSRIs: Prozac, Lexapro, Zoloft, Luvox, Celexa
	SNRIs: Cymbalta, Effexor XR
	
	Atypical antidepressants: Wellbutrin, Remeron
	
	Lamictal (lamotrigine)
	
	Tricyclic antidepressants: imipramine, nortriptyline, desipramine, amitriptyline, clomipramine
	
	Antidepressants + antipsychotics (e.g., Abilify) if problems with hallucinations or problems in reality
	
	Antidepressants + benzodiazepines (e.g., Ativan) if anxiety
	
	For nonresponders consider combined medication strategies: antidepressant + lamotrigine, SGA (e.g., Abilify), lithium, stimulants, or modafinil
	
	Electroconvulsive therapy (ECT)

Bipolar disorder (manic–depressive disorder)	SGAs: Risperdal, Abilify, Seroquel, Invega, Zyprexa, Geodon, Saphris (asenapine) Mood stabilizer: lithium (Eskalith, Lithobid), Tegretol/Equetrol/Carbachol (carbamazepine) or Trileptal (oxcarbazepine) Valproate (Depakote, Depakene sprinkles, valproic acid) Other anticonvulsants (Lamictal, especially if depressed; Neurontin, especially if anxious; Topamax; Gabitril) Older antipsychotics: Trilafon, Thorazine, Mellaril, others For nonresponders consider lithium and antipsychotic, two anticonvulsants, or two antipsychotics If agitation or anxiety, add benzodiazepine (e.g., Klonopin) If ADHD, consider Wellbutrin, stimulants, Intuniv (guanfacine), clonidine, modafinil

8
Autism Spectrum Disorder

Children vary widely in their mental and physical development over time. A group have what we call *developmental disorders*— either substantial delays in reaching developmental milestones or failure to reach those milestones. A child can have a developmental disorder in a very specific area, such as a problem with reading (developmental reading disorder), writing (developmental writing disorder), or processing verbal information (central auditory information processing disorder). Or the developmental disorder can be more global, affecting learning (intellectual disability), emotions, and speech and language (autism spectrum disorder [ASD]). Whereas a child who is speaking few words by age 2 may be within normal development, a similar problem in a 5-year-old flags a major problem.

The Disorder

ASD in the new DSM-5 diagnostic system includes what were previously referred to as pervasive developmental disorders and Asperger's syndrome. ASD is characterized by marked impairment in several areas of development, but what parents might find most noticeable and most disturbing is the child's apparent disconnection from the rest of the world. Many parents describe children with ASD as "living in their head" or "inhabiting their own little world." These children may seem distant, unemotional, passive, and withdrawn. Many parents report that their children seemed unresponsive to emotional interactions, cold, and aloof as early as infancy or toddlerhood. Mental health professionals now believe that ASD does begin in early childhood and is probably present prenatally, with a prominent genetic component.

Children on the autism spectrum often have very restricted interactive social skills. They simply don't seem to reciprocate or connect with others. Delayed or essentially nonexistent speech and language communication are very common, as is poor nonverbal communication. Children with ASD often don't make eye contact and can't read or interpret social cues, from smiles or expressions of anger to the more complicated "body language." Imagine how difficult it is for children to receive feedback from those around them without having the capacity to "read" these nonverbal cues.

These children generally have a limited repertoire of interests and activities, and some have a very active fantasy life. Though no one knows why, changes in their routine and surprises often elicit anger and anxiety in children and adolescents with ASD. Many of these children are described as rigid or inflexible—as having difficulty with transitions, especially if unannounced or impromptu.

Children with ASD often engage in repetitive actions, commonly called *stereotypic behaviors,* that may seem bizarre to onlookers. This behavior may include rocking, hair twirling, biting themselves, and head banging. Sometimes the stereotypic behavior is set off by the anxiety of a change in routine; often the child is apparently trying to stimulate herself. Again, we don't know exactly what is at work in stereotypic behavior.

Some children, like 13-year-old Ralph, have a higher-functioning type of ASD previously referred to as *Asperger's syndrome.* Ralph has long-standing ADHD but normal to seemingly advanced speech and language development (Ralph talks too much, which is called being "hyperverbal"). He does relatively well academically but has no friends or interest in making any. Ralph is very interested in police vehicles and spends his free time hanging out with the police and listening to their calls. Ralph's condition is known as a "high-functioning ASD" because his isolated disturbances are mainly in social interactions, and he has substantial speech and intellectual capacities, allowing him to function more easily in his world. Daytrana (the methylphenidate patch) improved Ralph's ADHD symptoms, and occupational therapy during elementary school has helped him function better. As he has matured, his ability to get along with his peers has improved too. Another stimulant formulation, Quillivant XR, has received attention for this group, as

> **occupational therapy:** A type of therapy that helps children attain the basic tools necessary to function. Kids work on using their hands to improve dexterity, doing coordination exercises, and expressing themselves with art.

it is a suspension whose dose can be carefully controlled to provide good ADHD control without undue side effects.

Often in adolescence, the child becomes more aware of his differences in social abilities compared to his peers. This difficulty in making and maintaining friendships can hit hard in adolescence, bringing on demoralization, anxiety, and depression in your teen with ASD. So, if your child is diagnosed with a variant of ASD, talk to the doctor about how to watch for these symptoms.

In the past, disorders like ASD were thought to be caused in part by cold, aloof parenting. Now scientists agree that no specific parenting or environmental factor appears to cause ASD. Scientific reports based on brain imaging pictures have suggested instead that abnormal neurological development is at the root of the problem. Multiple regions of the brain, and the size of its fluid cavities of the brain (ventricles), appear to be different in children with developmental disorders. Lower serotonin levels have also been reported in these children. Because children with these disorders may also have excessive anxiety and obsessiveness, depression, bipolar disorder, psychosis, and ADHD, it is important that the doctor carefully evaluate your child for co-occurring disorders. The child's daily functioning stands a good chance of improving once other problems are identified and treated.

ASD is thought to affect approximately 1 in 68 children, according to estimates from the Autism and Developmental Disabilities Monitoring Network of the U.S. Centers for Disease Control. More general studies conducted in Asia, Europe, and North America have identified individuals with ASD with an average prevalence of about 1%. Of interest, there has been an increase of more than 50% in the incidence of ASD over the past few decades. This increase has raised considerable controversy: Why has there been such a huge increase in the diagnosis of this disorder? Are we overdiagnosing it? Also being debated are the appropriate interventions and the claims about cause on which they are based: the use of diet and other peripheral treatments. Of note, there is a much higher incidence of gastrointestinal problems in individuals affected with autism, and this is currently an area of intensive scientific study. ASD is reported to occur in all racial, ethnic, and socioeconomic groups. It is almost 5 times more common among boys (1 in 42) than among girls (1 in 189).

The Treatment

Various forms of specialized behavior therapy continue to be the most popular nonpharmacological strategy for ASD. There is no specific standard medication regimen, so prepare yourself to be patient through the trial-and-error process that treatment of ASD often demands. However, medications can be very helpful in diminishing some of the core symptoms, such as irritability and anxiety; see Table 7. For instance, large multisite studies have demonstrated that SGAs are helpful for some aspects of ASD, particularly the irritability that is seen in many kids with ASD. Studies have shown that risperidone (Risperdal) and aripiprazole (Abilify) are effective in reducing autistic symptoms and self-injury, and both are FDA approved for treating autism. Recent work with cholinesterase inhibitors suggests that these agents may be selectively helpful in assisting these children with general cognition. In contrast, gastrin, secretin, and other peptide hormones that were supposed to be helpful in controlled trials failed. Moreover, there has been increasing focus on treating psychiatric disorders or prominent psychiatric symptoms that often accompany ASD, such as mood, anxiety, and attention deficit disorders. Often the treatments for the accompanying disorders (e.g., ADHD) are somewhat less effective for the co-occurring disorder, and the child may experience more side effects of the medication. Such is the case in treating children with ASD and ADHD with stimulants—unfortunately, the child commonly experiences less response of the ADHD and more side effects.

Twelve-year-old Chaka is a fairly typical example. Brought to me (T. E. W.) for help with the self-biting that accompanied her ASD, she also would stimulate herself by rocking and occasionally required a helmet as well because of her banging her head against the wall when her routine was changed. Her eye contact was limited, her speech development poor, and she engaged in little nonverbal communication. Physically she appeared immature, had small underdeveloped ears, and her eyes were close together. We tried Depakote, Inderal, clonidine, and Klonopin, all to no avail, despite their reported effectiveness in some cases. Finally she responded moderately well to Zoloft (sertraline), an antidepressant that belongs to the class of SSRIs, which are often used in these children.

While sometimes they are remarkably helpful, the problem with Zoloft and other individual drugs is that they reduce only some of the core symptoms and therefore cannot entirely resolve the impairment caused by ASD. The SSRIs Zoloft, Prozac, Paxil, Lexapro, Celexa, and Luvox, in addition to a tricyclic antidepressant called Anafranil, reduce the obsessive and compulsive activity, rigidity, anxiety, and irritability that often accompany ASD. They are not especially useful, however, with the communication or social interaction problems. Strattera has been reported by some clinicians to be helpful in reducing the anxiety and attentional issues in some kids with ASD and ADHD.

Two classes of medications, the alpha agonists (e.g., Intuniv/guanfacine and Kapvay/clonidine) and the atypical antipsychotics, also can be helpful for certain behaviors associated with the developmental disorders. Although they didn't work for Chaka, beta blockers, a class of medications that block a select group of norepinephrine receptors (molecules that are on nerve and other cells), such as propranolol, at generally high doses (up to 240 mg per day) and Intuniv (typically dosed 0.1–0.4 mg once a day) are increasingly reported to be useful in controlling the aggression of patients with developmental disorders, whether that aggression is directed at themselves (head banging or self-mutilating behavior) or others. Older work with Haldol and more recent work with Risperdal (risperidone), Abilify (aripiprazole), Geodon (ziprasodone), and Saphris (asenapine) has demonstrated their usefulness for youth with ASD. In a large multisite study of Risperdal, not only did the symptoms of ASD improve (particularly irritability), but there was a notable improvement in functioning. We treated Justin, a 7-year-old with ADHD, some mood concerns, and ASD. He had outbursts that limited his participation in mainstream classes and were unresponsive to ADHD treatment and SSRIs. Low-dose Risperdal (0.5 mg) was extremely helpful in controlling his outbursts (usually secondary to frustration) and allowing him to be in a regular classroom with additional support.

Self-mutilating behavior can sometimes be reduced by using naltrexone or ReVia at doses of 25 mg up to three times daily.

Children with ASD have a lot of problems with cognition and executive function. As described on page 135, executive functioning is like the secretary of the brain (or the function of the mother or father!)—helping the child organize, plan, execute, and follow through on a project. Obviously, executive function deficits make it extremely difficult for a child to conduct a normal life. Recent research has produced some preliminary data suggesting that Alzheimer's medications such as Namenda (memantine) may be selectively useful in assisting these children with general cognition and executive function in particular, but since little research is currently being conducted, it could be a long time before such medications become accepted for this use. In contrast, gastrin, secretin, and other peptides that were supposed to be helpful to children with ASD failed when tested in controlled trials.

For children who have severe irritability, moodiness, or depression, the antidepressants already mentioned may be helpful. And if the child's mood swings are substantial, a mood-stabilizing agent such as lithium, Tegretol/Equetrol, Trileptal, Depakote, Neurontin, or Lamictal may be beneficial. In children with prominent anxiety symptoms, for example around mealtimes, the Valium-like medications (benzodiazepines) such as Ativan and Klonopin may be useful. Children with ASD and ADHD or prominent ADHD-like symptoms benefit from the same medications as for ADHD—namely stimulants, antidepressants, and alpha agonists. It is notable that many children with ASD also have a seizure disorder and require an anticonvulsant. If your child is one of them, you need to talk to the doctor about potential drug interactions with other medications used to address behavioral concerns.

Over a decade ago, the U.S. federal government unveiled a 10-year interagency plan to address the growing rate of autistic disorders in American children. Goals target coordinated biomedical research, earlier diagnosis, and therapeutic methods. A goal listed as realistic in the plan is to develop effective treatments along with the Department of Education. One treatment modality that is currently under study, albeit more challenging, is the development of effective medications for these disorders. Meanwhile, however, there has been an increase in funding of and research on ASD.

Table 7. Pharmacotherapy of Autism Spectrum Disorder

No specific pharmacotherapy for the core disorder, although see below for problematic symptoms within the disorder (e.g., repetition, irritability)

Look for other disorders (ADHD, depression, anxiety)

Pharmacotherapy of repetitive behaviors

    Selective and nonselective serotonin reuptake inhibitors—Prozac, Zoloft, Luvox, Paxil, Anafranil, Celexa, Lexapro

    SGAs (Risperdal, Abilify, others)

For severe irritability

    SGAs (Risperdal, Abilify, others)

For aggression and self-abuse

    Beta blockers (e.g., propranolol), clonidine (Kapvay), guanfacine (Tenex/Intuniv)

    Benzodiazepines (e.g., Klonopin, Tranxene)

    Lithium, anticonvulsants (e.g., Tegretol, Valproate, Neurontin, Trileptal), naltrexone

9

Schizophrenia and Other Psychotic Disorders

The Disorders

Psychosis generally means abnormal thinking that includes substantial problems with reality awareness. Psychosis can occur in disorders such as schizophrenia, which occur in about 1% of adults but are quite rare in children (about 5% of adults with schizophrenia report the onset in adolescence), or in other disorders such as bipolar disorder (occurring in about one-quarter of bipolar kids). Your child would be diagnosed as having psychosis if he had either delusions or hallucinations. *Delusions* are false, implausible beliefs. *Hallucinations* are false perceptions involving any of the senses—visual (sight), auditory (hearing), tactile (touch), or olfactory (smell). Many children with psychosis have both. Fourteen-year-old Karin, for example, described hearing voices "outside of her head" (hallucinations) and also was convinced that someone was poisoning her food (delusion).

As in adults, psychotic disorders in children are categorized as functional or organic. Functional psychoses are mental illnesses, including schizophrenia, schizoaffective disorder, and severe forms of mood disorders in which the child suffers breaks in reality. Organic psychosis refers to damage to the brain or central nervous system as a result of medical illness, trauma, or drug use.

In children with either type of psychosis, imaging tests may show that certain areas of the brain are slightly smaller than in nonpsychotic children. Neuropsychological testing often shows profound abnormalities in a child's ability to ascertain, organize, perceive, manipulate, store, and recall information. In many cases, the brain's processing problem occurs far in advance of the breaks in reality. Although the causes of schizophrenia are not well defined, congenital (birth) brain malformations, fetal exposure to toxins or infectious agents, excessive drug (marijuana) use, and genetics are among the most likely contributors.

For parents the challenge is recognizing that a serious problem exists, requiring a full evaluation. Children are notorious for not telling their parents about their hallucinations or delusions. It is not unusual for me to find out during an evaluation that a child has been hearing voices for 2 years and has not told anybody. Often children don't know that the voices talking to them are abnormal or are afraid to tell others about them. When a psychosis begins or worsens, however, the child is likely to display severe behavioral problems, including having outbursts, acting strangely, or withdrawing. Often these children have difficulty with organizational skills such as orchestrating activities and completing schoolwork and may be failing academically and socially. Adolescents may use drugs or alcohol excessively to self-medicate. Children may also become severely withdrawn and paranoid.

Children who develop psychotic disorders may have had earlier symptoms of other psychiatric and neurological disorders. Some children start out with ADHD-like symptoms (see page 129), which progress in intensity and level of disorganization. In other children you may notice a "flat" mood, which is often followed by the onset of hallucinations. Yet others may feel mild weakness in an arm or leg and then begin to behave in bizarre ways. Most children with psychosis develop these uncharacteristic behaviors, often along with hallucinations (usually auditory). Unfortunately, these disorders typically continue through childhood, often getting worse as the child gets older. Many adolescents may smoke marijuana at or around the time of the worsening symptoms, further exacerbating their condition.

It is also important to note that if psychosis is part of another disorder, such as a mood disorder, the psychotic symptoms will largely be present during the active symptoms of the other disorder (e.g., manic symptoms of bipolar disorder). For instance, Drake was a 16-year-old with bipolar disorder who when manic thought he had magical powers to fly (by jumping off elevated surfaces). When he was not manic, he did not report any thoughts of thinking he could fly. Elsie was a 13-year-old girl with major depression who when very depressed became convinced everyone was plotting against her and was afraid to take her medication out of fear of being poisoned.

The Treatment

See Table 8 for a list of the medications used to treat psychosis in children. Antipsychotic drugs, also referred to as *major tranquilizers* or *neuroleptics,* are the standard treatment for psychotic disorders in children. Your child's doctor may prescribe any of a large number of antipsychotic medications, including the newer SGAs and others. Be aware, however, that these medications typically work better on the *positive symptoms*—active problems such as hallucinations, delusions, formal thought disorder (incoherence), and/or catatonic symptoms (stupor, negativism, rigidity, and posturing) or bizarre feeling states. In contrast, the *negative symptoms*—important elements that are missing from the child's emotional makeup—are not as likely to be improved by the antipsychotics, particularly the older-generation ones (haloperidol and others). Because of unresolved lack of emotionality, little speech and thought, lack of involvement in activities (*apathy*), inability to enjoy (*anhedonia*), and poor social functioning, many children with psychosis may have ongoing difficulties with day-to-day life.

A number of the SGAs, such as Abilify and Zyprexa, are FDA approved for the treatment of schizophrenia in adolescents. Therefore, when an evaluation uncovers a picture that suggests long-standing psychotic symptoms, such as those that indicate schizophrenia, many practitioners start children on Abilify, Risperdal, Zyprexa, or other newer antipsychotics. Clozaril is reserved for children who do not respond to multiple trials of older and newer antipsychotics. Because of side effects and variable effectiveness, the older antipsychotics such as Thorazine, Mellaril, Haldol, Stelazine, Trilafon, and others may still be useful as alternative agents if the SGAs are not effective or not tolerated.

Because antipsychotic medications are often used with other agents, it is important to be aware that they generally increase the blood levels of the other medications, such as increasing nortriptyline levels by 30%. Likewise, certain antidepressants (Prozac and others) may increase the blood levels of the antipsychotics.

With all of the antipsychotics, the child's weight needs to be monitored carefully, and at least yearly testing of the child's blood will need to be done to ensure the child is not developing blood sugar (glucose) or lipid (fat, cholesterol) abnormalities. If your child is receiving any of the antipsychotics, you need to work closely with her to ensure healthy eating habits and physical activity to help reduce the weight gain that is an unfortunate side effect of this class of medications. Sometimes your child's practitioner may prescribe metformin, a medication used for diabetes in adults, to help reduce excess blood sugar and/or weight gain related to the atypical antipsychotics. Not all of the new antipsychotics are equal in producing weight gain, however. For instance, reports indicate that risperidone and olanzapine may cause more weight gain than Abilify and Geodon. Children on the older antipsychotics, or even some of the newer ones (Abilify, Geodon), also need to be monitored for the development of potentially irreversible abnormal movements called tardive dyskinesia, which often start as involuntary tongue movements and lip smacking.

Parents can take comfort in the fact that children with psychotic problems such as schizophrenia have been helped greatly by our improved understanding of the disorder and the new generation of medications available for their treatment. Although you can anticipate that your child's problems are likely to continue into adulthood, providing the child with the new medications, psychotherapy, and a low-stress, structured environment should allow your son or daughter some normalcy in childhood and hope for the future. One should be comforted by the ongoing development of new medications for psychosis that is under way.

Table 8. Pharmacotherapy of Schizophrenia and Psychotic Disorders

SGAs: Abilify, Risperdal/Invega, Zyprexa, Seroquel, Geodon, Saphris (asenapine), Latuda, and others

    May be tried as first-line drugs of choice

    Clozaril reserved for children not responding to treatment

Older antipsychotics: Trilafon, Haldol, Thorazine, Stelazine, and others

    Caution with risk for tardive dyskinesia

For agitation, add high-potency benzodiazepines (e.g., Ativan, Klonopin, Xanax)

For children not responding to treatment

    Use atypical antipsychotic

    Switch antipsychotic class: from risperidone to Haldol, Thorazine to Trilafon, from Navane to Zyprexa

    Combine treatments

If mood swings present, antipsychotics + lithium, mood-stabilizing anticonvulsants

    If severe outbursts, antipsychotics + propranolol (and/or mood-stabilizing agent)

    If marked anxiety, antipsychotics + benzodiazepines (e.g., Klonopin, Ativan) or gabapentin (Neurontin)

    If depression, add lamotrigine (Lamictal), bupropion (Wellbutrin), lithium, low-dose SSRI

10
Disorders of Known Medical and Neurological Origin

Tics and Tourette's Disorder

Despite the fact that they are clearly medical or neurological in nature, a number of childhood behavioral problems end up being diagnosed and treated by mental health professionals. This happens in part because the major symptoms are psychiatric—rage, for example—and in part because certain psychiatric symptoms or disorders tend to occur along with them (OCD and ADHD, for instance, commonly appear with Tourette's disorder or autoimmune neurological disorders). Because psychotropic medications are commonly used to treat both the major symptoms of the disorders discussed in this chapter and the co-occurring psychiatric disturbances, it makes sense to consult a mental health practitioner if your child has these problems.

The Disorders

Tics are relatively common in children, with surveys indicating that approximately 15% of children will have them at some point. They range from the twitches and spasms known as *motor tics* to the verbal noises called *phonic tics*. Tics can also be *simple,* such as a twitch, or *complex,* including bending, grimacing, or shrugging.

Children whose tics last longer than 1 year are considered to have chronic tic disorders. We simply do not know why some tics last and some do not. We do know, however, that at least 50% of the tics that begin in childhood disappear by age 18.

If your child has not only motor tics but also phonic tics and other behavioral and psychological symptoms, the child's diagnosis will be Tourette's disorder. The child's phonic or vocal tics usually show up as coughing or throat clearing, but they may appear in the form that has gotten the most publicity: the shouting of swear words (*copralalia*). The phonic tics that Tourette's features have caused much misunderstanding about the disorder because at times they appear to be and may be willful.

Tourette's disorder begins in childhood and sometimes lasts throughout life. Its symptoms often fluctuate spontaneously over time. Stressors, such as starting the school year or simply discussing the child's tics, often accentuate them by raising the child's level of anxiety. Although children may have some ability to suppress their tics temporarily when they are specifically directed to do so, they usually have little long-term control over them.

Complicating the picture, it is not uncommon for disturbing emotional or behavioral patterns to surface, caused to some degree by comorbid disorders. In fact, you and your child's doctor will have to make treatment decisions on the understanding that in many cases these co-occurring disorders, not the primary tic or Tourette's disorder, are the major source of distress and disability. A growing research effort has been directed at unraveling the connections between tic and Tourette's disorders and the disorders with which they often co-occur—anxiety disorders, OCD, and ADHD:

- How are they related?
- Is any cause and effect involved?
- What genes cause tics or Tourette's disorder, and why do these tics often get turned on and off spontaneously?

Much of this interest has been aimed at the overlap of tic and Tourette's disorders with OCD. Studies at Yale and Harvard have uncovered two interesting interrelations:

- About one-third of the children with Tourette's disorder have significant obsessive–compulsive symptoms.
- A sizable number of children with severe tics or Tourette's disorder have a relative with OCD, leading researchers to believe that these two disorders are genetically connected.

Similarly, interesting associations with ADHD have been identified in other research:

- Approximately half of children with Tourette's disorder have ADHD.
- ADHD appears earlier in life than tics.
- Many of the behavioral problems and impairments in these children are related to the ADHD and not the tics.
- The use of stimulants may or may not worsen tics.

The Treatment

Cognitive-behavioral therapy and behavioral modification can be very useful in diminishing many of the aberrant behaviors that may emerge or in helping children identify and fight their complex tics, such as repetitive writhing, standing up and turning around, and touching body parts in a specific manner. Cognitive-behavioral therapy may help the child identify early urges that lead to these behaviors, what sets the behaviors off, and how the child can "relax" herself and, to some degree, control these repetitive acts. Pharmacological approaches to tics and Tourette's disorder have evolved greatly since the 1990s; medications used are listed in Table 9. Unfortunately, because the order in which medications for tics and Tourette's are tried and their availability have changed so dramatically during that time, many practitioners are not up to date on the current treatments.

The alpha agonists (blood pressure medications) clonidine and, to a lesser extent, guanfacine have become the first line of treatment for tics and Tourette's disorder. They work quite well—two-thirds of children respond favorably—but you can expect an accurate evaluation of their effectiveness in your child to take 2–4 weeks. The necessary dose varies greatly, so the doctor will probably start your child on a low dosage and increase it depending on response and side effects. Both immediate-release (clonidine and guanfacine) and extended-release agents (Intuniv and Kapvay) now exist in this class; all are helpful.

The tricyclic antidepressants—desipramine, nortriptyline, imipramine, amitriptyline—have also been found useful in controlling tics and Tourette's disorder. As with the alpha agonists, dosing should be started low and increased to typical "full" dosing based on side effects and response. Both classes of drugs are particularly helpful for the large group of children with Tourette's disorder and ADHD.

When more conventional treatments fail to help children with Tourette's disorder, the atypical SGAs, including Risperdal, Geodon, Abilify, Seroquel, and Zyprexa, are being used. Despite their good treatment record, however, antipsychotics have a couple of significant drawbacks: They have limited effects on the frequently associated disorders such as OCD, and they carry significant risk for the development of both short- and long-term adverse effects. For example, the SGAs often result in weight gain and may cause blood sugar and blood lipid (metabolic) problems. Clinicians also still use the older antipsychotics such as Haldol and Orap (pimozide), given their effectiveness and the fact that Orap is FDA approved for Tourette's in kids. These medications also need to be monitored for both short- and long-term side effects, including the development of tardive dyskinesia (see page 275). For these reasons, before starting the SGAs or older antipsychotics, I advise that you should try other pharmacological interventions. Children who also have OCD may need additional pharmacotherapy with serotonergic drugs such as Anafranil or the SSRIs, such as Luvox or Prozac (which alone have little effect on tics). Children with ADHD plus tics may need a medicine for the tics like clonidine and one for the ADHD like a stimulant. Strattera and desipramine also have demonstrated improvement in tics in children with ADHD and tics.

> **serotonergic:** Related to serotonin, the chemical messenger in the nervous system that affects mood, anxiety, aggression, and sleep.

Temporal Lobe Epilepsy, Complex Partial Seizures

The Disorder

Juan, age 15, was admitted to a psychiatric hospital for irritability, hypochondriasis, and "bizarre thoughts." An examination revealed that he had multiple hallucinations—distortions, bizarre smells, and tastes—as well as unreal perceptions, such as the feeling of having been somewhere before (*déjà vu*) and the feeling of being outside of his body (*depersonalization*). Eighteen-year-old Dominick had been hospitalized four times, all for severe rage attacks. Both have a type of seizure disorder called *complex partial seizures,* or *temporal lobe epilepsy* (TLE). TLE involves seizures—abnormal electrical activity in the brain—but unlike the grand mal seizures that we think of when epilepsy is mentioned, temporal lobe epilepsy does not make children shake and lose consciousness. These seizures occur deep in the brain substance located at about the level of the ears, in the region called the *temporal lobes*. This region of the brain is related to emotion, perception, and memory, and seizures here affect the major communication lines within the brain. TLE causes emotional and behavioral disturbances in the form of periodic heightened states such as marked moodiness or rage, leading to outbursts for no apparent reason. The disorder appears in children of all ages. Children with this type of seizure may report variable psychic symptoms. Many of them involve perceptual distortions. Visually they might include seeing objects as bigger or smaller than they are or seeing shadows in the periphery, or side, of their visual fields. These distortions can also affect the senses of smell and taste. Like Juan, children report abnormal smells such as burning tires and metallic tastes. Feelings of *déjà vu* are related to disturbances in memory. These somewhat bizarre experiences can occur steadily or wax and wane.

> **psychic:** Related to a wide array of perceptual and emotional states, such as heightened emotions or rage.

TLE is not a common disorder and is not easy to diagnose. Only a thorough history that turns up the types of symptoms just described is likely to lead an evaluator in the right direction. Once TLE is suspected, an electroencephalogram (EEG) should be completed to look for abnormal brain electrical activity. To help elicit seizure activity, the EEG may need to be completed both while the child is awake and while he is asleep. This type of EEG is called a *sleep–awake EEG* and generally requires keeping your child awake all night, or at least awakening the child after he has slept only from midnight until 3:00 A.M. If your child has to undergo a sleep–awake EEG, be prepared for the "fun and excitement" of forcing him or her to remain awake while terribly sleepy. Some practitioners have moved to 24-hour EEGs to enhance the ability to "catch" a seizure occurring.

In Juan's case, a sleep–awake EEG showed abnormal seizure activity in the temporal lobes and led to pharmacological treatment. In Dominick's case, the EEG was normal, but a 24-hour EEG revealed periodic seizure activity on the left side of the brain in the temporal lobe. These seizures coincided with the marked anger attacks Dominick recorded in a diary.

In cases of an abnormal EEG, some children are asked to have a brain imaging scan. Whereas the EEG may identify abnormal electrical activity in the brain, brain imaging tests—MRIs—can uncover problems with the brain substance itself (tumors, birth malformations, artery problems, etc.).

The Treatment

Medications for children with temporal lobe epilepsy include the older anticonvulsant medications Tegretol/Equetrol (carbamazepine), Depakote (valproic acid), Trileptal (oxcarbazepine), Neurontin (gabapentin), and Lamictal (lamotrigine). These seizures commonly require higher doses of the anticonvulsant agents, which means the child's blood levels of some of the medications must be monitored closely. Juan's symptoms were markedly improved with Tegretol, and in Dominick's case the same drug eliminated his rage attacks altogether.

If your child does not respond to a single agent, other anticonvulsants may be tried, or two anticonvulsants may be necessary. If the child has hallucinations, the doctor may want to add an antipsychotic medication to the anticonvulsants. The anxiety-breaking medications (benzodiazepines), such as Klonopin (clonazepam), may be helpful if your child has prominent anxiety. Interestingly, Klonopin has been used at higher doses of 6–12 mg daily for seizures and in fact is FDA approved for use as an anticonvulsant in children.

As with other seizure disorders, the doctor should reassess your child periodically and should discontinue medication if the child's symptoms are gone and the child's EEG is normal. Most often, TLE continues into adulthood, which means your child will need ongoing anticonvulsant treatment. Dominick's treatment continues to be effective 5 years after he began taking Tegretol.

Organic Mental Disorders and Brain Injury

The Disorders

Sadly, a significant number of children suffer some sort of brain damage that causes emotional or behavioral disorders. Generally these problems are called *mental disorders due to medical conditions*. These disorders can be congenital, which means they occur at birth for no apparent reason, they can be caused by in utero trauma (such as fetal distress), or they can be caused by birth trauma. At any later point in the child's life, they can be caused by encephalitis (infection of the brain), meningitis (inflammation of the lining of the brain), toxicity (drugs or exposure to harmful agents), or blunt trauma (such as occurs during a sporting event, bicycle, or motor vehicle accident).

Be assured that the vast majority of concussions that affect children are not severe and will resolve fully with time. More severe concussions and brain injuries are often referred to as traumatic brain injuries (TBIs), which were receiving much media attention as of 2016 due to their association with sports like football and with military combat. They are increasingly recognized as preventable, and both the public and medical practitioners are increasingly aware of the need to examine injured individuals for TBIs. TBI is often associated with headaches, double vision, dizziness, coordination issues, cognitive ("thinking") impairment, and personality changes. The good news is that most TBI resolves with time; however, reinjury after an initial concussion may happen more easily and may also lead to a longer course of healing fully after a TBI. It is noteworthy that practitioners are now appreciating it may take months for a child's brain to heal fully from a TBI. We treat Adam, a 20-year-old college student, who suffered a sports-related concussion in high school and had two subsequent concussive episodes. He now has some postconcussion symptoms (headaches, arousal problems, attention problems, slowed thinking) that have responded to care in not reinjuring himself and low-dose stimulant medication (see page 185).

Children with brain injury are known to exhibit a wide array of behaviors, such as disinhibition (acting out of control, being exceedingly silly, or overreacting), rage attacks, temper tantrums, aggression, and panic reactions, as well as cognitive dulling and slowness, coordination issues, and isolation or withdrawal.

The Treatment

How these children are treated depends on the specific symptoms or problems the child has. The more common symptoms are cognitive, and sometimes very-low-dose stimulants may be helpful, with the child monitored carefully for the appearance of "acting out" or moodiness during treatment. For externalizing or acting-out problems behavioral modification should be tried first. This form of therapy may be very helpful in reducing specific symptoms. Medications found helpful for aggression and acting out include low doses of the atypical antipsychotics and the mood stabilizers (lithium, Tegretol, Depakote), Valium-like medications (benzodiazepines such as Klonopin), alpha agonists/blood pressure medications (guanfacine, clonidine), and rarely Trexan or ReVia (naltrexone). For severe cases, especially those in which children are harmful to themselves or others, multiple medications may need to be prescribed. Plan to keep a diary documenting outbursts and other "target" behaviors during medication trials. Many children have some issues that existed before the brain injury and may benefit from continued treatment with medications after the healing process appears to be complete. For others, careful tapering of the medications after a period of stable mood and emotions may be useful, with close monitoring of the child's emotional and behavioral state.

Table 9. Pharmacotherapy of Tics and Tourette's Disorder

Kapvay, Catapres (clonidine)

Tenex, Intuniv (guanfacine)

Strattera (atomoxetine)

Tricyclic antidepressants: desipramine, imipramine, nortriptyline

Klonopin (clonazepam) and other benzodiazepines

High-potency antipsychotics: Risperdal (risperidone), Haldol (haloperidol), Orap (pimozide), others

Combined pharmacotherapy for treatment nonresponders or children with other disorders: clonidine + Zoloft (sertraline), desipramine + Concerta (extended-release methylphenidate; watch for possible tic worsening with stimulants), clonidine + stimulants

11
Other Mental Health Disturbances Affecting Children and Adolescents

Eating Disorders: Anorexia and Bulimia

The Disorders

Anorexia nervosa (commonly called *anorexia*), bulimia nervosa (commonly called *bulimia*), and binge-eating disorder occur in 0.3%, 0.9%, and 1.6% of the population, respectively, and are complicated eating disorders that affect mainly girls and young women, although some boys and older men and women suffer from the disorder as well. Eating disorders often begin in later childhood and adolescence (the most frequent onset is at ages 12–13), and recent research shows that adolescents with eating disorders often have symptoms of both anorexia and bulimia at the same time.

Anorexia is defined by profound weight loss or the inability to maintain a body weight higher than 15% below the "ideal body weight" (the suggested weight for the height and age of the child). People with anorexia report feeling and looking fat (they have a distorted body image), even though to others they often appear frail or very thin. Anorexic girls often do not begin to have their menstrual periods or lose their periods (*amenorrhea*) during their episodes of decreased eating. These children and adolescents are obsessed with issues surrounding food and may exercise excessively.

Bulimia is characterized by repeated episodes of overeating (bingeing), intermixed with attempts to vomit (purge), abuse laxatives, or exercise excessively. Bulimic young people, usually girls, are preoccupied with body weight, as are anorexics, but unlike anorexics they do not necessarily feel or perceive that they are overweight. In fact, most bulimics range from normal weight to slightly overweight. Often stress and feelings of hopelessness or depression will worsen bulimia. Binge-eating disorder is characterized by episodes in which the person eats excessive levels of food in an obsessive way and feels totally unable to exert the control to stop. There is a growing consensus among researchers that adolescents often suffer from a combination of components of the various eating disorders, such as both purging and restricting food.

In both anorexia and bulimia, co-occurring disorders are very common. Depression, anxiety, PTSD, and personality issues often accompany eating disorders, and it is possible to see traits of both anorexia and bulimia simultaneously in one child. Although the neurobiological connection is not well worked out as of 2015, children with eating disorders appear to have disturbances in the brain neurochemicals serotonin and dopamine and in the *opioid* (pain control) system.

Although it is most likely to occur in adolescence, it is not uncommon to see anorexia in children as young as 7 years old and into adulthood. The prognosis for children with anorexia or bulimia is generally good. Although the treatment of anorexia has improved, a child's obsessiveness about food and distorted body image may continue to some degree into adulthood, and children who succeed in gaining weight customarily report feeling uncomfortable and distressed and require encouragement and counseling. There appear to be better outcomes over time for bulimia and binge eating than for anorexia. As they grow into young adulthood, many binge eaters and people with bulimia will harbor the urge to binge or purge during periods of stress but will not act on their urges.

The Treatment

Nonpharmacological treatments for anorexia include a multifaceted approach including family and individual psychotherapy (e.g., focused cognitive-behavioral therapy) as well as nutritional counseling. These are often very helpful in identifying family and individual dynamic issues as well as educating the family about the frequently long-standing condition. Various members of your family, including your child, other children, and you and your significant other, may very well require therapy. Often including the family in the treatment assists greatly in normalizing eating behavior, reducing stress in the family, and providing support for the adolescent. Specific types of cognitive-behavioral therapy have been shown to be helpful in eating disorders. The SSRI antidepressants (Prozac, Zoloft, Celexa, Luvox, and Paxil) have been shown to be somewhat effective and may be worth trying. These antidepressants may help primarily by reducing urges, craving, and obsessions, but they sometimes cause the unwelcome side effect of actually increasing weight loss. If an antidepressant is prescribed for your child, be vigilant for further weight loss.

Identification and treatment of co-occurring disorders such as anxiety or depression may hold out hope for improving the condition and quality of life for a child with anorexia. For children with severe anxiety, the benzodiazepines (Valium-like medications) may be beneficial. Less commonly, children with anorexia may require antipsychotics to help improve their profound distortions in thought.

For bulimia, nonmedication treatments are similar to those used for anorexia. As with anorexia, therapy and medications are often combined, although teenagers with bulimia may respond better to medications than those with anorexia. The tricyclic antidepressants (desipramine, imipramine, amitriptyline) and the SSRIs (Zoloft, Prozac, Luvox, Celexa, and Paxil) may be helpful in reducing the binge-and-purge cycles. For children with prominent mood swings along with bulimia, the doctor may prescribe lithium, Depakote, Trileptal, Neurontin, or other mood stabilizers.

More recently, sibutramine (Meridia), Vyvanse, Effexor, and Topamax have been shown to be effective in reducing binge eating (sibutramine) and bingeing/purging (Topamax) in those with bulimia and are worthy of consideration. Sally is a 17-year-old high school senior who reported bingeing and purging daily for 1 year. She had a history of depression that was not currently problematic. Psychotherapy plus Topamax at 100 mg daily was very effective in helping stop her bulimia. Binge eating is treated with the use of Vyvanse (a long-acting stimulant), SSRI antidepressants, treatment of anxiety, and the use of Topamax to help reduce the obsessiveness related to the binge cycles.

Alcohol and Substance Abuse

The Disorder

Many adolescents and, to a lesser extent, children have tried alcohol and/or drugs at some point in their lives. Studies indicate that over half of high school seniors have used alcohol and marijuana, and approximately 25% have smoked cigarettes. A smaller group of approximately 10–15% have used cocaine, amphetamines, and inhalants. Prescription drug abuse has been emerging as a major problem for adolescents and most commonly involves painkillers such as OxyContin or Vicodin, sedatives such as benzodiazepines (e.g., Klonopin or Ativan), and stimulants such as Ritalin or Adderall. What makes a child start using cigarettes, other drugs, or alcohol is not entirely known. Availability, community and personal values, level of self-esteem, peer pressure, parental substance use, and a host of other issues appear related. In addition, studies indicate that a family history of alcoholism or drug abuse puts children at about a fourfold risk for substance abuse. For instance, a well-known historical study based in Sweden indicated a ninefold risk for alcoholism in the sons of fathers with alcoholism. Other studies have shown that juvenile-onset substance abuse runs in families, is highly heritable, and is often accompanied by conduct (delinquency) and mood disorders. In fact it is now clear that approximately three-quarters of adolescents with a substance abuse disorder also have a psychiatric disorder and that untreated psychiatric disorders result in higher risk for cigarette smoking and substance abuse.

Determining the difference among normal use, misuse, and abuse can be difficult. *Use* generally means infrequent to occasional use of a substance commonly used by others in the community with little direct harm to the adolescent. *Misuse* indicates a pattern of use with some negative consequences. *Use disorder* is a more serious problem in which the child has begun to lose control of the substance ("needs to get high"). An alcohol or drug use disorder is diagnosed when there is an established and often continued pattern of substance use despite legal, interpersonal, or medical consequences. Direct evidence of a use disorder includes blackouts, substance use prior to or during school, substance use alone or with strangers, driving while intoxicated, and consumption in dangerous situations. Changes in school or work performance, fights, irritability, and a lack of interest in activities or lack of motivation are indirect evidence that your child may be involved in substance abuse. A more serious disorder is evident when the child demonstrates a daily pattern of excess substance use for which there are more serious consequences, such as school failure or legal problems. Adolescents with more severe use disorders may become physiologically addicted and may have difficulty stopping their substance or alcohol use because of disturbing withdrawal symptoms or psychological dependence. Rey is a 16-year-old boy with ADHD whom I (T. E. W.) treated. He had been in and out of treatment for years, and his parents brought him in because of delinquent acts such as stealing from them, a change in his peer group, and a sudden academic decline. When questioned, Rey revealed that 6 months earlier he had tried painkillers belonging to his grandparents and was now buying them on the street and had just started sniffing heroin—hence the abrupt change in his personality and need for funds to supply his now daily habit.

Cigarette use is one of the most common substance use problems in adolescents in general and in those with psychiatric disorders in particular. Young people who smoke tend to have higher rates of mental health problems, and conversely, higher rates of cigarette use tend to be seen in psychiatrically impaired youth. It's important to mention your child's nicotine use (including chewing tobacco and electronic cigarettes) to the doctor not only to address the child's addiction but also because of the potential for drug interactions—nicotine can increase or decrease the amount of the prescribed medication in the child's system. We and others have also shown that nicotine may prime the brain to use *more* drugs and alcohol later in life.

The psychiatric conditions most often seen with substance problems in children are conduct disorder, ADHD, oppositional defiant disorder, depression, bipolar disorder, and, to a lesser extent, anxiety and panic disorders. In many cases the psychiatric problem precedes the substance problem, leading to conjecture that many children "self-medicate" their symptoms by using substances. In addition, children with psychiatric problems may not have the foresight or inhibition it takes to resist getting involved with alcohol or drugs. This appears to be the case with ADHD. The myth that taking stimulant medications for ADHD leads to later substance abuse persists to this day, even though it seems more and more certain that it is the impulsivity of ADHD that often leads these kids to use alcohol or illegal drugs. Data from a recent large Swedish study in over 25,000 adolescents and young adults indicate that stimulant treatment of ADHD reduces not only criminality but also drug-related issues. Moreover, longer-term prospective clinical trials continue to show a reduction in cigarette smoking and drug and alcohol use disorders in treated individuals compared to those who are not receiving treatment for their ADHD.

The Treatment

There is no unifying treatment for alcohol or drug problems. Initially, both you and your child need to understand what substances are being misused and what risks that misuse brings. Following that, it is important to take several measures:

- Monitor your child to deter further use. Random saliva or urine toxicology screens to detect illicit substances in your child's body, provided by the child's practitioner or school, can be useful. When teens complain that requiring drug tests demonstrates a lack of trust in them, I find it helpful to comment that it is "the disorder of addiction" that is distrusted, not necessarily the child. For kids who refuse or are unable to provide a urine sample for analysis, saliva testing is advised.
- Provide additional structure yourself or arrange for it to be provided by your child's school and after-school programs.
- Look into support groups such as Al-Anon, Alcoholics or Narcotics Anonymous, and Rational Recovery for teens and their families.
- Seek appropriate psychotherapy. Research indicates that family therapy, cognitive-behavioral therapy, and coping skills training (how to deal with life stressors) are the most effective types of psychotherapeutic intervention for adolescent substance abusers.

For cigarette use, apply the same cessation techniques that adults use and also reduce your child's access to cigarettes. Use of the nicotine patch initially and then nicotine gum or lozenges alone or in concert with Zyban (bupropion) can be somewhat effective in helping an adolescent stop smoking cigarettes or using snuff. A nicotine-based medication called Chantix (varenicline) is also effective in stopping cigarette smoking but remains relatively untested in kids and should be monitored carefully due to the possibility that it may increase a child's depression. Unfortunately, many insurance policies will not cover the cost of a prescription (upward of $400–500). If you decide to try Chantix, I recommend paying privately for the medication (perhaps a few pills at a time) because of the serious long-term problems associated with untreated cigarette smoking and the effectiveness of this medication.

The pharmacotherapy that your child's doctor devises will be aimed at reducing the child's craving and diminishing the child's underlying psychiatric disturbance. Medications that reduce cravings include those used to replace dangerous street drugs (and accompanying high-risk behavior). Buprenorphine, for example, is an orally administered medication that can help adolescents who are addicted to heroin or painkillers and can be prescribed for those 16 and older by specially trained and licensed practitioners. More recently, a naturally occurring agent called "NAC" (*N*-acetylcysteine) has been shown to be helpful for reducing marijuana craving. The SSRIs and Wellbutrin have been used in adults with limited effectiveness in reducing drug cravings. Naltrexone has also been shown useful in reducing alcohol consumption in adults with alcoholism and has some data suggesting it also works in teens (if they take it!). If adherence to treatment with the oral form of the naltrexone is problematic, a once-a-month injection called Vivitrol is available and can be very helpful; it may help with either alcohol abuse or opioid/heroin/painkiller addiction. We typically recommend Vivitrol as an early treatment for adolescents who are having difficulty staying away from painkillers or street narcotics such as heroin.

Most pharmacotherapy in adolescents with substance use disorders is aimed at the underlying or co-occurring disorders, such as ADHD, which occurs in about one-quarter of the teenagers with a significant drug or alcohol habit, and depression, which occurs in about half of them. It's not always clear, however, whether these other conditions are primary or secondary disorders. Depression, for example, can just as easily be a product of substance abuse and will disappear once the child has been sober or abstinent for a certain period of time.

Often, then, your child's doctor may wait until the child has been sober for 1–4 months before diagnosing or initiating medication treatment for a majority of disorders. For some conditions such as bipolar disorder or schizophrenia, it may be necessary to start medication before the child stops abusing the substance. Studies show that treating a substance-abusing adolescent with bipolar disorder with agents directed at the bipolar disorder (see page 161) reduces the substance abuse. If your child has developed a substance problem while on medication, most doctors will not restart the medication until the child has been "clean" for 1 month. Make sure your child gets the message directly and clearly from the doctor: *No substance abuse while taking prescribed medication.*

Beyond that caveat, the timing of treatments is done on a case-by-case basis and depends on a thorough evaluation of the child's functioning with family, peers, and school. Julia had been using LSD and marijuana daily, and I (T. E. W.) suspected that her depression had been a cause—not a result—of her substance abuse because of what else I learned about her: she had "fallen in with the wrong crowd," and although her school performance was low, it had not always been that way. After engaging in group therapy, Julia had successfully stopped using drugs for 4 months, but she continued to appear depressed, with low energy and sadness, and so she was treated with a very low dose (37.5 mg of the extended-release medication daily) of the antidepressant Effexor. Her mood improved, she reunited with her old friends, and she subsequently performed well academically for the next year with no substance use.

There are no special rules for treating underlying psychiatric problems in cases of substance abuse, although we have more established algorithms for treating adolescents with substance abuse and other disorders. For example, in a substance-abusing adolescent with bipolar disorder, one should treat bipolar disorder. Such is probably the case for depression, which is now seen as not entirely secondary to the effect of substances of abuse on the brain. ADHD is a mixed bag, the recent consensus being to stabilize the addiction and then treat the ADHD relatively rapidly. As for anxiety and OCD, doctors typically recommend behavioral treatments, then SSRIs.

Your child's practitioner may take one of these approaches:

- Young people with ADHD benefit from the traditional regimens, including Strattera, Wellbutrin, the tricyclic antidepressants, the alpha agonists, and the extended-release stimulants. Should kids who have a recent history of drug or alcohol problems be placed on the stimulants? This is a common concern, but since these medications are the best studied and most effective agents for ADHD, their use in "high-risk" groups is acceptable as long as the children are monitored closely. Your child's doctor might consider initially using a stimulant with a lower abuse potential such as Vyvanse, Concerta, Metadate CD, or Ritalin LA, and then other stimulants.

- Co-occurring depressive disorders are best treated with antidepressants, including the SSRIs (Prozac, Zoloft, Paxil, Celexa, Lexapro, and Luvox), Wellbutrin, Remeron, Serzone or trazodone, Effexor, and less commonly the tricyclic antidepressants (nortriptyline, imipramine, and others).

- Children with bipolar disorder will require atypical antipsychotics and/or mood stabilizers, which should be started as soon as the diagnosis is made—even if the adolescent is still abusing drugs or alcohol—as mentioned above. Since tight monitoring is essential with the mood stabilizers, I recommend using the antipsychotics as first-line agents for treating the bipolar disorder in substance-abusing adolescents.

- Adolescents with a history of substance abuse in whom anxiety is a problem can be tried on nonaddictive anxiety-breaking compounds such as Buspar, the SSRI or tricyclic antidepressants, Remeron, Effexor, and more distantly the Valium-like benzodiazepines.

To ensure your child's safety, frequent discussions with your child's practitioner are paramount. Adequate monitoring by you, the doctor, and other caregivers is necessary to make sure your teen is not using substances, to evaluate the effectiveness of the medication, to check compliance, and to assess for potential drug interactions. Although most medications are safe when combined with periodic alcohol or drug use, the literature has included a number of cases in which children developed delirium, severe blackouts, agitation, and medical complications after mixing them with street drugs. For example, our research group reported that using marijuana while taking nortriptyline or desipramine caused severe delirium in a number of patients. While this has not been studied systematically, there appears to be good relative safety in the combined use of the stimulants (methylphenidate and amphetamine-based compounds), Wellbutrin, Strattera, mood stabilizers, and atypical antipsychotics with the major substances of abuse: alcohol and marijuana.

If you suspect your child is using a particular drug while receiving a prescribed psychotropic, in addition to your child's physician you may wish to contact the U.S. Poison Control Centers for information about potential drug interactions and suggested instructions.

Sleep Disturbances

The Disorders

Sleep disturbances are common in children, and it is perfectly normal for them to occur temporarily during certain developmental stages. They are, however, often reported by parents whose children have psychiatric disorders. Sleep disorders may also lead to behavioral and cognitive symptoms that could be construed as psychiatric. Children who have poor sleep often have problems with arousal (staying awake), cognition (thinking), and mood.

Some disturbances that affect sleep itself appear to be related to psychiatric disorders, such as a reduction in sleep related to depression or a manic episode in a child with bipolar disorder. Another group that often has these sleep disturbances is children with ADHD. Although this is not well documented in laboratory sleep studies, reports from parents indicate that children with ADHD have difficulty falling asleep, sleep poorly, and have difficulty awakening. Children with sleep apnea or prominent snoring may be at increased risk for behavioral problems. Conversely, some children with depression may oversleep both at night and during the day.

Other disturbances involve abnormal behavior or events during sleep—nightmares, sleep terrors, sleepwalking, and sleep talking. These disturbances occur during various sleeping states and may be related both to the underlying psychiatric disorder and to its treatment. Children with mood disorders may report violent, scary dreams. The use of certain medications such as clonidine may produce nightmares; however, few medications are related to sleepwalking. Obstructive sleep issues that may disrupt a child's sleep can be identified by monitoring for excessive snoring by the child.

The Treatment

Evaluation of the nature of the sleep disturbance is the first step. Let your child's doctor know if your child is snoring—a referral to an ear, nose, and throat doctor may be necessary to assess for blockages that are causing the nightly obstruction. Initially, you should try to improve your child's sleep hygiene. Structure and routine are a great help: eliminate caffeinated beverages (certain colas, tea, hot chocolate), reduce activity around bedtime, and try playing soft music or relaxation tapes to help your child go to sleep easily. Make sure your child avoids strenuous activity prior to bedtime. Whereas some children find the computer relaxing, others become stimulated by it and should avoid contact with the computer prior to bedtime. Awaken children early and avoid letting them take daytime naps. One 8-year-old patient of mine (T. E. W.) with ADHD was in the habit of going to bed at 9:00 P.M. but would not fall asleep until midnight; then he would nap for up to 2 hours every day after school. After about 2 weeks of keeping him from napping (no small task!), his parents saw his sleep cycle return to normal. While it is common to let kids sleep very late on weekends, it may be difficult for the child who sleeps until noon on Sunday, for example, to go to bed that night by 9:00 P.M. to get up early Monday for school.

Correction of an underlying psychiatric disorder can assist in reducing a sleep problem. For example, 16-year-old Sam, who has bipolar disorder, says his first sign of becoming manic is a change in his sleep cycle. Whereas Sam usually sleeps for 8 hours, when feeling manic symptoms, he sleeps for only 3–4 hours and feels fully rested. In these cases his Seroquel is increased, with additional medication given at night to help him sleep. Increasingly, it is becoming recognized that correction of sleep is essential for stabilization in psychiatric disorders.

Medications for sleep problems should not be used without careful thought and a hypothesis about what is causing or exacerbating the sleep problem. Over-the-counter medications such as antihistamines (Benadryl, Dimetapp, and others) may be useful on an as-needed basis for passing sleep problems. Dosages ranging from half a teaspoon (12.5 mg) to 1 teaspoon (25 mg) in a child or 2 teaspoons (50 mg) in an adolescent are generally effective. Although usually quite safe, they may cause excessive morning sedation and dry mouth, and the child often becomes tolerant of the medication's sleep-producing effects.

Melatonin has been reported to be useful in controlled studies in children. Studies show that melatonin helps both in the short and longer term. Most children seem to respond favorably to lower dosing (half of an adult dose, roughly 1.5–3 mg at night), but some may require full adult doses. While some practitioners may recommend that your child take the medication at 6:00 to 7:00 P.M., others believe it should be administered 1 hour prior to the time of sleep. Like other *soporifics* (sleep-inducing agents), melatonin may cause morning sedation; otherwise, no major side effects have been reported. Because of the variability in the available preparations, I recommend finding a trusted brand from a reputable store and staying with it (if effective).

Clonidine is commonly prescribed for sleep, particularly if the sleep problem is related to ADHD or other psychiatric disorders. Generally it is started at half a tablet (0.05 mg) and increased as necessary, which should be supervised by your doctor. In our clinic, we reported on a study in which children received clonidine safely for up to 3 years, with the majority of parents reporting an excellent continued response. Some children with nightmares benefit from a related medication, low-dose prazosin (Minipress) (e.g., 1–2 mg).

Other agents include the Valium-like medications such as Ambien, Klonopin, and Ativan. These medications may cause marked daytime sedation, disinhibition, and nightmares and are generally not used over the long haul. More recently, sleepwalking, sleep talking, and binge eating have been associated with the use of this class of medications, and although these problems are infrequent, children should be monitored for them. In addition, these medications should be avoided in cases of substance abuse, since they may be addictive, although there are few data to indicate a problem with everyday use in young people.

Sedating antidepressants such as amitriptyline or imipramine (25–75 mg) or Remeron (7.5–15 mg) can be useful not only for promoting sleep but also to help treat bedwetting, ADHD, and anxiety. These medications can be used on a regular basis or as needed.

Some children develop a sleep problem only in response to their medication. Most notable are the stimulants, which are notorious for producing insomnia (difficulty in sleeping). In those cases, earlier administration of the medication or a reduction in the dose may alleviate the problem. If the daytime medication is very effective and needs to be given, another medication at bedtime may be beneficial. Bedtime doses of melatonin, clonidine, Remeron, and amitriptyline have been reported to be useful in stimulant-induced sleep problems associated with ADHD.

For children who have severe, unremitting sleep problems or sleep problems related to psychotic disorders (bipolar disorder or schizophrenic illness), the antipsychotics may be necessary. Most commonly, Seroquel, Thorazine, Zyprexa, or Risperdal is used and may cause confusion, heaviness, excess sedation, and abnormal muscle movements. Since long-term use may cause blood metabolic problems (e.g., sugar or lipid accumulation) and irreversible involuntary muscle movements (tardive dyskinesia), especially with the older agents (Thorazine, Mellaril), this class of medications should not be used unless other treatments have proven ineffective or psychosis is present.

Enuresis

Bedwetting (*enuresis*) in children is not uncommon, with up to 15% of 11-year-old boys still having difficulties with this problem. There is often a family history of bedwetting, generally in the father. Bedwetting is thought to represent an immature neurological system and not the presence of major mental illness. Bedwetting without a known medical cause such as infection usually responds to maturity or nonpharmacological therapies such as behavior modification. A number of commercial products that take a behavioral approach to reducing nighttime bedwetting are available.

Pharmacological treatment relies on two very different agents: a synthetic hormone or a tricyclic antidepressant. With both agents, relief is generally immediate, but discontinuation will lead to return of the bedwetting. Antidiuretic hormone desmopressin (ddAVP) has been shown to be effective for the treatment of bedwetting, although the medication is expensive. Previously the ddAVP nasal spray was frequently prescribed; however, the FDA has advised against using this form of the medication because of problems with blood salt (sodium) levels and seizures. The tablet form, however, remains a safe and viable form of the medication. While it is relatively free of side effects, certain medical conditions may also make it inadvisable to use this medication. Imipramine is also FDA approved for bedwetting at doses of 25–50 mg nightly and works both short and long term. Imipramine is generic and hence a less expensive alternative to other treatments.

Trials off medication should be attempted periodically, since enuresis may remit spontaneously. Medications may also be used intermittently when the child is involved in sleepovers and overnight camps where the embarrassment of bedwetting may be significant. While medications are effective in two-thirds of children, bedwetting typically resumes when they are discontinued.

Part III

The Psychotropic Medications

This section presents detailed information on the medications referred to in Parts I and II—how the medications work, which disorders they are used to treat, typical dosage ranges and other information on administering the drug, and side effects to watch for. Tables will sum up important facts and provide a handy cross-reference of brand (marketed name) and generic (chemical) names for each medication.

Questions that parents ask time and again in our offices reveal that there is much confusion over the terms used to categorize and name these drugs:

- "How can a drug called a stimulant be right for my hyperactive son?"
- "Why would you prescribe an antidepressant for my daughter when we both agree she's not suffering from depression?"
- "Why does it make sense to give my 10-year-old something designed to treat high blood pressure or epilepsy?"
- "Can you explain—in English—what a serotonin norepinephrine reuptake inhibitor is?"

These are all valid questions and honestly plague some practitioners too. Medications with psychoactive properties used to treat behavioral and emotional difficulties are globally referred to as *psychotropics*, but beyond that the terminology becomes quite confusing.

Most of the compounds you are about to read about are classified generally by their effectiveness in treating adult disorders—antidepressants for depression, antipsychotics for psychosis, mood stabilizers for mood disorders, and anxiolytics for anxiety. Others are named for the effect they have on behavior—the mood stabilizers, for example—or for their similarities to other compounds, as in the case of the stimulants. More specific medications are named for their chemical structures (tricyclic antidepressants) or how they work in the brain (selective serotonin reuptake inhibitors, alpha agonists).

To complicate matters further, a number of medications are considered one type of compound but are used for another problem. For example, clonidine and guanfacine are antihypertensives—that is, they lower blood pressure—but are used in psychiatry to treat tics and ADHD and more recently have been referred to as alpha agonists to reflect how they work on the brain to bring about change (they bind to the alpha [and beta] receptors). While the tricyclic antidepressants (named based on their chemical structure) are commonly used for ADHD, enuresis (bedwetting), and anxiety, they are rarely used for depression in youth these days.

Why use these labels to head the following chapters if they are so misleading? First, because realistically they are what you will encounter in discussions with all mental health professionals. Even more important, though, understanding these classifications will help you become an informed collaborator in your child's care. In today's health care environment, it's quite likely that your child will have different practitioners over the years. The more you understand about your child's medication history—"No, John was constantly giddy on Ativan, so I'd be worried about trying Klonopin" or "Yes, we'd be willing to try Prozac, but you should know that Zoloft didn't help"—the more you can preserve continuity of care for your child. Keeping track of each drug's classification on a medication log (see page 294) will help maintain a clear picture of your child's course of treatment.

Don't let the chemical structures, mechanisms, or names of the medications intimidate you—just remember to write down the names of the medications (brand and generic) that your child will be taking, and when you have *any* question about a medication being prescribed for your child, ask the prescriber, the pharmacist, and anyone else who is participating in the care of your child.

12
The Stimulants and Nonstimulants for ADHD

You may already know more about the stimulant medications than any other drugs used to treat psychiatric disorders in children. Not only are they the most commonly used and well-studied psychotropic agents in children and adolescents today, but they continue to receive a lot of attention in the popular press. Increasingly, and throughout the world, the nonstimulants used to treat ADHD are also becoming very well known—for their effect not only on ADHD but also on ADHD plus other conditions (e.g., tics).

The Stimulants

The stimulants have been around since their usefulness was first described in 1937 in the United States, and today over one million children in this country alone are being treated with these medications. Perhaps because of their prevalence, the stimulants continue to be in the news. Reports ranging from stunting of growth to stimulation of aggression or initiation of substance abuse have left many parents hesitant to authorize stimulant treatment of their children with ADHD. As a parent making important health decisions for your child, you should know that much of the hype about aggression originated in individual cases rather than in broad cross-sections of young patients. In a number of those cases, the teenagers involved had not been taking the stimulants within a year of the incidents reported, so there is no cause-and-effect link. Similarly, cardiovascular risks were debated in 2006 but should not be a concern for children without existing heart disease (see the details later in this chapter)—in fact, as of 2015 we have carefully examined and agree with the now large literature on this subject concluding that these medications do not cause heart problems.

If you decide on a trial of stimulants for your child, the medications the prescriber is most likely to name are:

- Methylphenidate: Ritalin LA, Metadate CD, Concerta, Focalin XR, Daytrana, Quillivant/QuilliChew, Aptensio

- Amphetamines: Dexedrine, Adderall XR, Vyvanse, Evekeo XR, Dyanavel XR

The stimulants are available in less expensive generic preparations (e.g., Concerta, Adderall XR), with the newer stimulants available only in branded form (e.g., Daytrana, Vyvanse).

The stimulants are under strict control by the Drug Enforcement Administration and are classified as schedule II (see the box on page 205). This means you will have to be prepared to get your prescriptions rewritten monthly or bimonthly and to provide a photo ID at the pharmacy. Of note, various mail-order prescription services allow a 3-month supply of a stimulant; however, your doctor may be limited to prescribing a 2-month supply by various state and federal regulations. Contact your insurance carrier to see how many months it will cover at one time.

How the Stimulants Work

The stimulant medications, while they are in a child's bloodstream, appear to normalize biochemistry in the parts of the brain involved in ADHD. Specifically, they enhance nerve-to-nerve communication by making more neurotransmitters available to boost the "signal" between neurons. The stimulants work by blocking the recycle mechanism of the sending nerve cell, leading to an accumulation of the neurotransmitter, which is then available to pass on the signal. The neurotransmitters that are released more effectively when a child takes stimulants are dopamine and norepinephrine. Some recent work also suggests that glutamate and GABA may be involved in ADHD.

You may wonder why, if they all enhance nerve-to-nerve communication, there is such a selection of stimulants for the doctor to choose from.

Drug Enforcement Administration Drug Scheduling

The Drug Enforcement Administration (DEA) "schedules" a drug based largely on its abuse potential (*liability*), either by the individual taking the medication or by others who may steal the medication, diverting it from its proper use. Prescribed medications that are watched very carefully and require special prescribing practices are considered *schedule II or III*. Among more frequently prescribed psychotropic medications, schedule II compounds include Ritalin, Concerta, Metadate, Dexedrine, and Adderall. Different federal, state, and local laws govern the use of schedule II compounds, but generally prescriptions for them must be issued either monthly or bimonthly and patients have only 3–30 days to fill the prescriptions. Thought to be less likely to be abused, schedule III and schedule IV compounds are prescribed medications that are also watched carefully but allow for refills and more latitude in the time allotted to fill the prescription. Schedule III compounds include some painkillers. Schedule IV compounds include the benzodiazepines (Valium, Klonopin, Ativan, Tranxene, others) and narcotic painkillers (such as Percocet).

Because the laws applying to schedule II, III, and IV drugs come from several levels of government, how pharmacies handle these prescriptions varies from location to location. For example, some pharmacies will allow a 2-month prescription of Ritalin, whereas others allow for only 1 month's supply. Likewise, some pharmacies require two forms of identification to fill a prescription, whereas others need only one. Try to remain patient with the rules and feel free to ask the pharmacist about any laws and regulations he or she is obligated to follow in filling your child's prescription. Another complicating factor is that each doctor's office has different monitoring requirements for patients who are receiving controlled substances: some require monthly check-ins, although most practitioners require less frequent visits. Some prescription services and more recent federal legislation allow for up to 90 days' administration at a time, but each state differs on this, insurance may not pay for more than 30–60 days, and many practitioners do not feel comfortable giving more than a monthly prescription of a controlled substance.

> **How can a stimulant possibly make my son less active?**
>
> I can see why you would be skeptical, and many parents are—we all think of stimulants as medications that keep us awake and aroused. The low to moderate oral doses used to treat ADHD actually make most people—whether they have ADHD or not—more attentive, less distractible, and less active. The "stimulant" name came from studies many years ago in which high doses of the medication given to rodents in laboratory tests actually "stimulated" their physical activity.
>
> The response to stimulants is considered "nonspecific"—that is, those with ADHD get much more improvement in their attention than those without ADHD; however, the stimulants have been misused by college students and others who don't have ADHD, largely as "study buddies."

The fact is that one class (methylphenidate vs. amphetamine) may have a slightly different mechanism of action from the other. This means that, despite their similarities, different stimulants may reduce your child's ADHD symptoms to different degrees. Don't be discouraged, then, if a trial of Ritalin or Concerta has disappointing results in your child; he may respond very well to Vyvanse, Adderall XR, or Dexedrine instead. Be patient and be prepared for some experimentation—strategies to try when your child does not respond to a medication are in Table 10.

How Effective Are the Stimulants?

The stimulants are among the best-studied medications, with their safety and effectiveness in ADHD assessed, as of 2015, in well over 350 controlled studies of more than 6,000 patients over 50 years. *The research has shown that, all told, the stimulants are effective in approximately three-quarters of those with ADHD—children, adolescents, and adults included—and offer the following benefits:*

- Diminish the inattention, distractibility, overactivity, and impulsivity that disrupt the lives of children and adults with ADHD.

- Improve parent–child interactions, peer relationships, academic performance, and classroom behavior.

Table 10. What to Do If Your Child Does Not Respond to the Stimulant Medications

Symptoms	Intervention
Worsened or unchanged ADHD symptoms (impulsivity, hyperactivity, inattention, distractibility)	• Increase stimulant dose. • Change timing of administration. • Change preparation (extended to short-acting). • Substitute stimulant (e.g., Concerta to Adderall XR). • Add another medication (Intuniv or Kapvay). • Consider alternative treatment (Strattera, alpha agonists [Intuniv or Kapvay], antidepressant like Wellbutrin).

Problematic side effects	• Assess whether side effect is medication-induced.
	• Determine when side effect is occurring (peak vs. wear-off).
	• Consider changing:
	  1. Timing of dose (give earlier or later in day)
	  2. Preparation (e.g., short-acting to extended-release or patch)
	  3. Type of stimulant (e.g., Vyvanse to Concerta)
	  4. Manufacturer (generic to brand)
	• Use adjunctive medication (e.g., melatonin, clonidine, Remeron, for sleep).

Marked rebound	• Change preparation to an extended-release or patch form. • Change timing of administration. • Add another small dose of like medication 30 minutes prior to rebound symptoms (e.g., 2.5 mg of Ritalin to Concerta). • Consider adjunctive clonidine or guanfacine in afternoon or Intuniv in morning; Strattera or tricyclic antidepressant in afternoon. • Consider alternative treatment.

(cont.)

Table 10 (*cont.*)

Symptoms	Intervention
Development of, or use with, tics or Tourette's disorder	• Assess continuation of tics off stimulant. • If tics stop, try stimulant again. • If tics worsen with stimulant, discontinue stimulants. • Use alternative treatment (Strattera, clonidine [Kapvay], guanfacine [Intuniv], tricyclics). • If ADHD symptoms continue, cautiously reintroduce stimulant. • Consider use with adjunctive treatment (Strattera, clonidine, guanfacine, desipramine, Risperdal, Geodon, Haldol, Orap).
Emergence of marked sadness, anxiety, agitation, irritability	• Assess timing when the side effect appears for toxicity (at peak effect 1–2 hours after taking) or withdrawal (during the wear-off phase, 6–12 hours later). • Reduce or change dosing. • Evaluate for return of ADHD symptoms. • Evaluate for another psychiatric disorder (e.g., depression, particularly if mood symptoms develop later in day during wear-off). • Change preparations or substitute type (Vyvanse or Adderall to Concerta). • Discontinue stimulants. • Consider alternative treatment (Strattera, antidepressant).

Note. In each case, determine if the stimulant is helpful. If there has been no response, reevaluate the dose and consider trying either another form of the stimulant or, if tried, another type of medication.

- Are effective for boys and girls and for those of all ages, from preschool through adulthood (although preschoolers and those with severe cognitive disabilities and ADHD respond less well and with more side effects). Clinical experience has confirmed the research here.
- Are effective long-term.

- May be sufficient as a sole treatment. In two earlier government-funded studies, for example, after 2 years of follow-up, methylphenidate was still very effective in reducing the core ADHD symptoms, and additional multimodal treatment (parent training and psychotherapy) did not add substantially to the medication's already significant effect.

↪ **Take-Home Point:** If your child responds well to medication, additional psychotherapy may not automatically be warranted (although specific psychotherapies can be useful for some components related to ADHD).

The Prescription

Among the most commonly prescribed and best-known stimulants are methylphenidate and amphetamine-based products.

Preparations on the shorter- and longer-acting ends of the spectrum are available for all of the stimulants, and they all have approximately the same efficacy

We typically do not recommend the use of methamphetamine for ADHD.

(see Table 11). In general, you'll probably see the effect on your child's attentiveness and behavior within 30–60 minutes after the child takes any stimulant (once a correct dose is reached via the process described on page 213). For shorter-acting stimulants (e.g., Ritalin) these effects usually peak between 1 and 4 hours after the drug is taken. This relatively short "behavioral half-life" naturally requires multiple doses to sustain the child's response over the waking hours. Many parents opt for longer-acting or extended-release stimulants so their child does not have to go to the school nurse for a dose of the stimulant. Slow-release preparations usually have a peak clinical effect 1–6 hours after administration, with continuation of the effect for up to 12 hours, meaning one dose given in the morning may last the whole school day.

Be aware that dosing equivalents for short- and long-acting stimulants varies:

- 10 mg of Dexedrine is roughly equivalent to 10 mg of the short-acting tablet.
- 36 mg of sustained-release Concerta is roughly equivalent to 10 mg of regular Ritalin stretched out through the day.

Table 11. The Preparation and Strength of the Stimulants

Generic name	Brand name	Sizes and preparation	Duration (estimate) of action/form
Methylphenidate	Ritalin	5, 10, 20 mg; tablets	4 hours/tablet
Extended release	Ritalin SR	20 mg; tablets	6 hours/tablets
Extended release	Ritalin LA	10, 20, 30, 40 mg; capsules	8 hours/capsule
Extended release	Concerta	18, 27, 36, 54 mg; capsules	12 hours/capsules
Extended release	Metadate CD	10, 20, 30, 40, 50, 60 mg; capsules	8 hours/capsule
Extended release and short acting	Methylin	2.5, 5, 10 mg; chewable tablets	4 hours/tablet
		5 mg/1 tsp and 10 mg/1 tsp; suspension	
Extended release	Daytrana	10, 15, 20, 30 mg; patch	Variable duration—12-hour approval
Extended release	Quillivant	25 mg/1 tsp suspension	12 hours
Extended release	Aptensio XR	10, 15, 20, 30, 40, 50, 60 mg; sprinkle	12 hours
d-Methylphenidate			
Extended release	Focalin	2.5, 5, 10 mg; tablets	5 hours
	Focalin XR	5, 10, 15, 20 mg; capsules	8–12 hours
Dextroamphetamine	Dexedrine	5, 10 mg; tablets	4 hours/tablet or spansule
		5, 10, 15 mg; spansules	
Extended release	Vyvanse	20, 30, 40, 50, 60, 70 mg; capsules	12 hours

Medication		Sizes and preparation	Duration (estimate) of action/form
Generic name	Brand name		
Amphetamine compounds	Adderall	5–30 mg; tablets	6 hours/tablet
Extended release	Adderall XR	5, 10, 15, 20, 25, 30 mg; capsules	12 hours/capsule
Extended release	Dyanavel XR	2.5 mg/ml or 12.5 mg/1 tsp; suspension	12 hours

Note. 5 cc = 5 ml = 1 tsp. Not all stimulant doses and preparations will be available at all pharmacies. Often, a less frequently used stimulant preparation may need to be ordered by your pharmacist. Some of the stimulants are generic (usually available less expensively for either private full pay or for copays).

- Focalin is twice as potent as regular Ritalin (in other words, 10 mg of Focalin = 20 mg of Ritalin).
- To complicate matters further, amphetamine (Vyvanse, Dexedrine, and Adderall) is about twice as potent as methylphenidate, so 20 mg of methylphenidate is equivalent to 10 mg of amphetamine.

The best solution for stimulant timing problems may be to try another preparation of the stimulant; and if that doesn't work, consider mixing preparations (such as a short-acting methylphenidate and a sustained-release preparation like Concerta) or using the methylphenidate patch (Daytrana), but arriving at the appropriate combination demands collaboration and communication.

Take-Home Point: As a parent, you need to get feedback on how your child is doing at various points in the school day and then pass on that information to the prescribing doctor.

The parents of 7-year-old Ken, for example, knew that their son had severe behavioral difficulties on the school bus and both behavioral and attentional problems in school. The bus drivers and teachers were able to tell them that the 10 mg of short-acting Ritalin Ken was taking helped his school bus ride and earlier hours in school, but the driver and teachers all noted a marked deterioration from around noon until 2:00 P.M., as well as on the return bus ride. Together Ken's parents and practitioner decided on a change to 20 mg of Metadate CD and agreed to watch him closely. Ken's parents reported to the doctor that the new prescription helped Ken considerably in the later hours at school and on the bus ride home but left him without medication effect in the afternoon to do homework. This time around, they tried a combination of 20 mg of Metadate CD in the morning and 5 mg of regular Ritalin in the afternoon on days he had work to do, which gave Ken consistent improvements throughout the school day—and he was able to eat dinner and sleep without difficulty.

> Most children are now being prescribed the new extended-release preparations of methylphenidate (e.g. Concerta, Ritalin LA, Metadate CD, QuilliChew/Quillivant, Daytrana) or amphetamine (Adderall XR, Dyanavel XR, Vyvanse), which provide sustained treatment of ADHD throughout the school day.

With the increasing interest in treating ADHD throughout the entire day, extended-release preparations of stimulants (Concerta, Ritalin LA, Focalin XR, Metadate CD, QuilliChew/Quillivant, Vyvanse, Adderall XR, Daytrana [methylphenidate transdermal system, or MTS]) are the stimulants of choice. Ritalin, Dexedrine, and

---

Can't we try Adderall with my daughter to find out for sure if she has ADHD?

When a child's problems elude diagnosis, it is tempting to use a "proven" treatment to come up with answers. As in all of medicine, though, a response or lack of response to a treatment cannot be relied on to diagnose ADHD. For instance, one-quarter of those with ADHD do not respond to stimulants, so not responding to a stimulant (what the doctor may describe as *treatment refractory*) does not necessarily mean the child does not have ADHD. And as above, some individuals without ADHD who are given stimulants will be able to concentrate better—but that does not mean they actually have ADHD.

Adderall, in contrast, may be given only at the times or in the situations when the symptoms of ADHD cause the child the greatest problems. Parents often consider the school hours the crucial times for medication. But before you choose to withhold medication after school, you should review the problems ADHD may be causing outside school. When medication is withheld, any interpersonal, family, and peer problems caused by ADHD may continue to plague your child during his or her free time. Also, many kids find that difficulty concentrating affects the extracurricular activities and sports in which they participate; continuing their medication after school greatly benefits their athletic performance and enjoyment. Even sporadic events like long car rides may be easier for your child with the medication's help.

> **Take-Home Point:** In the final analysis, whether to administer stimulants continuously on evenings, weekends, and holidays is an individual decision that should be based on how severely and pervasively your child's social and family life is impaired. Remember, however, that attention is fundamental to navigating life.

That decision can also be based on what you observe in your child when medication is initiated. The exact nature of the positive effects and side effects your child experiences may help you decide not only whether to give the medication continuously but also how to schedule the doses. If, for example, the appetite suppressant effects of the stimulants are a problem for your child, it may be a good idea to administer the medicine during or after breakfast. Giving methylphenidate products (e.g., Concerta, Ritalin) with food does not appreciably alter your child's body's ability to absorb the medication properly. In contrast, studies consistently show some delay in the absorption of amphetamine compounds (e.g., Adderall), which translates into taking longer for the medication to work if given with a high-fat meal.

Getting to the Right Dose

To arrive at the proper dose, the prescriber will start with a low dose and gradually increase it until positive effects are observed by you and the child's teachers or until developing side effects signal that a higher dose would be harmful. The starting dose for the short-acting stimu-

> **Can't we try Adderall with my daughter to find out for sure if she has ADHD?**
>
> When a child's problems elude diagnosis, it is tempting to use a "proven" treatment to come up with answers. As in all of medicine, though, a response or lack of response to a treatment cannot be relied on to diagnose ADHD. For instance, one-quarter of those with ADHD do not respond to stimulants, so not responding to a stimulant (what the doctor may describe as *treatment refractory*) does not necessarily mean the child does not have ADHD. And as above, some individuals without ADHD who are given stimulants will be able to concentrate better—but that does not mean they actually have ADHD.

lants (Ritalin and Dexedrine) is generally 2.5–5 mg per day and for extended-release stimulants 10–20 mg given in the morning and increased with the smallest increment every few days. If prominent wear-off is occurring at midday, most prescribers should suggest switching from an immediate-release to an extended-release stimulant. The wide array of literature on the stimulants also suggests that in some cases more medicine may be better than less medicine for controlling both the attentional and behavioral ramifications of ADHD.

Dosing and types of medication vary surprisingly within families. For example, Shelly is a 12-year-old girl with ADHD who is doing well on Vyvanse, receiving 30 mg in the morning. Her 8-year-old brother receives 36 mg of Concerta in the morning and sometimes a 5-mg dose of Ritalin in the late afternoon.

blood level: The amount or concentration of medication in the blood. Synonymous with serum or plasma concentration.

Side Effects

You can expect your child to experience some side effects while taking stimulants, but the most common ones often can be managed. Table 12 lists these side effects and what you can do about them. While your child is beginning a trial of stimulants, start a medication log, as described on

Table 12. Some Management Strategies for Common Stimulant-Related Side Effects

Side effect	Management
Loss of appetite (anorexia), weight loss	• Monitor weight closely; may see initial loss of appetite that improves with use (e.g., 4–6 months into treatment). • Give stimulant with meals. • Add calorie-enhanced snacks (e.g., instant breakfast, frozen yogurt). • Don't force meals.
Difficulty falling asleep (insomnia)	• Encourage good sleep hygiene (e.g., waking at same time daily, no caffeine, reducing activity prior to sleep). • Administer stimulants earlier in day. • Change to shorter-acting forms (e.g., Concerta to Metadate CD). • Discontinue afternoon or evening dosing. • Consider melatonin, low-dose clonidine or guanfacine, periactin, Remeron, or imipramine at bedtime.
Dizziness	• Hold next doses and talk to your child's practitioner. • Check blood pressure and heart rate. • Have your child drink more fluids; have snack midday. • Change to alternate/extended-release form (Adderall XR, Ritalin LA, Concerta, Vyvanse).
Rebound phenomena	• Change to extended-release or patch form. • Overlap stimulant dosing (usually by 30 minutes). • Add short-acting stimulant 30 minutes before rebound. • Consider additional treatment (low-dose clonidine/guanfacine or Strattera).

(cont.)

Table 12 (*cont.*)

Side effect	Management

Irritability, sadness, moodiness, agitation	• Evaluate when it occurs.
	  • Peak (may be too much medication)
	  • Wear-off (see "Rebound" above)
	• Reduce dose.
	• Change to another preparation.
	• Assess for another problem such as depression.
	• Consider adjunctive treatment (fish oil, antidepressants, lithium, anticonvulsants) for another problem.

Growth problems	• Monitor. • Compare with parental height history. • Attempt weekend and vacation holidays. • Refer to pediatrician. • Change to nonstimulant treatment (Strattera, nortriptyline, clonidine, guanfacine, Wellbutrin).
Heart symptoms: palpitations (heart pounding), dizziness, almost passing out, chest discomfort/pain	• Stop medication, notify practitioner immediately. • Consider referral to specialist (e.g., cardiology).

page 99, and record the details of the effects you observe. Don't forget to note when these problems are occurring. The timing of side effects can give your child's doctor important clues to what might be causing the effects and how the treatment should be altered.

➤ **Take-Home Point:** Side effects that occur 1–2 hours after taking the medication are likely related to the *peak effect* of the medication, whereas those that occur 6–12 hours after your child takes the medication may relate to *wear-off* from the stimulants (such as tiredness).

The most commonly reported short-term side effects of the stimulants are:

- Appetite suppression
- Sleep disturbances
- Headaches
- Stomachaches

Appetite Suppression

Parents naturally worry about this, particularly since there has been an ongoing debate over whether long-term stimulant use stunts growth in children. See page 221 for a discussion of this subject.

Sleep Disturbances

Sleep disturbances can be marked and may diminish the daytime effectiveness of these medications. If your child is having sleep problems on the stimulants, earlier timing of the stimulant, a reduced dose, or a change from a long- to a short-acting form may be necessary. On the other hand, if the child is responding quite well to the stimulant, the doctor may suggest adding a low dose of another medication—clonidine, Remeron, or imipramine—instead. Studies support the use of melatonin for sleep-related issues in children, and parents of children who take melatonin to help them sleep have reported no known drug interactions with the stimulants.

Irritability

Sadness or irritability as well as worsening of the ADHD during wear-off (called *rebound phenomena*) also appear, but less frequently. Irritability or sadness occurring 1–2 hours after dosing may indicate too much medication. Bill had a good response to Dexedrine tablets but had mood symptoms 1 hour after taking each dose. He did very well by simply switching to Adderall. Irritability 4–12 hours after dosing may signal withdrawal. Rebound phenomena can occur in some children between doses, creating uneven and often disturbing symptoms. The good news is that the advent of the extended-release stimulants has virtually elimi-

> **My daughter was diagnosed with ADHD 7 years ago, and she still needs medication. At first it was all pretty simple (if not easy); Concerta was pretty much the drug of choice. Now so many different new medicines are available—how do I know which one would be best for her?**
>
> What is similar and what is different among all the medications for ADHD on the market today may be confusing, especially if your child's doctor isn't scrupulously up to date. While Concerta, Metadate CD, Focalin XR, Ritalin LA, and Daytrana are all methylphenidate, Adderall XR, Vyvanse, and Dexedrine are amphetamines. Metadate CD and Ritalin LA work for about 8 hours, while Concerta, Daytrana, Vyvanse, and Adderall XR work for up to 12 hours (the effect from the Daytrana patch may last longer than 12 hours if it is left on for more than 9 hours). See Table 11 for comparisons among them all. Then, in consultation with your child's doctor, determine which advantages are most desirable for your child's academic/occupational/social needs and balance those benefits against any side effects experienced.

nated problems with wear-off or rebound. The overlapping of doses or a change to longer-acting preparations may help reduce both withdrawal symptoms and rebound phenomena. Treatment with 10 mg of Ritalin twice a day improved 14-year-old David's academic performance and behavior significantly, but his mother reported that David was isolating himself when he got home from school and acting "depressed and angry." David's afternoon problems went away when we changed him to Focalin XR. Another strategy could have been to add 2.5 mg or 5 mg of the Ritalin or Focalin when he got home from school to "smooth out" the wear-off from the Ritalin.

Other Side Effects

Although headaches and stomachaches are among the most commonly reported side effects, they occur less frequently than appetite suppression, sleep disturbances, and irritability. Less frequent side effects of the stimulants in children also include repeated movements (such as picking the nails or skin), dizziness, staring spells, and fatigue. Stimulant-associated hallucinations are extremely rare and often signal too high a dose or another underlying problem—stop the medication and notify your child's doctor immediately if this should occur.

Drug Interactions

For information on drug interactions with the stimulants, see Table 13. Although we don't advocate that adolescents use drugs of abuse when treated for their ADHD, results from controlled clinical trials are comforting in indicating a lack of severe drug reactions reported between stimulants and marijuana, alcohol, or other drugs of abuse.

When Disorders Overlap

Some concerns linger over whether the stimulants cause or worsen tic disorders (involuntary muscle spasms) and seizures. Since both of these problems coexist with ADHD in a substantial number of children, you would be wise to keep current with developments on these fronts. Many professionals now feel that stimulants merely bring out a vulnerability for underlying tics but don't often cause them outright. In part this theory is based on the excess overlap of tics and ADHD: half of children with tics or Tourette's disorder have ADHD, and 15% of children with

---

What's the best way to find out how the stimulants are working at school?

As described on pages 88–89, asking a favorite teacher or guidance counselor to give you weekly feedback about your child's behavior and attention will not only provide you with invaluable information but also engage the school system in your child's care. Although some practitioners find the use of teacher report forms that you can get from your practitioner's office or online (e.g., *schoolpsychiatry.org*) helpful in dissecting treatment effects, our group prefers frequent parent e-mail or voice contact with the school during the medication initiation phase to ask about ADHD symptoms and other behavioral issues the child may have and find out how the child is responding to treatment.

Table 13. Potential Drug Interactions of Stimulants with Commonly Used Drugs

Medication	Comments
Decongestants Pseudoephedrine, phenylephrine (Actifed, Sudafed)	Can increase both medications' effects; start with lower doses of decongestant.
Antihistamines (Benadryl, Dimetapp)	May diminish effectiveness of stimulants.
Strattera (atomoxetine)	No noted interaction.
Tricyclic antidepressants	May increase both medications' effects.
Anticonvulsants	May infrequently increase or decrease anticonvulsant level.
Prozac (fluoxetine) and related antidepressants; Wellbutrin (bupropion)	No noted interaction.
Antibiotics	No noted interaction.
Antipsychotics, anxiety-breaking agents	No noted interaction.

ADHD have tics unrelated to the stimulant treatment or the ADHD. A cautious approach for children with ADHD and tics would be to try non-stimulant treatments such as clonidine (Kapvay and others), guanfacine (Intuniv and others), tricyclic antidepressants, or atomoxetine (Strattera) first. Then, if nothing else works for the ADHD, stimulants can be used as long as the child is observed closely for worsening of the tics. If any worsening occurs, immediately take the child off the stimulant medication to see if the stimulants were a direct cause of the worsening. Our own clinical experience agrees with the longer-term studies that suggest some children with tics can still benefit from stimulants as long as they are monitored carefully.

You may read in the package insert that comes with the medication or on the Internet that stimulants should not be used if your child has a seizure disorder because the stimulant might increase the frequency of seizures. This issue is of utmost importance, since a number of children with seizures also have ADHD. However, scientific investigations of both absolute seizure rates and brain wave recordings (EEGs) in stimulant-treated children simply do not support this contention. You should also know that many pediatric neurologists use stimulants in children treated for their seizure disorders without reports of worsened seizures. Generally children should be treated for both disorders, which means prescribing stimulants for the ADHD and the appropriate anticonvulsant agents (such as Dilantin, Lamictal, Depakote, Tegretol, or others) for the seizures.

The Effects of Long-Term Stimulant Use

Questions about whether children taking stimulants over long periods suffer impairments in height and weight growth have been asked for the past three decades. Unfortunately, this subject is still shrouded in myth. While early and uncontrolled reports prematurely alarmed parents, the most recent information suggests that the vast majority of these children ultimately achieve normal height and weight as young adults. In other words, they may be slightly shorter as children but catch up as they mature.

> **Take-Home Point:** By nature of their ADHD, these children may mature and grow at a later stage (usually later adolescence) of their life.

Additionally, the most recent data derived from large multisite studies seem to indicate that stimulants may have a very subtle effect on both weight and height, lasting for only up to 2 years. Children tend not to gain weight over the first 6–9 months of treatment with the stimulants (and with Strattera, coincidentally). Over 2 years, data are indicating that children weigh about 3–5 pounds (1.4–2.3 kg) less and may be 0.1–0.5 inches shorter compared to the "normal growth chart" from the Centers for Disease Control and Prevention. Of significance, those children who are already short and thin demonstrate essentially no effect of treatment, whereas those who are the largest and heaviest display the most effect. It may be that extended-release methylphenidate preparations lead to less effect on growth than multiply dosed short-acting agents or amphetamine—this clearly requires further study. In clinical practice, we've had very good results from using stimulants in children with short stature who subsequently receive treatments such as growth hormone for their size—the stimulants do not appear to interact adversely with their growth.

There *is* a small group of children with ADHD who have a definitive reduction in weight and growth that is attributable to stimulants, but it occurs when the children stop eating, lose weight, and therefore simply don't grow. As a parent, you should keep tabs on your child's growth while she is taking any medication. If your child is taking stimulants,

---

My son says he hates to take his medicine, and he has several reasons for feeling this way: He doesn't want to think of himself as being "different," he doesn't like to swallow pills, and he hates having to go to the school nurse for his midday dose. How can I make this easier for him when I know (and he does too) how much better he does on the medication?

Virtually all kids will want to stop their medication for some reason. First, it's important to discuss the child's disorder with him and help him vent his frustration about what he is dealing with and about needing treatment. One point we make is that "normal" is a statistical concept—all children have some issue and are different in some manner.

In terms of midday dosing, forms of medication are available that should make your lives easier. Today there are osmotic-release capsules (in which water from the intestine slowly enters the capsule chamber, causing the medication to be "pushed" out a laser-drilled hole in the capsule) and beaded technologies (allowing you to sprinkle extended-release medication on food for kids who have problems taking medications—e.g., Adderall XR and Ritalin LA). There is also the methylphenidate patch (Daytrana), and there are long-acting suspensions and, finally, dissolving tablets that don't need to be swallowed. Ask your doctor and pharmacist about the availability of your child's medication in these alternative forms, some of which are also available as generics and may cost less in copays.

watch for a substantial decrease in appetite or a weight loss and take the following precautions:

1. Make sure your child's doctor does a before-treatment assessment and takes height and weight measurements two or three times a year. Your child's height and weight can be charted on growth charts that you can access online at the American Academy of Pediatrics website (*www.aap.org*) or purchase, or that may be available from your child's practitioner.

2. If a decrease in weight is noted during the early phase of treatment, caloric supplements or foods rich in calories (all of the food you don't dare eat!) may be helpful in counteracting the daytime appetite suppression. Data from studies with Adderall XR and Concerta indicate that it's common to see a transient effect on weight (i.e., no gain) over the first 6–9 months of treatment followed by resumption of normal weight gain.

3. If stimulant-induced delays or reduction in growth are noticed, talk to the doctor about drug holidays—weekends/holidays/vacation periods where children are taken off their stimulants. Studies have demonstrated that stimulant-related effects on growth may be lessened by these periods off the medication. However, the benefits of drug holidays need to be weighed against the sometimes negative effect of medication discontinuation (i.e., untreated ADHD).

4. If the height and weight growth problems are severe, they may require switching your child to an alternative treatment. We have found, for instance, that children often gain weight when placed on nortriptyline for their ADHD.

In the mid-2000s, you may have heard about reports of catastrophic problems such as stroke and sudden death in children and adults receiving the stimulants methylphenidate and amphetamine for ADHD. In fact, though, given the number of patients taking stimulants, the rate of stroke and cardiac issues is no higher in those taking stimulants than in those not taking them. Given that lack of association, and because children have a very low risk of heart problems, the FDA has required only that package inserts advise against stimulant use in children with existing heart disease and other known cardiovascular problems. (The risk of a problem in kids with structural cardiac issues who receive stimulants is probably similar to the elevated risk for a catastrophic event in a student athlete not receiving any medication.)

What emerged from the close examination of this issue was the importance of screening for cardiac defects that may predispose a child to a slightly higher risk of a catastrophic outcome if he uses a stimulant. Your child's doctor should ask you the questions put forth by the American Heart Association, including (1) whether your family has a history of sudden cardiac death prior to age 30; (2) whether your child has a history of structural cardiac defects; and (3) whether your child has ever complained of dizziness, chest pain, syncope (passing-out episodes), or palpitations that are not explained by something else that is going on. If you are aware of any of these problems, however, don't wait for your child's doctor to ask the questions; bring the problems to the doctor's attention. Also ask your doctor if you should consult a pediatric cardiology specialist. As part of the screening process, the American Heart Association and American Academy of Pediatrics consider it reasonable for a child's doctor to *consider* performing an electrocardiogram (ECG), *but not mandatory.*

Despite the stimulants' many years of use, we still have no systematically obtained information to disentangle the ways in which medication for ADHD prevents or causes impairment much later in life. The consensus in the field continues to be that assertive treatment of any disorder will result in lessening of the impairment caused by not treating the disorder over time. An example of this is a host of studies that demonstrated significant reductions in criminality, depression, anxiety, cigarette smoking, and substance abuse in youth with ADHD being treated with stimulants.

Take-Home Point: Of note, these studies also suggest that the protective effects occur only when the child continues to take the medication.

Strattera (Atomoxetine)

The first FDA-approved nonstimulant medication for ADHD, Strattera (atomoxetine) is approved for the treatment of ADHD in children, adolescents, and adults. Strattera has been studied extensively not only for use in ADHD itself but also for ADHD plus other psychiatric conditions. As of 2015, there are more than 30 controlled studies including children, adolescents, and adults demonstrating Strattera to be very useful in the treatment of ADHD by itself. Many studies of Strattera in specific groups of people with ADHD are under way.

Strattera is mechanistically similar to the older tricyclic antidepressants. It makes more norepinephrine (and dopamine) available for nerve-to-nerve communication. Unlike the stimulants, Strattera has no abuse potential and is not a scheduled medication. Your child's doctor can write prescriptions with renewals and can call this medication in to a local pharmacy for your child.

Strattera is among the first-line agents for ADHD. Studies also indicate that it is useful in children and teens who do not respond to stimulant medications and in those who are intolerant of their adverse effects. Strattera has been demonstrated to be helpful in all subtypes of ADHD.

One of the most intriguing applications of Strattera is for the child who has the common co-occurrence of anxiety, tics, or substance abuse with ADHD. Studies show that Strattera is helpful not only in treating the ADHD under these circumstances but also in improving the anxiety or tics. Strattera has also been useful in reducing the prominent oppositional symptoms often occurring in kids with ADHD. Since Strattera is free of abuse liability (and presumed diversion to other kids), it is an ideal candidate for adolescents who have a history of or are at risk of using substances of abuse. One study in recently abstinent adult alcoholics showed improvements in ADHD and reductions in heavy alcohol use in the group receiving atomoxetine. No serious side effects have arisen in conjunction with alcohol or marijuana.

Getting to the Right Dose

Strattera is readily absorbed in the gastrointestinal tract and peaks in the serum soon after administration. Dosing is typically from 40 to 80 mg per day in children. Don't be in a hurry to go to full dosing too rapidly—we have found that it may lead to sedation, which is not a problem when starting the medication slowly. In children and adolescents weighing less than 154 pounds (70 kg), Strattera should be started at a total daily dose of 0.5 mg per kg (around 25 mg at night) and increased after 2 weeks to 1.2 mg per kg per day (around 50–80 mg in the morning). In older adolescents or adults, it can be started at 40 mg at night and increased after 2 weeks to 80 mg and then ultimately to a maximum of 100 mg in those who have not had a maximal effect. Some children do better with twice-daily administration of Strattera (especially for after-school issues). No blood monitoring of Strattera levels or other blood tests are necessary.

Drug Interactions

Strattera is broken down (metabolized) in the liver (hepatic system), and there are some potential drug-to-drug interactions, so you should ask your child's doctor before starting other medications. Likewise, if your child is on Strattera, remind the doctor of the potential for a drug interaction.

Side Effects of Strattera

Strattera is generally well tolerated. Short-term side effects reported include:

- Excessive tiredness (especially when first started—it gets better)
- Insomnia
- Stomachaches
- Headaches
- Nausea
- Vomiting
- Weight loss/appetite suppression

There are other, infrequent side effects:

- Irritability or aggression (infrequent but not rare)
- Hepatitis (liver problems, rare)
- Suicidality (rare)

A black-box warning of potential suicidality exists on Strattera in children, although in our opinion the risk is very minimal, and Strattera remains a very safe, useful drug for the treatment of ADHD. No specific child appears more likely than others to develop any of the side effects noted here, but of course you should monitor your child for any of these problems and immediately contact your child's practitioner if any arise.

Other Nonstimulants

In general, the nonstimulants are somewhat less effective than the stimulants; however, they tend to cover ADHD throughout the day with minimal effects on appetite or sleep.

Antihypertensives/Alpha Agonists

There are two medications that were developed as antihypertensives in adults—and more recently reclassified as alpha agonists—based on their nerve cell effects on norepinephrine. These medications are clonidine (Catapres, Kapvay) and guanfacine (Intuniv, Tenex), and both are now FDA approved for ADHD. Both of these agents are available in generic shorter-acting versions as well as longer-acting branded versions. Clonidine is a relatively short-acting compound, lasting about 6 hours in children and often requiring two to four administrations daily to maintain clinical effectiveness. A longer-acting form (Kapvay) can be administered once or twice a day. The daily dose range of clonidine is from 0.05 mg to 0.4 mg.

Guanfacine is longer-acting than clonidine, with usual daily dose ranges from 0.5 mg to 3 mg. A once-daily preparation of guanfacine has been developed (Intuniv). Both agents improve attention and hyperactivity/impulsivity.

The alpha agonists have been used not only for the treatment of ADHD but for associated motor and vocal tics, aggression, and sleep disturbances, particularly in younger children. Sedation is the most commonly seen side effect with both clonidine and guanfacine, but it tends to improve with time and can be minimized by starting these medications at very low doses initially until the sedation improves. Other side effects include mood symptoms, slowing of the heart rate, dizziness, and, if stopped abruptly at relatively higher doses, a transient increase in your child's blood pressure.

More recently, clonidine (Kapvay) and guanfacine (Intuniv) have also been FDA approved *in combination* with stimulant medications for

ADHD. A number of combination studies using clonidine or guanfacine and stimulants (see the previous page) have been conducted in children with ADHD or ADHD plus tics. Interestingly, the combination of medications was more effective than either agent alone in improving ADHD as well as controlling ADHD plus tics. Side effects of the combination resemble those of the alpha agonists alone—sedation, slowed heart rate, and dizziness.

Useful Second-Line Nonstimulants

A number of the following medications are not FDA approved for ADHD but have been shown in research studies and in clinical practice to be useful second- or third-line agents. Bupropion (Wellbutrin, Zyban) is an adult antidepressant with indirect dopaminergic and noradrenergic effects. Bupropion has been shown to be effective for ADHD in children and adults. Less rigorous studies have shown it to be helpful for individuals with ADHD and depression as well as ADHD and less severe bipolar disorder. Given its use in reducing cigarette smoking and improving mood and the fact that it doesn't require monitoring or have significant side effects, bupropion is often used as an agent for complex cases of ADHD—for patients with substance abuse or a mood disorder. Treatment should be initiated at 75–100 mg and increased upward every week up to 300 mg in children and 450 mg (XL preparation) in older children or adults. The medication is generic and available in immediate-release, sustained-release (given twice daily), and once-a-day versions (XL). Side effects include activation, irritability, insomnia, and, rarely, seizures.

The tricyclic antidepressants—imipramine (Tofranil), desipramine (Norpramin), and nortriptyline (Pamelor, Aventyl)—block the reuptake of neurotransmitters, including norepinephrine. These medications are often considered third-line treatments and are effective in controlling behavior and attention impairments associated with ADHD. They are particularly useful in stimulant failures or when oppositionality, anxiety, or tics co-occur within ADHD. Dosing of the tricyclic antidepressants starts with 25 mg daily and is titrated upward slowly to a maximum of 50–200 mg a day, depending on the specific medication and the weight of the child. Unwanted side effects include sedation, weight gain, dry mouth, and constipation. As minor increases in heart rate and nondangerous slowing of electrical impulses through the heart can occur, your doctor may request an ECG for your child before starting the medication and 2–3 months into treatment (if you elect to continue the medication).

Provigil

Currently modafinil (Provigil, Sparlon), a wake-promoting agent that is FDA approved for narcolepsy, is not approved for ADHD, although it has been shown to be helpful for the treatment of all aspects of ADHD, mainly in children. Given that it works somewhat differently from stimulants and nonstimulants, it may be that it is particularly useful for certain attentional issues associated with ADHD, such as helping to stimulate motivation, that remain problematic with current treatment. One lesson learned during studies is that higher doses (higher than 200 or 300 mg per day) are typically necessary in children and adolescents. Routine side effects are similar to those of the stimulants, with reduced sleep and appetite, as well as headaches, the most commonly reported effect. Rarely, a serious skin rash (Stevens–Johnson syndrome) may occur, so be sure to report any rash to your child's practitioner.

13
The Antidepressants

The antidepressants are a wide, diverse group of medications so named because they are all used to treat adults with depression. In children, they also have different benefits: They have been shown scientifically to help children and adolescents with anxiety disorders, OCD, tic disorders, ADHD, and bedwetting (enuresis). Ironically, the effectiveness of certain antidepressants in children with depression is not as clear.

The main classes of antidepressants are the SSRIs; the atypical antidepressants such as Wellbutrin, Effexor, Remeron, and trazodone;

Why don't the antidepressants work as well for depression in children as they do for adults?

We are not at all sure why some antidepressants are not effective for depression in children and adolescents but seem to be effective in adults. Some notable observations suggest that in the studies testing these compounds most of the children in the trial noted relief of their depression including those receiving the inactive placebo. Because the response to placebo was so good, it was difficult to show a difference between the placebo (inactive medication) and the active medication. Some researchers have suggested that depression in youth may be very different at the neurotransmitter level from what is seen in adults. Since we think the medications work by altering neurotransmitter levels, this would help explain why some medicines work better in adults than in children.

the tricyclic antidepressants; and the MAOIs, which are rarely used in children. Effexor XR and Cymbalta are sometimes referred to as SNRIs because of their actions on both serotonin and norepinephrine. Table 14 lists these medications, and the text in this chapter describes each group separately.

The Selective Serotonin Reuptake Inhibitors

The SSRIs are the most commonly used antidepressants for children. They include:

- Prozac (fluoxetine)
- Paxil (paroxetine)
- Lexapro (escitalopram)
- Celexa (citalopram)
- Zoloft (sertraline)
- Luvox (fluvoxamine)

Many parents are hesitant to use these widely publicized medications, especially Prozac, because of claims that they cause violence or suicidal thoughts. In our clinic, we have used SSRIs in large numbers of children and found them highly effective with little incidence of violence or other serious behavioral problems. In extensive research they have also had an excellent track record.

As to suicidality, this controversy is related in part to black-box warnings on labels that approximately 4% of young people receiving SSRIs in multiple studies of depression have emergent suicidal thoughts, compared to 2% in those who received a placebo. There is more on this issue under "Side Effects," on page 236, but it is important to note that the worsening of depression after starting SSRIs is something you should watch for. Hal, now age 15, was 9 when treated with Prozac for OCD, at which time he developed depression about 2 weeks after starting the medication. Interestingly, the depression improved after stopping the Prozac. Yet 5 years later he did develop a depression off all medication. Prozac and Lexapro are FDA approved for the treatment of depression in adolescents, for instance.

Table 14. The Preparation and Strengths of the Antidepressants

Generic name	Brand name	Sizes and preparation
\multicolumn{3}{c}{Selective serotonin reuptake inhibitors}		
Fluoxetine	Prozac	10, 20, 40, 60 mg; capsules and tablets
		20 mg/1 tsp; suspension
Escitalopram	Lexapro	5, 10, 20 mg; tablets
		5 mg/1 tsp; suspension
Citalopram	Celexa	10, 20, 40 mg; tablets
		2 mg/cc; solution
Sertraline	Zoloft	50, 100 mg; tablets
		20 mg/cc; suspension
Fluvoxamine	Luvox	25, 50, 100 mg; tablets
Paroxetine	Paxil	10, 20, 30, 40 mg; tablets
		20 mg/1 tsp; suspension
\multicolumn{3}{c}{Tricyclic antidepressants}		
Desipramine	Norpramin Pertofrane	10, 25, 50, 75, 100, 150 mg; tablets
Nortriptyline	Pamelor	10, 25, 50 mg; capsules
	Aventyl	10 mg/1 tsp; oral suspension
Imipramine	Tofranil	10, 25, 50, 75, 100, 150 mg; tablets and capsules
Amitriptyline	Elavil	10, 25, 50, 75, 100, 150 mg; tablets
Protriptyline	Vivactil	5, 10 mg; tablets
Maprotiline	Ludiomil	25, 50, 75 mg; tablets
Clomipramine	Anafranil	25, 50, 100 mg; tablets

Note. 5 cc = 5 ml = 1 tsp.
*The monoamine oxidase inhibitors are not recommended for children or adolescents.

Medication		
Generic name	Brand name	Sizes and preparation
Atypical antidepressants		
Venlafaxine**	Effexor	25, 37.5, 50, 75 mg; tablets
		37.5, 75, 150 mg; extended-release tablets
Desvenlafaxine**	Pristiq	50, 100 mg tablets
Duloxetine**	Cymbalta	20, 30, 60 mg; capsules
Vortioxetine	Brintellix	5, 10, 15, 20 mg; tablets
Trazodone	Desyrel	50, 100, 150, 300 mg; tablets
Vilazodone	Viibryd	10, 20, 40 mg; tablets
Nefazodone	Serzone	50, 100, 150, 200, 250 mg; tablets
Bupropion	Wellbutrin	75, 100 mg; tablets
		100, 150, 200 mg; sustained-release (twice daily) tablets
		150, 300 mg; extended-release (once daily) tablets
Mirtazapine	Remeron	15, 30 mg; tablets
Doxepin	Sinequan	10, 25, 50, 75, 100, 150 mg; capsules
		10 mg/cc; solution
Monoamine oxidase inhibitors*		
Phenelzine	Nardil	15 mg; tablets
Tranylcypromine	Parnate	10 mg; tablets

**Also referred to as SNRIs.

Based on large, multiple-site studies of these agents in kids, the SSRIs are considered the first line of pharmacological treatment for depression, OCD, selective mutism (not speaking in certain settings), and certain other anxiety disorders. Because of their effects on the body, these medications have fewer sedative, cardiovascular (blood pressure and ECG changes), and weight-gain side effects than other antidepressants. Although similar in their effect of making more serotonin available in regions of the brain, the SSRIs vary from one another in their chemical structures, breakdown rates in the body, and side effects. Often, when one SSRI proves ineffective for a child, another may be very effective.

Dosage

The suggested daily doses of SSRIs for children have been similar to those for adults, but this is changing. A study that our group did with the makers of Prozac showed that 10 mg per day, versus the adult dose of 20 mg per day, was sufficient. For instance, children ages 6–12 who require Prozac for depression, anxiety, or OCD should have this medication started at no more than 10 mg daily and increased slowly as necessary. We have found that very low doses tend to be tolerated better and are sometimes remarkably effective—particularly for those who do not have the full-blown disorder. Given what we know from how the medications are broken down in children's blood, it seems prudent to start younger children on one-quarter to one-half the starting dose for an adult.

Prozac lasts a long time in the body, approximately 7–9 days, whereas most of the other SSRIs last about one-half to one day. That is why it takes 1 month to reach a consistent blood level of Prozac and up to 2 months after discontinuing Prozac for it to leave the blood entirely. For the same reason, the shorter-acting SSRIs are the better choice for children who have the potential to become agitated or to swing toward mania because of the antidepressant effects. Children who are more likely to switch from depression to bipolar disorder include those with a family member with bipolar disorder, those with sudden onset of their depression, those with psychosis (hallucinations), and those who are already agitated. Should the medication need to be stopped, the shorter-acting medications will leave the bloodstream quickly and thus cut off any disabling effect. Be careful, though; some of the short-acting ones can have some nondangerous but quirky side effects if stopped suddenly (paroxetine for one).

The dosage range depends on which medication is prescribed for your child. In general, though, doses of the SSRIs are lower for depression and anxiety and relatively higher for OCD. We've found that the solutions or suspensions of the antidepressants can be invaluable for starting the medication, as you can give very low doses initially quite easily and increase in very low increments without breaking tablets or capsules. For instance, we successfully treated 5-year-old Ethan for severe moodiness that did not respond to environmental and parent involvement with 2 mg of liquid Prozac (that's right, one-tenth of an adult dose!). Younger children (under 12 years) should be started at relatively lower doses of these medications than adolescents. For example, before puberty children should be started at 5 mg of Prozac or Luvox; in contrast, adolescents can start at 10 mg per day, like adults. Although more or less equally effective, Zoloft and Luvox require higher dosing than Lexapro, Celexa, and Prozac because the former two are less potent (see page 232). Here are some guidelines:

- Prozac is typically dosed from 5 to 40 mg daily and is available in both capsule form (10 and 20 mg) and a liquid preparation (20 mg per 5 cc, which is equivalent to 1 teaspoon).
- Lexapro is generally dosed from 2.5 to 20 mg and comes in 10 mg tablets that can be broken.
- Celexa is dosed generally from 5 to 40 mg daily and is available in 10, 20, and 40 mg tablets and 10 mg per 5 cc suspension.
- The range of Zoloft dosing is from 50 to 200 mg daily. Zoloft comes in 50 mg and 100 mg tablets, which are scored and easily broken in half, and 20 mg per cc suspension.
- Luvox is dosed from 50 to 300 mg daily and also is available in scored 50 mg and 100 mg tablets.

All of the SSRIs can be given once daily, although parents sometimes note that their children respond better and tolerate the medications more fully when the shorter-acting compounds Zoloft and Luvox are prescribed in split doses twice a day. The SSRIs are generally administered in the morning, with the exception of Luvox, which may cause sedation and, if so, is better tolerated when given at night. Luvox is an excellent choice for depressed, obsessive, or anxious children who have marked sleep problems and can benefit from the sedative properties of the drug, usually noted 1–8 hours after administration.

Side Effects

The most common side effects of these medications include:

- Agitation
- Stomachaches and diarrhea (gastrointestinal symptoms)
- Irritability
- Activation
- Headaches
- Sleep disorders

In one study we did, we reported that emotional and behavioral side effects such as panic symptoms or activation emerged in 20% of kids taking the SSRIs. On average, these side effects were relatively minor, started 3 months into treatment, and typically abated with discontinuation of the SSRI. We also found that almost half of those kids who had a reaction to one SSRI (e.g., Prozac) had another reaction to a different SSRI (e.g., Zoloft).

Kids on more than 40 mg of Celexa (citalopram) should be checked to ensure they do not have electrical changes in their ECG showing something called prolonged QTc. The QTc is a combination of waveforms on the ECG that shows the heart's electrical system is "resetting" properly.

Since October 2004 the black-box warning mentioned above has called attention to the increased suicidality (suicidal thoughts and behavior) in children and adolescents taking SSRIs for depression. Although the risk is small, and no actual suicides occurred in the tests that resulted in the warning, parents and doctors must take this risk into account and weigh it against the potential benefits to the depressed child or teen. *Of interest, recent data suggest that the reduction in use of SSRIs because of the black box has resulted in an increase in the overall suicide rate in teenagers, clearly pointing out the risk–benefit ratio of this class of medications for a serious condition, namely depression.* The association is less clear, but note that kids receiving these medications for OCD, anxiety, and other reasons appear also to be at risk for these behavioral side effects. Talk to your child's doctor to make sure you understand the signs of suicidal behavior to watch for. Also, don't take your child off an antidepressant abruptly or without consulting the doctor.

↳ Take-Home Point: The risk of increased suicidal thoughts from SSRIs must be weighed carefully against the risks of suicidality from untreated depression.

Some SSRIs alter the liver's ability to break down other medications, so *be sure to ask your child's doctor about the safety of taking any other medications, including over-the-counter preparations.* For example, Prozac is well known to increase blood levels of other medications, such as tricyclic antidepressants and some medications used to control seizures. The FDA also cautions against the use of common antihistamines such as Tavist and certain antibiotics (like erythromycin) with some of these medications because of a theoretical drug interaction. To date, for children with seasonal allergies (hay fever), Claritin, Allegra, or Zyrtec appears to have the least such interaction.

With the exception of checking an ECG if your child is receiving more than 40 mg of citalopram, your child does not need to have cardiac monitoring or blood tests before or during treatment with the SSRIs. The drugs are largely free from cardiovascular side effects, and blood levels of these medicines, vital signs, or routine blood monitoring are not used in clinical practice.

Other Antidepressants

Several other antidepressants effective in adults are used frequently in children and adolescents. These medications are atypical in that their chemical structures and mechanism of action are different from the other antidepressants.

Wellbutrin (SR, XL) (Bupropion)

Wellbutrin (bupropion) is a unique antidepressant. The Wellbutrin molecule looks similar to the stimulant preparation amphetamine, and the compound also resembles it in its effect on dopamine neurotransmission in the brain. This drug is helpful for ADHD and depression and is particularly useful in depressed children who have bad mood swings or in those in whom there are concerns about mania or behavioral activation with a medication. Bupropion may also be very helpful for ADHD or mood problems in adolescents with substance use problems. This medicine is also FDA approved to help with smoking cessation in adults (called Zyban).

Wellbutrin works rapidly, peaking in the blood after 2 hours and lasting 8–14 hours. The usual dose range in children is from 37.5 to 300 mg per day in two or three divided doses. The sustained-release preparation (100, 150, and 200 mg) can be given once or twice daily. A new extended-release form (150 mg and 300 mg) can be given once in the morning and is preferred and available as a generic, and therefore typically used by practitioners.

Bupropion is relatively free of drug interactions with prescribed or over-the-counter medications. Bupropion is commonly used with a stimulant, for example. The major side effects in children include irritability, decreased appetite, insomnia, and worsening of tics. Irritability is often a flag that the dose needs to be reduced. Short-acting Wellbutrin also has a somewhat higher rate of drug-induced seizures (4 in 1,000 individuals) relative to other antidepressants, particularly in higher doses or in patients with untreated preexisting seizures or with bingeing and purging problems (bulimia). No ECG or laboratory monitoring is necessary during Wellbutrin therapy.

Effexor XR (Venlafaxine)

Effexor (venlafaxine) is similar to the SSRIs in that it enhances serotonin in certain areas of the brain by blocking its reuptake, but it also possesses some *noradrenergic* properties. It is thus known as an SNRI (*serotonin–norepinephrine reuptake inhibitor*). While clinical use suggests that Effexor, like Paxil, is helpful for depression in kids, it has not been systematically shown in clinical trials

> **noradrenergic:** Pertaining to the adrenergic nerves. Noradrenaline (synonymous with *norepinephrine*) is involved in many of the body's "automatic" activities, such as heart rate control, as well as being involved in anxiety, mood, and inhibition control.

to beat placebos. Moreover, more infrequent cases of fleeting suicidality were seen in the Effexor group compared to placebos. Therefore, as with any medication, careful observation of your child for side effects while initiating and during the earlier phases of treatment is paramount.

An isomeric (chemical) form of Effexor, called Pristiq, produced in 50- and 100-mg tablets, is now available. To date, however, it remains unstudied in children.

Effexor is dosed from 12.5 mg up to a total of 225 mg daily in twice-a-day split dosing. An extended-release (XR) tablet is available and preferred, allowing once-a-day dosing. The medication's potential side effects are nausea during the initial stages of treatment, agitation, stomachaches, headaches, and, at higher doses, blood pressure elevation. No specific blood monitoring is required, but you should discuss the potential drug interactions with the doctor before your child starts on this drug.

> **split dose:** A dose meant for a single administration that is divided up for a two- or three-times-a-day regimen. Synonymous with *divided dose*.

Desyrel (Trazodone)

Trazodone is a relatively short-acting compound lasting about 12 hours. In children and adolescents, trazodone is dosed from 25 to 200 mg and is generally given at night. Because of the sedative properties of trazodone, it has been used very successfully as a sleep agent at doses of 25–50 mg nightly. Common side effects of these medications include sedation, agitation, dry mouth, constipation, and confusion at higher doses. In males, trazodone has been relegated to a second- or third-line drug of choice because it has been reported infrequently to cause the potentially serious difficulty of painful, sustained erections (priapism). No ECG or blood monitoring is necessary with trazodone.

Remeron (Mirtazapine)

Remeron is a unique antidepressant with serotonergic activity, used for depression in adults. Because of its sleep-promoting effects, Remeron is commonly prescribed for youth with depression and/or difficulty going to sleep (see page 197). The dosage is generally 7.5–15 mg nightly. Side effects include excess sedation, heaviness, and upset stomach.

Cymbalta (Duloxetine)

Cymbalta (also an SNRI) shares similarities with venlafaxine (Effexor) in that it has both serotonergic and noradrenergic reuptake blockade effects. In studies in adults (there are no child depression studies to report on at this time), it is well tolerated and a very efficacious antidepressant. Cymbalta has recently been approved by the FDA for generalized anxiety in children and has been increasingly used in the treatment of children with anxiety disorders and depression. It also appears to be helpful for chronic pain situations. Watch the Internet and sources of reliable science reports for continued updates on its use in kids.

New and Untested in Children

A number of very new antidepressants are now available for adults but remain virtually untested in children for both effectiveness and safety. These include Viibryd (vilazodone), which has similarities to trazodone and Serzone, and Brintellix (vortioxetine), which affects serotonin and has some similarities to venlafaxine.

The Tricyclic Antidepressants

The tricyclic antidepressants include:

- Amitriptyline (Elavil)
- Imipramine (Tofranil)
- Desipramine (Norpramin)
- Nortriptyline (Pamelor)
- Doxepin
- Clomipramine (Anafranil)
- Protriptyline (Vivactil)

These medications are used primarily for ADHD and tic disorders and less frequently for anxiety and depression. They all act on children (and adults) in similar ways. Called *tricyclics* because of their chemical structure (three rings), they appear to work by making more of the neurotransmitters available for nerve-to-nerve communication. Different antidepressants also have different side-effect profiles. Desipramine, for instance, because it causes less blockade of a body and brain chemical called *histamine* (as in "antihistamine"), causes less sedation and dry mouth in children than other medicines in this class, such as imipramine.

Dosage

To start, the doctor will probably prescribe a 10-mg or 25-mg dose, often at night, and increase it slowly every 4–5 days by 10–25 mg. Current practice, which varies from doctor to doctor, suggests that when an effective dose is reached, blood levels and an ECG should be obtained. Typical dose ranges for the tricyclic antidepressants are from 25 to 150 mg daily.

Side Effects

The tricyclic antidepressants are one option for children who suffer from insomnia or tics when their ADHD is treated with stimulants—11-year-old Gail found 25 mg of nortriptyline twice a day very effective in controlling her ADHD and allowing her to sleep better than she did on Metadate CD or Dexedrine—but these drugs also have side effects of their own. Common short-term adverse effects of the tricyclic antidepressants include dry mouth, constipation, sedation, headaches, vivid dreams, stomachaches, rash, and blurred vision. Gail reported dry mouth and occasional nightmares. Since the tricyclic antidepressants reduce the production of saliva and lead to a dry mouth, they may also promote tooth decay.

There are lingering concerns about cardiac risks associated with tricyclic antidepressants in children. The issue arose following several case reports of sudden death in children who were being treated with desipramine almost 20 years ago. One evaluation of this issue concluded that children who are taking desipramine may have a slightly increased risk of sudden death, but not much higher than that of children who are not taking medication. Parents should know, however, that the data evaluated were imprecise, and the reports were plagued by uncertainty. The sad fact is that a number of unfortunate children die each year for unclear reasons, probably underlying congenital cardiac problems,

> **What can I do for the dry mouth that bothers my daughter so much?**
>
> I suggest keeping a water bottle by your child's bed and allowing her to take sips of water throughout the day. Encourage your children to avoid candy with sugar, since it will increase the potential for cavities. Other treatments include over-the-counter agents for dry mouth such as Biotene.

and the link suggested in these cases may simply have been a coincidence resulting from the fact that at that time many children were being treated with desipramine. This is not to say the tricyclic antidepressants have no effect on the heart. In fact, minor effects on the ECG are seen often, most commonly a speeding up of the heart (*tachycardia*) and slowing of the electrical impulses through the heart (*conduction delays*). Although this varies from practice to practice, many doctors have an ECG completed prior to starting a tricyclic antidepressant and order follow-up ECGs occasionally throughout treatment. If your child has a preexisting cardiac problem outside of a common heart murmur, you may want to ask your pediatrician about a consultation with a pediatric cardiologist before initiating treatment with a tricyclic antidepressant. Far and away the greatest risk brought by tricyclic antidepressants is overdose. Because of the lethality of tricyclic antidepressant overdose, you must carefully store the medication so it is inaccessible to all the children in your family.

Take-Home Point: The tricyclics are useful for some children, but the danger of overdose makes safe storage of the medications paramount.

More novel treatments that use older medications for children include lamotrigine (Lamictal) and ketamine. Lamictal, discussed in the section on mood disorders, is an antiseizure medication that has FDA approval for the treatment of depression in adults with bipolar disorder. It has also been useful in a number of children with depression alone. Because of a real risk for severe rash, the medication must be started slowly (e.g., 12.5 to 25 mg initially, increased no faster than 25 mg per day) and the dosing schedule must be adhered to strictly. Effective dosing is typically 100–200 mg per day. Ketamine has been purported in largely less rigorous trials to be useful for severe depression. Its reported benefits are that at very low doses, inhaled or given intravenously, it improves depressive symptoms very quickly (within days) and is safe from abuse and its "psychogenic" effects and can help reset a severe depression. More studies are necessary before recommendations can be made.

14
The Mood Stabilizers

The name of this class of medications describes what these drugs do: control the volatile emotional and behavioral swings that plague those with mood or severely disruptive and/or aggressive disorders. It is not surprising, then, that this group of drugs is still a common choice for children with bipolar disorder, or manic–depression, and that these medications also are used often in children who suffer from significant mood swings, overactivity, severe reactivity, and aggressiveness. Interestingly, however, there is a dearth of controlled data showing them to be truly effective for unstable mood and/or severe aggressiveness in children and adolescents. In contrast, multiple controlled trials now support the effectiveness of the second-generation (atypical) antipsychotics in adolescents with bipolar disorder or irritability/aggression as part of other disorders (such as ASD). A number of atypical antipsychotics have also received FDA approval for bipolar disorder in teens. See Chapter 17 for more on the antipsychotics.

The most common of the mood stabilizers is lithium, followed by various anticonvulsants (see Table 15).

Lithium Carbonate

Lithium carbonate (Cibalith, Eskalith, Lithobid, Lithonate, Lithotabs) is one of the mainstays of treatment for juvenile bipolar disorders and for those with aggression and agitation as part of other disorders. Lithium is a salt, and it bears chemical similarities to sodium, potassium, cal-

Table 15. The Preparation and Strengths of the Mood Stabilizers Most Commonly Used in Children and Adolescents

Medication		
Generic name	Brand name	Sizes and preparation
Lithium salts	Lithobid, Lithonate, Lithotabs, Eskalith, Cibalith	150, 300, 450 mg; tablets 8 mEq/1 tsp; suspension (= 300-mg tablet)
Carbamazepine	Tegretol, Carbachol, Equetrol	100, 200, 400 mg; tablets 100 mg chewable tablets 100 mg/1 tsp; suspension
Lamotrigine	Lamictal	25, 100, 150, 200 mg; tablets 100 mg/1 tsp; suspension
Oxcarbazepine	Trileptal	150, 300, 600 mg; tablets
Valproic acid	Valproate, Depakote, Depakote ER, Depakene sprinkles	125, 250, 500 mg; tablets and capsules 250 mg/1 tsp; suspension
Gabapentin	Neurontin	100, 300, 400 mg; capsules 400, 600, 800 mg; tablets
Topiramate	Topamax	25, 100, 200 mg; tablets

Note. 5 cc = 5 ml = 1 tsp.

cium, and magnesium, which occur naturally in the human body. In fact, before its toxicity at high doses became apparent, lithium was used as a salt replacement for adults with high blood pressure. (Imagine the mellowing after-dinner effects on adults who salted their steak with lithium!) Although we don't know exactly how lithium works (as is the case with most psychotropic agents), it appears to operate at a cellular level, altering hormones and neurons.

In children and adolescents, lithium lasts about 18 hours in the bloodstream. Unlike the majority of psychotropic agents, lithium is broken down (metabolized) and cleared (excreted) exclusively in the kidneys. Children and adults break the drug down in a similar fashion, though children's excretion of lithium is faster and more efficient.

Dosage

It's important to monitor the amount of lithium in the child's blood to help in dosing for effectiveness and to avoid side effects and even toxicity. As with other medications, your child will have to be on the same daily dose for 5–7 days before reaching a "steady-state level" that will give an accurate reading of how much lithium is in the bloodstream. Samples for blood lithium determination should be drawn from the child approximately 12 hours after the last dose of lithium. Generally, lithium levels are drawn in the morning, with no lithium given to the child until after the sample is taken. If lithium is administered directly before a blood sample, the blood reading can be reported as falsely high. Usually your child's blood will be drawn from a vein (venipuncture), but for children in whom this method is a problem, some medical facilities offer finger stick measurements and saliva lithium levels.

The usual lithium starting dose ranges from 150 to 300 mg in twice-a-day dosing. In some children, lower doses are sufficient to control mood and behavior, but some children may require more than 1,800 mg per day (up to six tablets) for adequate control of their mood. There is no firm agreed-on therapeutic blood lithium level in pediatric psychiatry. Suggested guidelines include levels of 0.6–1.5 milliequivalents per liter (mEq/L) for children with marked current problems and levels of 0.4–0.8 mEq/L for maintenance or prophylactic (protective) therapy. *Nevertheless, as with any other intervention, the lowest effective dose and/or serum level should be used.* For example, we've treated a 14-year-old girl with bipolar disorder who did well on 150 mg twice daily with a blood level of only 0.4 mEq/L. Slow- or controlled-release lithium preparations are available (Lithobid, Lithotabs).

> The lowest effective dose of lithium and any other medication should always be used.

Side Effects

Lithium has a number of important side effects. The more common short-term side effects include:

- Gastrointestinal symptoms such as nausea, vomiting, and upset stomach
- Central nervous symptoms such as tremor, sleepiness, and, rarely, memory impairment
- Kidney symptoms, including increased urination (polyuria), leading to increased drinking of fluids (polydipsia)

An important point is that lithium essentially "tricks" the kidneys and produces a mild state of dehydration, which is why you will see your child drinking water so frequently. You should allow your child unlimited fluid and make arrangements for the school to do the same. To reduce the risk for weight gain and dental issues, we recommend that water be made available at will regularly to your child. Lithium can accumulate quickly in your child's blood, sometimes to a toxic level, during dehydration states. Toxic levels of lithium can damage the kidneys. Problems with walking or talking, tiredness, and seeing "weird colors" (especially around lights) are all signs of toxicity. *If your child is vomiting, has sustained diarrhea, or is not taking in a reasonable amount of fluid, contact the child's doctor.* In our practice, we often ask parents to reduce the dose of lithium by half or not give the lithium until the child is feeling better and taking in fluids appropriately. Be particularly mindful of your child's hydration state in warm climates and during strenuous exercise.

Take-Home Point: Parents need to guard against dehydration in children taking lithium.

Long-term use of lithium may alter your child's metabolism, causing substantial weight gain. Watch your child's diet and encourage exercise to control the weight gain. Other long-term side effects are decreased thyroid effectiveness, leading to hypothyroidism (low thyroid), and possible kidney damage. Information collected over the last 15 years, however, suggests that maintenance lithium therapy does not lead to serious kidney problems, at least in adults. Children should be checked by blood test to see how their thyroid and kidneys are working before lithium treatment is started, and these tests should be repeated approximately every 6 months while the child is on lithium.

Particular caution should be exercised if your child suffers from

> **How can we be sure our daughter gets the medication she needs when she keeps hiding the tablet in her cheek?**
>
> This is, unfortunately, a common ploy of children who, for whatever reason, do not want to take their medication. First, try to understand what in particular is keeping your child from taking the medication. Often it is an issue involving side effects, or it may be the taste or texture of the medication. For these children—and for those who have difficulty swallowing capsules or tablets—medications are available in liquid form (often referred to as a "suspension") or as dissolving tablets, patches, and beads or sprinkles (small beads that can be mixed in with food). For example, lithium is available in a liquid form, lithium citrate. The liquid dose is roughly 1 teaspoon (5 cc), which is equivalent to the typical 300-mg tablet. There are also newer types of tablets, such as Risperdal Consta and Saphris, that dissolve in your child's mouth and are helpful for kids who have problems swallowing tablets or those who hide or "cheek" their medications.

serious neurological, kidney, or heart disease. In addition, you should contact your child's practitioner if your child requires repeated nonsteroidal anti-inflammatory agents such as ibuprofen (Advil, Motrin). Also, be sure to mention to any practitioner who may be starting your child on another medication that the child is on lithium, since there are a number of potential drug interactions. Often a repeat lithium level will be done if another medication with a potential drug interaction leading to increased blood lithium levels is added.

Tegretol/Carbachol

The anticonvulsants, also the treatment of choice for organic disorders such as seizures, temporal lobe epilepsy, and brain injury, work as mood stabilizers by reducing abnormal firing of nerve impulses in the limbic regions (the emotional center) of the brain. The anticonvulsant medication Tegretol (carbamazepine) has been used to treat certain types of seizures in children for over 25 years and is often used in place of lithium or as a second-line drug of choice for mood instability and aggressiveness.

Dosage

Tegretol is usually given in twice-a-day dosing and stays in the blood for about 16 hours. To reduce stomach irritation, it is commonly given with meals. The typical starting dose is 100 mg (in chewable form) to 200 mg daily up to a typical dose of 400–800 mg per day, depending on the amount in the blood and its effectiveness. The amount in the blood usually necessary to produce favorable effects without causing an excess of side effects is 4–12 mEq/L. Unfortunately, many children require higher doses and blood levels on the high side to maintain stability of their mood. Since the amount of medicine your child takes and the amount that is actually in the blood varies among individuals, close blood level monitoring is necessary. Tegretol is broken down extensively by the liver, and the amount in the blood may be either increased or decreased by other medications. Because of these complications and some potentially serious side effects, your child's blood should be monitored before starting on Tegretol, generally after 6 weeks, and then at least twice a year, for liver and blood counts as well as to check Tegretol levels.

Side Effects

The side effects that Tegretol may cause are unfortunately fairly broad in scope. The most common short-term side effects include:

- Drowsiness
- Nausea
- Vomiting
- Dizziness
- Blurred or double vision, particularly at higher doses and blood levels

In addition, Tegretol may reduce the number of white blood cells and therefore your child's ability to fight infection. A simple blood test to determine the white blood cell count is advised any time your child develops a serious sore throat or other infection. Reactions such as liver toxicity and skin disorders, including a serious rash involving the skin, inside of the mouth, and the palms of the hands (Stevens–Johnson syndrome), have been reported but appear to be rare.

Lamictal

Lamictal is another mood stabilizer, also used for complex partial seizures, that has been FDA approved for the treatment of depression in bipolar disorder in adults. Lamictal is also used frequently to treat depression in youth with bipolar disorder because it does not activate mania. Increasingly, it is being prescribed as a single medication for depression in kids as well as often added to other medications for bipolar disorder, such as an antipsychotic like Abilify (see Chapter 17). Like Depakote and Tegretol, Lamictal has a number of drug interactions, so your child's blood levels of certain other medications that may be affected should be monitored.

Dosage

In adults, typical dosing of Lamictal is 150–250 mg twice daily. Dosing for childhood mood instability has not been established, although we typically use between 100 and 300 mg daily. *Adherence to the dosing requested by your child's treater is very important.* The dose of Lamictal should be increased very slowly in weekly increments by no more than 25 mg. Many practitioners start the medication at 12.5 mg and increase it in 12.5-mg increments rather than 25-mg increments. Unfortunately, if your child misses multiple doses (e.g., more than 3 days), call your doctor—you may need to restart it at the lowest dose.

Diana is a 14-year-old girl with bipolar disorder. She noted feeling depressed but did not manifest mania on 1 mg of Risperdal twice daily with 1,000 mg of Depakote ER every morning. An increase in both the Risperdal and Depakote was not helpful. Lamictal was started at 25 mg and increased to 100 mg over 4 weeks. She noted a dramatic improvement in the depression as well as reduced overall irritability. Over time, her Depakote was discontinued, and she remained well controlled on Risperdal and Lamictal.

> **Take-Home Point:** Lamictal can be an effective additional or single medication for treating the depression of bipolar disorder in children without activating mania. Lamictal needs to be dosed upward slowly to avoid a serious rash.

Side Effects

The dose of Lamictal must be increased slowly to avoid the risk of a skin rash, which is one of the major side effects. The rash associated with Lamictal can be of two major types: (1) a more minor rash, typically on the trunk of the child, that occurs in up to 1 out of 10 children, and (2) a very serious rash, necessitating emergency care, that affects areas of the body including the mouth, hands, and feet, with blisters and loss of skin. It is important to give Lamictal on a regular basis and not to miss doses. Missing doses and/or "restarting" Lamictal seems to increase the likelihood of a rash. Blurred and double vision, tiredness, and dizziness are other major side effects.

Valproic Acid

Valproic acid (brand names Valproate, Depakene, and, most common, Depakote), an anticonvulsant-class agent (treats seizures), is FDA approved for the treatment of bipolar disorder in adults but is also, although less commonly, used to treat bipolar disorders in children and adolescents. Depakote is broken down by the liver and lasts 8–16 hours in the blood. A typical blood level is between 50 and 100 mEq/L, although some doctors will push blood levels to 130 mEq/L for children who have seizures that don't respond readily to treatment, severe mood instability, or behavioral outbursts. Children are generally started on 125–250 mg daily, and from there the dose is increased as necessary to achieve a therapeutic blood level. Another form of valproic acid, Depakote ER, can be given once or twice a day in children and, like Depakote, is helpful for bipolar disorder. Since Depakote ER is slightly less potent, it needs to be prescribed in higher amounts than Depakote.

Dosage

The ultimate dosage will vary greatly from child to child, depending on how each one breaks down the medication. Complicating the dosing further, Depakote will actually increase its *own* breakdown. Therefore, to arrive at a safe but effective blood level of the drug, many doctors request frequent blood levels during the initial phases of treatment. Your child will definitely need to have a blood test to determine blood counts and liver function before treatment begins and approximately every 6 months during treatment with the drug. Some children may require more than 1,500–2,000 mg a day to sustain a reasonably effective level of Depakote.

Side Effects

Common short-term side effects include sedation, nausea, dizziness, loss of appetite, and weight gain. Rarely, Depakote may cause a reduction in the blood count or may cause a mild and generally nondangerous inflammation of the liver (hepatitis), which is often picked up only on routine blood studies and resolves spontaneously. The risk of serious liver problems appears to be increased when Depakote is used with other antiseizure medications, particularly in children under age 10. Depakote may also rarely cause a painful swelling of the pancreas, and some practitioners will ask about symptoms (e.g., pain, fullness) and/or request blood tests to monitor the pancreas.

Valproic acid has been reported to be associated with polycystic ovary syndrome, a condition characterized by painful ovarian cysts, increased testosterone, and obesity. In fact, many doctors avoid its use in adolescent girls. Another look at the data complicates the issue in that being obese and having bipolar disorder are the biggest risk factors for this uncommon condition and that other medications share a similar risk for causing obesity—and possible polycystic ovaries. Excessive weight gain, growth of hair, abdominal pain, and/or irregular periods should signal you to contact your child's doctor. Another concern is the use of this medication in pregnant women; there is growing evidence of potential cognitive delays or problems in the unborn baby. Hence, some practitioners require adolescent or adult women using these medications to use two birth control methods; some have stopped prescribing them in women with childbearing potential.

Other Anticonvulsants Used for Mood Stabilization: Trileptal, Topamax, Neurontin, Gabitril

A newer generation of anticonvulsant medications that are also mood-stabilizing medications has been used in children and adolescents with aggression, agitation, self-injurious behavior, and, most commonly, severe moodiness and bipolar disorder. While these medications are currently undergoing testing for their efficacy and tolerability in juvenile bipolar disorder, controlled data derived from studies of adults and smaller open studies in kids indicate that Trileptal (oxcarbazepine), Topamax (topiramate), and Neurontin (gabapentin) may be useful agents to add to the arsenal of medications used for kids. While we use these in clinical practice, it is important to note that none of these medications has been demonstrated effective in treating bipolar disorder in kids in research studies or has FDA approval for this use.

Trileptal is a sibling medication of Tegretol (carbamazepine) that has been somewhat helpful for the management of less severe aggression and manic symptoms of bipolar disorder, although one study did not show it to be better than placebo. Trileptal is dosed starting with 150–300 mg daily and increased in twice-a-day dosing to a typical dose of 1,200 mg per day in a younger child and up to a maximum of 2,400 mg per day in an adolescent. As with other anticonvulsants, it may take from 4 to 6 weeks to see the full therapeutic benefit of Trileptal unfold.

Trileptal has few drug interactions. Side effects most commonly include nausea, dizziness, and tiredness. Your child should have her blood checked for sodium level, as this medication rarely can cause a reduced blood sodium level (hyponatremia).

Topamax (topiramate) is another anticonvulsant that has been predominately used for stabilization of weight in children who have drug-induced weight gain with the medications for bipolar disorder. Often Topamax is added to an antipsychotic or anticonvulsant regimen with good effects at doses of 25–100 mg twice daily to keep weight off, as well as assist youth who have gained massive amounts of weight due to their medications. We have seen some children shed significant weight when treated with Topamax in addition to their other medications. Moreover, some data in adults suggest that Topamax is a viable treatment for bulimia. It has also been used for the treatment of addictive behaviors in adolescents (see Chapter 11).

Side effects of Topamax include dulling of thinking processes at relatively higher doses (more than 100 mg per day) that can limit its use. Rarely Topamax can cause children to overheat—in part related to the lack of sweating. Parents should observe children on this medication during strenuous activities in the heat to ensure that they are adequately hydrated and do not appear overheated. Other side effects are more of a nuisance in nature and include sedation and dizziness. A blood test for your child's acid-base status should be completed infrequently.

Little is known about use of the seizure-treating medication Keppra for behavioral disturbances; however, Neurontin used to be touted as an agent that is helpful for bipolar disorder but without substantial side effects. Unfortunately, no clinical trials have been completed in children, and numerous controlled trials in adults have failed to demonstrate efficacy compared to placebo for bipolar disorder. Despite these negative findings, largely because of its very benign side-effect profile, clinicians continue to use Neurontin in less severe cases of bipolar disorder or more mild moodiness. Like lithium, Neurontin is broken down by the kidneys, so there is relatively little chance of drug interactions with the bulk of medications, which are metabolized by the liver. It appears to be extremely well tolerated and does not require intensive blood monitoring. Dosing of Neurontin usually starts at 300 mg twice daily up to 600–900 mg twice daily, with dizziness and sedation the most common side effects.

Also relatively new on the anticonvulsant scene and just being tried in children with bipolar disorder or marked moodiness is Gabitril. Like Topamax, it is FDA approved for adolescents for seizures but is being used in children as well. The maximum recommended daily dose of Gabitril is 32 mg. Since dosing information is based on adolescents with seizures, dosing of these medications should start low and be increased slowly until a positive effect of the medicine is noted or the maximum allowable dose is reached. Gabitril may cause dizziness, tiredness, and an unstable gait. Also like Topamax, Gabitril may interact with other drugs, so be sure to inform your child's primary-care doctor that your child is receiving these agents.

15

The Anxiety-Breaking Medications

Like the mood stabilizers, the anxiety-reducing medications (listed in Table 16) are categorized by the effect they have in children. Also called *anxiolytics,* they are used to treat the wide range of anxiety and panic disorders that share the predominant symptoms of worrying, nervousness, obsessing, and anxiety. They are also used as additional treatment for tics and for sleep.

Although they are classified as antidepressants, your child's practitioner will probably elect to try an SNRI (e.g., Cymbalta) or SSRI (e.g., Luvox, Zoloft, Paxil) for your child's anxiety as a first-line agent,

anxiolytic: A class of medications used to reduce ("lyse") anxiety.

as explained in Chapter 6. The SSRIs are often used because of how long they work (i.e., long duration of action), treatment of co-occurring depression, low abuse potential, favorable side effects, and long-term safety data. Cymbalta is FDA approved for anxiety in children. See Chapter 13 for details on SNRIs and SSRIs. Less frequently, your child's practitioner may elect to use a very-low-dose antipsychotic (see Chapter 17)—particularly if your child also has severe mood instability as part of his clinical picture.

Because of their safety and effectiveness, benzodiazepines are also used for uncomplicated juvenile anxiety disorders. In some children who have severe anxiety conditions or a co-occurring disorder, combined

Table 16. The Preparation and Strengths of Anxiety-Breaking Medications

Generic name	Brand name	Sizes and preparation
\multicolumn{3}{c}{**Antihistamines**}
Diphenhydramine	Benadryl	25, 50 mg; tablets
		25 mg/1 tsp; suspension
Hydroxyzine	Vistaril, Atarax	25, 50 mg; tablets
		2 mg/1 tsp; suspension
Chlorpheniramine maleate	Chlor-Trimeton	2, 4, 8 mg; tablets
\multicolumn{3}{c}{**Benzodiazepines (partial list)**}
Clonazepam	Klonopin	0.5, 1, 2 mg; tablets
Lorazepam	Ativan	0.5, 1, 2 mg; tablets
Alprazolam	Xanax	0.25, 0.5, 1 mg; tablets
Triazolam	Halcion	0.5, 1, 2 mg; tablets
Oxazepam	Serax	15, 30 mg; tablets
Diazepam	Valium	2, 5, 10 mg; tablets
Clorazepate	Tranxene	3.75, 7.5, 15 mg; capsules
\multicolumn{3}{c}{**Atypical**}
Buspirone	Buspar	5, 10, 15 mg; tablets
Zolpidem	Ambien	5, 10 mg; tablets
Zaleplon	Sonata	5, 10 mg; tablets
Eszopiclone	Lunesta	1, 2 mg; tablets

Note. 5 cc = 5 ml = 1 tsp. Antidepressants such as duloxetine (Cymbalta) and sertraline (Zoloft) are frequently used for the treatment of anxiety in children.

treatment (such as an SSRI antidepressant or an atypical antipsychotic and a benzodiazepine) may be necessary.

The Benzodiazepines

A common class of medications used to treat anxiety is the benzodiazepines. Among medications in this class of agents are Valium (diazepam), Librium (chlordiazepoxide), Ativan (lorazepam), Xanax (alprazolam), and Klonopin (clonazepam). The newer-generation benzodiazepine-like medication includes Buspar (buspirone).

The benzodiazepines act mainly on the central nervous system (brain), affecting a type of receptor called the *GABA receptor*. Barbiturates (*sedatives*) and alcohol have similar effects on this receptor, which is why all three are considered sedative in nature and can be used to stop withdrawal from one another. For instance, it is common practice to use Librium or Serax (oxazepam) to treat symptoms of withdrawal from alcohol.

> **sedative:**
> A sleep-producing agent.

Dosage

In general, the benzodiazepines all have similar effects on anxiety, and the level of all of them peaks in the blood in 1–3 hours following a dose. Where they differ is in their sedative side effects and their strength. Panic attacks and various types of anxiety (e.g., severe generalized anxiety) require a lot of antianxiety medication, so the stronger (more potent) benzodiazepines have been used increasingly in young people. The *high-potency* benzodiazepines, Xanax and Klonopin, are effective and safe treatments for anxiety and panic disorder with and without agoraphobia (difficulty leaving the house or being confined in limited spaces). Klonopin is a long-acting benzodiazepine given one to three times a day (usually twice a day) with a typical daily dose of 0.5–3 mg. Klonopin may take up to 2 hours to work. Xanax and Ativan, other high-potency benzodiazepines, work faster (within 30 minutes) but wear off more quickly and consequently are dosed more often during the day. A long-acting form of Xanax is now available and lasts most of the day. The typical dose of Ativan and Xanax is 0.5–3 mg daily, similar to Klonopin. The intermediate-acting, midpotency benzodiazepines (Valium, Tranxene) work within 30 minutes and are also given three or four times a day because of the wear-off. Typical dosing is 2.5–20 mg daily.

Side Effects

In general, serious toxic effects of the benzodiazepines are virtually nonexistent when the medications are used appropriately. The most commonly encountered short-term side effects are sedation, drowsiness, and decreased mental *acuity* (sharpness). Children may also have a paradoxical response to the benzodiazepines: instead of becoming less anxious or sedated (if used for sleep), they may get agitated and disinhibited. Disinhibited children may be silly, agitated, talkative, and overactive, become more anxious, or sleep poorly (insomnia). Generally, if your child is the unlucky one to have this reaction, it will last for only a couple of hours. We recommend that parents try a very low dose of a benzodiazepine during a weekend morning to ensure that their child does not "disinhibit"—and if the child does, he has the whole day to recover. Rarely, benzodiazepines can cause or initiate a depression. With the exception of the small potential risk for dependence in children, the benzodiazepines have no known long-term, adverse effects. No baseline laboratory tests are necessary, and there is no need for blood monitoring with treatment.

> **disinhibition:** Loss of normal restraint or censorship of impulses and urges.

Long-term use of these medications may lead to tolerance, however. When the child's body gets used to the medication, more of it may become necessary to reduce the symptoms of anxiety. Stopping the medication abruptly, especially at higher doses, may lead to withdrawal. Withdrawal symptoms include agitation, edginess, sweating, and anxiety. More severe symptoms may include increased blood pressure, confusion, and seizures.

> **tolerance:** The loss of a response, either behavioral or physical, to a medication over a sustained period of time.

Take-Home Point: The good news is that tapering off the drugs rather than stopping them abruptly can easily prevent withdrawal symptoms.

> **The pharmacist tells me my son's prescription is for a schedule IV controlled substance, and now I'm worried that he'll get addicted to his medication. Should I be concerned?**
>
> Medications like benzodiazepines can produce both physiological (body) and psychological dependence. However, addiction is generally a danger only when these substances are misused or abused. Given that there is little abuse of these medications by children taking them legitimately, your child has a very small likelihood of becoming addicted to any of the benzodiazepines. If your child's doctor prescribes an anxiety-breaking medication over a period of more than 6 months, you need to balance the very small chance of addiction against the risk of not treating your child's anxiety or panic disorder. Young people whose anxiety is not treated may try to medicate themselves by turning to alcohol and street drugs. Another consideration when having medicines like benzodiazepines around the house is to keep them stored safely to ensure others don't steal them, including "friends" of your adolescent.

Buspar

Buspar (buspirone) is also an anxiety-breaking compound. Buspirone may be effective in the treatment of aggressive behaviors in children with developmental disorders, including pervasive developmental disorders. Often Buspar is used in conjunction with the SSRIs (like Prozac) for anxiety or to boost the antidepressant's effect on depression.

Unlike the benzodiazepines, Buspar does not have anticonvulsant, sedative, or muscle-relaxant properties. Instead, the anxiety-breaking effect of Buspar may relate to reduction in serotonergic neurotransmission. Side effects include sedation, spaciness, confusion, and disinhibition. Buspar is used at a dose range of 5–15 mg three times a day and does not require blood monitoring.

Take-Home Point: Clinical experience with Buspar suggests that it is not as effective as typical benzodiazepines; however, it also has significantly fewer side effects and a lower potential for abuse or dependence.

Antihistamines

Antihistamines such as Benadryl are commonly used over-the-counter medications that parents can give their children for short-term or intermittent control of minor to moderate anxiety. Benadryl, which is usually dosed at 12.5 mg to 25 mg once or twice a day, may cause tiredness. Some parents prefer to use Benadryl if their child's anxiety occurs at night around bedtime both to help the anxiety and to help the child fall asleep. Over time, the medication often stops working for the treatment of anxiety.

16

The Alpha Agonists and Other Antihypertensives

The alpha agonists—clonidine and guanfacine—are so named because they work pharmacologically on the brain's alpha-adrenergic system. They are also referred to as antihypertensives because they are used to treat high blood pressure in adults. In children and adolescents, they are used psychiatrically to treat ADHD, tic and Tourette's disorders, mild moodiness, sleep problems, and, less frequently, developmental disorders such as ASD. These medications may also reduce behaviors that place children at risk for harming themselves or others, such as severe outbursts or aggressivity. The alpha agonists are commonly used in combination with other agents such as the stimulants—a safe combination that has been approved by the FDA. The alpha agonists have also been used with antipsychotics, mood stabilizers, and antidepressants. The alpha agonists and other antihypertensives are listed in Table 17.

Clonidine

Clonidine (Catapres) and clonidine extended release (Kapvay) have become increasingly prominent in the psychopharmacological treatment of children, in part because of their wide range of usefulness and relative safety. In addition to ADHD and sleep disturbances, clonidine is now considered a first-line treatment in Tourette's disorder and other tic disorders. In addition, reports indicate that clonidine helps control aggression in children and adolescents with autism spectrum illness and other,

Table 17. The Preparation and Strengths of the Commonly Used Alpha Agonists and Other Antihypertensives

Generic name	Brand name	Sizes and preparation
Alpha agonists		
Clonidine	Catapres	0.1, 0.2, 0.3 mg; tablets
		1, 2, 3 mg; skin patch
	Kapvay	0.1, 0.2 mg; extended-release tablets
Guanfacine	Tenex	1 mg; tablet
	Intuniv	1, 2, 3, 4 mg; extended-release tablets
Prazosin	Minipress	1, 2, 3 mg; tablets
Antihypertensives (beta blockers)		
Propranolol	Inderal	10, 20, 40, 60, 80 mg; tablets
		20, 60, 120 mg; sustained-release tablets
Nadolol	Corgard	20, 40, 80, 120, 160 mg; tablets

less well-described developmental disorders. A series of studies has shown the added utility of clonidine with methylphenidate (a type of stimulant) for the treatment of youth with tic disorders or Tourette's disorder and ADHD. Other studies have shown the usefulness of the extended-release preparation of clonidine, Kapvay, in combination with stimulants (e.g., Adderall XR, Concerta, and others) to treat ADHD that has responded only partially to the stimulants alone. Clonidine works by dampening one of the major chemical transmitter systems in the brain, the adrenergic nervous system. More specifically, it affects the release of norepineph-

adrenergic nervous system: The complex set of nerves that use norepinephrine-based messengers and connect extensively with multiple organs in the body, including the heart, lungs, and hormone-producing glands.

rine, and hence nerve-to-nerve communication, in certain areas of the brain.

Dosage

Clonidine is a relatively short-acting compound, working for about 4 hours in children, so some kids need to take it up to four times a day. Kapvay generally lasts 6–8 hours and is given once to twice daily. The amount necessary for effective treatment of tics and ADHD varies substantially among children, however. Clonidine comes as 0.1-, 0.2-, and 0.3-mg tablets, and therapy is usually started at the lowest possible dose of half or one-quarter of a 0.1-mg tablet, depending on the size of the child, and increased depending on the child's positive response and any adverse effects. Kapvay comes in 0.1- and 0.2-mg tablets.

At first it's best to give clonidine in the evening or before bed, since it often causes sedation. In fact, the drug can be very helpful to children with sleep disturbances commonly associated with ADHD or the stimulants used to treat it. For sleep, children usually benefit from the short-acting clonidine and require at least half of a 0.1-mg tablet about 30 minutes before bedtime. A study from our group showed that clonidine was extremely helpful for over 80% of children with sleep problems after 3 years of follow-up, but apparently children develop some tolerance to its sedating properties, since the average dose after 3 years was 0.15 mg (one and a half 0.1-mg tablets).

One drawback of having to take clonidine several times a day is that your child may suffer ups and downs. That's why some families have opted to use Kapvay once or twice a day. An alternative designed to solve this problem is a skin patch (*transdermal* preparation), available in all three strengths, that can be worn around the clock. Unfortunately, skin irritation at the site of the patch is quite common, severely limiting this form of delivery.

> **transdermal:** Absorbed through the skin.

Side Effects

The sedation that can be so helpful with sleep problems is the most common short-term side effect of clonidine. If your child is severely sedated, reducing the dose to a quarter of a tablet may be necessary, but be aware that sedation usually subsides with continued treatment. Clonidine can

> **My son has a much smoother day with the clonidine skin patch, but what can I do about the nasty rash he's developed where the patch goes?**
>
> These skin patches very commonly cause an inflammation (*dermatitis*) wherever they are placed on the skin. Often the skin is pink under the patch, which is not of concern (a raised, very red and sore area would flag a potential problem). Two ways to avoid mild inflammation are to move the patch to another spot on the body every day or to apply 0.5% hydrocortisone ointment or Benadryl ointment (diphenhydramine), which can be purchased over the counter, to the skin area before putting the patch on your child. As with most patches, the use of cotton soaked with olive oil to gently remove old adhesive will protect against the skin breaking down.

also produce irritability and depression. At doses of 0.4 mg daily and up, it may cause confusion. Over a decade ago, there was a report that three children receiving combinations of clonidine and other medications died for unclear reasons. However, further information indicated that there were many other extenuating circumstances surrounding the deaths, leading many experts to the conclusion that clonidine was not the main culprit. Clonidine itself is not known to be associated with long-term serious adverse effects. Surprisingly, despite being a powerful blood pressure medication in adults, clonidine has little effect on children's blood pressure. *However, abrupt withdrawal of clonidine has been associated with a temporary increase in the blood pressure, so slow tapering is advised.* In addition, caution should be exercised when clonidine is used with propranolol or other beta blocker agents, as it might be to treat severe behavioral outbursts, for children having marked sleep problems along with outbursts, or for children with blood pressure problems who need to be treated for hyperactivity/impulsivity and aggression associated with ADHD and/or comorbid conduct problems—because an adverse interaction has been reported.

Take-Home Point: Clonidine should be tapered gradually to avoid high blood pressure.

Tenex/Intuniv

Guanfacine (Intuniv or Tenex) is another alpha agonist used to treat adult blood pressure that has little effect on children's blood pressure when given daily. Both Intuniv (guanfacine extended release) and Tenex (guanfacine) have emerged as useful agents for ADHD, tic and Tourette's disorders, and, to a lesser extent, nonspecific aggression. Intuniv, which is FDA approved as a once-daily treatment for ADHD, appears to be effective for all aspects of ADHD but may be particularly useful for co-occurring oppositional or tic problems with ADHD. Guanfacine (both Tenex and Intuniv) appears to operate in the same areas of the brain as clonidine, affecting similar nerve-to-nerve communication. Because guanfacine binds to a specific receptor type in the brain (alpha-2A), it may cause less sedation than clonidine. As with clonidine, studies have shown its usefulness and tolerability when combined with Ritalin-like medications for the treatment of kids with ADHD plus tic disorders.

> **Take-Home Point:** Guanfacine may be particularly useful in combination with methylphenidate-type stimulants.

Dosage

Tenex and generic guanfacine are shorter acting and are typically given two or three times daily. We currently are using doses of the short-acting Tenex (guanfacine) that range from 0.5 mg (half of a 1-mg tablet) twice daily to 1 mg two to three times daily. Intuniv (extended-release guanfacine) is available in 1-, 2-, 3-, and 4-mg tablets that are dosed once in the morning. Typical dosing in children is from 1–4 mg daily, although recent research indicates that in some adolescents doses of up to 7 mg may be necessary for optimal ADHD control.

Side Effects

The side effects of Tenex are similar to those of clonidine. In work with the once-daily form of guanfacine, Intuniv, sedation or tiredness was the most common issue. Because sleep is so problematic with ADHD (or its treatment), Intuniv may be helpful with sleep problems, but often less so than clonidine. If your child is severely sedated, reducing the dose to a quarter or half of a tablet may be necessary, but be aware that sedation usually subsides with continued treatment. Tenex and Intuniv can also produce irritability and rarely depression and, like clonidine, should be tapered when stopping to avoid any potential cardiovascular effects. As with all medications we use in children, tell your doctor about any heart problems or complaints such as chest pain, dizziness, or fainting episodes that your child may have before starting the medication. Some doctors will order an ECG to be sure there are no underlying undetected issues prior to starting this class of medications (this is optional).

Because both clonidine and guanfacine (including Intuniv) can lower heart rate and blood pressure, it is recommended that your child's doctor (and you) monitor your child for dizziness, almost or actually passing out, and/or fatigue that may signal a heart disturbance. It is also recommended that the doctor (and you) check your child's heart rate and blood pressure periodically.

Propranolol and Other Beta Blockers

The beta blockers are commonly used in medicine to control blood pressure and, to a lesser extent, behavior. Although not systematically investigated in children, beta blockers have been reported to be helpful in individuals with anxiety, brain injury, and severe impulse and control problems. Propranolol has also received considerable attention for its usefulness in the overactivity (*akathisia*) sometimes induced by the stimulants or antipsychotics, in phobias such as fear of speaking in front of others, and in self-abusive behaviors.

Propranolol is one of the most frequently prescribed and oldest beta blockers. Other medications of the beta blocker type that are similar to propranolol include atenolol, pindolol, and nadolol (although atenolol and pindolol are not commonly used for children). Propranolol works by blocking areas of the adrenergic nervous system, specifically the set of receptors called the *beta-adrenergic receptors,* at multiple sites in the body. This in turn dampens the nerve-to-nerve communication. Propranolol also crosses the blood–brain barrier, and this probably accounts for some of its usefulness in reducing certain behaviors.

What are the differences between clonidine and guanfacine?

In general, these two medications share many characteristics but also have differences that will help determine which one is chosen for your child. An extended-release, once-daily preparation of guanfacine (Intuniv) is FDA approved for ADHD, and a twice-daily extended-release form of clonidine (Kapvay) is also FDA approved for ADHD. In treating ADHD, guanfacine may have a slightly better effect on attentional difficulties, while clonidine may have more effect on hyperactivity or aggression. Clonidine (other names: Catapres, Kapvay) is approximately 10 times more potent (stronger) than Tenex (short-acting guanfacine) or Intuniv (long-acting guanfacine), but Tenex/Intuniv causes less sedation and irritability.

Clonidine comes in 0.1-, 0.2-, and 0.3-mg tablets and is often started with half of a tablet once or twice a day, increased to 0.2–0.4 mg per day (often 0.1 mg three or four times a day if using short-acting clonidine or 0.1–0.2 mg twice daily if using Kapvay). Tenex comes in 1-mg tablets, and the typical starting dose is half a tablet twice daily; for Intuniv, the extended-release form, the starting dose is 1 mg daily, increased to 4 mg daily for best effect (slightly higher dosing may be necessary in adolescents). Tenex is dosed up to 1 mg four times a day safely and effectively; the once-daily form is dosed from 1 to 4 mg in the morning. Interestingly, Intuniv can be administered either in the morning or at night—both times of administration result in effectiveness throughout the day.

The major side effects of both clonidine and guanfacine include sedation, tiredness, and, rarely, agitation. Like clonidine, guanfacine (Tenex or Intuniv) should not be discontinued abruptly due to the risk of a transient rebound upward swing in your child's blood pressure. Children taking the alpha agonists (clonidine or guanfacine) should be monitored for low heart rate. Guanfacine and clonidine are commonly used with stimulants for youth with ADHD who are not responding to stimulants alone, ADHD plus tics, aggression, or sleep difficulties.

Dosage

Propranolol is relatively short-lived, working for only about 4–6 hours after being taken. Dosages vary among children but usually start at 10 mg daily and increase as necessary every week to 2 weeks up to a maximum of approximately 200–300 mg per day with careful attention to side effects at higher doses.

Side Effects

Short-term adverse effects of propranolol are usually not serious and generally disappear when the medication is stopped. Nausea, vomiting, constipation, and mild diarrhea have been reported. Children also report vivid dreams, depression, and, rarely, hallucinations. Propranolol can cause slowing of the heart and reduced blood pressure, particularly at higher doses, so your child will need to have periodic blood pressure and pulse (vital sign) checks, which can be done at home. Be sure your child's doctor knows about any cardiac problems the child has, because propranolol should be avoided with certain cardiac conditions. Propranolol may also cause worsening of some breathing problems (high airway resistance, wheezing) and thus should not be used in children who have asthma. Propranolol should also be used cautiously in children with diabetes, since it may mask any underlying emergency warning signs of dangerously low blood sugars. No long-term effects from continued use of propranolol are known, but gradual tapering is recommended to prevent a rebound swing in your child's blood pressure.

➤ **Take-Home Point:** Propranolol should be used cautiously for children with cardiac conditions and should be tapered gradually.

17
The Antipsychotics

The antipsychotics are the only drugs available that treat psychosis effectively, but they are also more commonly used to treat other disorders in children, such as substantial mood swings (mood *lability*), tics or Tourette's disorder, and severe agitation or aggression, when more standard treatments have failed. Also called *major tranquilizers* or *neuroleptics,* these drugs have a history of substantial side effects. That is why they are generally reserved for more severe disorders and disturbed behaviors in children, and those that don't respond to other medications. Therefore, it is wise for you and your child's doctor to choose them only with a clear understanding of what they are being used for and the proposed length of time your child will be receiving them.

The second-generation, atypical antipsychotics (Risperdal/Invega, Zyprexa, Seroquel, Abilify, Geodon, Latuda, and others) are FDA approved and considered the drug of choice for psychoses such as schizophrenia and the impairments in reality sometimes seen with depression or bipolar disorder (manic–depression) in kids. The newer-generation antipsychotics are now considered the first line of defense for the treatment of youth with severe and out-of-control moodiness (e.g., bipolar disorder). In fact, at the time of printing, there were at least five SGAs that were approved by the FDA for the treatment of children and adolescents with bipolar disorder, including Risperdal, Zyprexa, Seroquel, Abilify, and Saphris. Given the generally positive controlled medication trial results this class of medications has produced, more FDA approval seems likely to emerge for other medications within this class.

Invega, for example, seems to have similar efficacy to risperidone (Risperdal) and may be tolerated more easily (in terms of weight gain in particular), so it is being used by some physicians as an alternative to Risperdal when Risperdal has been helpful but weight gain has been a problem. Because it may last longer, it also is sometimes used to deal with breakthrough symptoms of bipolar disorder or irritability in the afternoon. The atypical antipsychotics are generally reserved as second-line drugs of choice for the treatment of Tourette's disorder and less clear diagnostic groups with severely disruptive, self-injurious, or aggressive behaviors.

Take-Home Point: Because of their side effects, antipsychotics are usually reserved for more severe problems in children.

One problem you should be aware of when an antipsychotic is chosen for one disorder is that it may still fail to address a commonly co-occurring disorder. Haldol (haloperidol) and Orap (pimozide), for example, are prescribed when Strattera, clonidine, guanfacine, and the tricyclic antidepressants fail to improve Tourette's disorder. While they can be very useful in reducing tics, they may have only limited effects on the obsessive–compulsive disorders and ADHD that often accompany Tourette's disorder. Similarly, while they may be useful in treating the severe agitation, rage attacks, racing thoughts, and sleep problems associated with mania in an adolescent with bipolar disorder, they may not improve the child's ADHD or anxiety.

Another cautionary note on how and when to choose antipsychotics: These drugs have also traditionally been used to control symptoms of agitation, aggression, and self-injurious behaviors in children with developmental disorders, including intellectual disability and ASD. Tradition, however, should not always rule. Here it is prudent to try medications with fewer side effects, including guanfacine or clonidine, first. If you and the doctor do conclude that an antipsychotic should be tried, know the differences among them: while a more sedating, lower-potency agent such as Thorazine, Mellaril, or Seroquel may be beneficial for the more agitated child or adolescent, a more potent agent such as Abilify, Risperdal (risperidone), or Trilafon may be helpful for children who are having active hallucinations. Because of the potential downside of these medications (see the information on side effects on page 274), we don't recommend the use of this class of medications for "nonspecific behavioral disruptive disorders." These medications are so effective nonspecifically that some practitioners use them for any behavioral problems. We strongly urge you to have a clear understanding of all diagnoses being treated prior to starting these medications.

Take-Home Point: Treatment should be guided by a diagnosis, but this is particularly important when considering antipsychotics. A thoughtful diagnosis will reveal whether a medication with fewer or milder side effects might be effective.

The antipsychotics share much in their pharmacological profiles and in how well they treat psychosis, behavioral control, and other psychiatric disturbances. However, as shown in Table 18, they differ substantially in their strength (potency) and side effects (especially with regard to muscular spasms and sedation). The major classes of the older, traditional antipsychotic drugs used clinically are:

- The weaker, or low-potency, compounds (requiring higher dosages), such as Thorazine (chlorpromazine) and Mellaril (thioridazine)

- The medium-strength compounds such as Stelazine (trifluoperazine), Navane (thiothixene), Trilafon (perphenazine), and Loxitane (loxapine)

- The strong, high-potency agents such as Haldol (haloperidol), Prolixin (perfenazine), and Orap (pimozide)

There are also the newer antipsychotic agents, or SGAs, described above. The SGAs are preferred by most practitioners, given (1) the growing FDA approval of this class of medications in children and adolescents, (2) more extensive data on this class of medications, and (3) their longer-term safety compared to the older antipsychotics in terms of a potentially irreversible side effect called tardive dyskinesia (described further on page 275). Be aware, however, that our patients have had variable responses to the newer antipsychotics or have not been able to tolerate them well (e.g., have experienced weight gain) and have responded nicely to the older-generation antipsychotics. It's important to know as much as possible about the individual drugs before agreeing to any prescription of antipsychotics for your child.

Table 18. Preparation and Strengths of Antipsychotics Commonly Used in Children and Adolescents

Medication		
Generic name	Brand name	Sizes and preparation
Second-generation (atypical) antipsychotics		
Aripiprazole	Abilify	2, 5, 10, 15, 20, 30 mg; tablets
		10, 15 mg; dissolving tablets
Risperidone	Risperdal	0.25, 0.5, 1, 2, 3 mg; tablets
Paliperidone	Invega	1.5, 3, 6, 9 mg; capsules
Quetiapine	Seroquel	25, 50, 100, 200, 300, 400 mg; tablets
Olanzapine	Zyprexa	2.5, 5, 7.5, 10, 15 mg; tablets
Ziprasidone	Geodon	20, 40, 60, 80 mg; capsules
Asenapine	Saphris	2.5, 5, 10 mg; tablets under the tongue (dissolving)
Lurasidone	Latuda	20, 40, 60, 80, 120 mg; tablets
Clozapine	Clozaril	25, 50, 100 mg; tablets
High-potency antipsychotics		
Haloperidol	Haldol	0.5, 1, 2, 5, 10, 20 mg; tablets
		2 mg/cc; suspension
Pimozide	Orap	2 mg; tablet
Fluphenazine	Prolixin	1, 2.5, 5, 10 mg; tablets
		5 mg/cc; suspension
Medium-potency antipsychotics		
Trifluoperazine	Stelazine	1, 2, 5, 10 mg; tablets
Perphenazine	Trilafon	2, 4, 8, 16 mg; tablets
		5 mg/cc; suspension
Thiothixene	Navane	1, 2, 5, 10, 20 mg; tablets
		5 mg/cc; suspension
Loxapine	Loxitane*	5, 10, 25, 50 mg; tablets
		5 mg/1 tsp; suspension

Note. 5 cc = 5 ml = 1 tsp.
*Brand name not available; limited availability of generic.

Medication		
Generic name	Brand name	Sizes and preparation
Low-potency antipsychotics		
Molindone	Moban	5, 10, 25, 50 mg; tablets
		4 mg/1 tsp; suspension
Mesoridazine	Serentil	10, 25, 50, 100 mg; tablets
		25 mg/1 tsp; suspension
Thioridazine	Mellaril	10, 25, 50, 100, 200 mg; tablets
		5, 6, 20 mg/1 tsp; suspension
Chlorpromazine	Thorazine	10, 25, 50, 100, 200 mg; tablets
		5, 6, 20 mg/1 tsp; suspension

The traditional antipsychotics such as Mellaril appear to work by blocking specific dopamine receptors (dopamine 2 type). Some of the side effects of these drugs result from their blocking other receptors as well: histamine, which results in the dry mouth and sedation characteristic of antihistamines; and the cholinergic system, which results in an increased heart rate and constipation. The SGAs have less effect on other receptors and affect different dopamine receptors and serotonin receptors (see page 276).

Dosage

These are the usual dosage ranges for the antipsychotic drugs:

- 25–300 mg daily for the lower-potency agents such as Seroquel, Geodon, Latuda, Mellaril, Thorazine, and Clozaril
- 4–40 mg daily for the midpotency agents such as Abilify, Zyprexa, Saphris, Trilafon, and Stelazine
- 0.5–6 mg daily for the high-potency agents such as Risperdal, Haldol, Prolixin, and Invega

Antipsychotic medications last a relatively long time in the blood and do not need to be given more than twice a day.

Most antipsychotic preparations are available in either tablet or capsule form. In addition, at least one compound from each class of antipsychotics is available in a liquid concentrate. Several compounds, including Geodon, Thorazine, Haldol, and Prolixin, are available in injection form (injectable/intramuscular). Haldol and Prolixin are also available in an oily suspension (Decanoate), which is administered as an intramuscular injection that lasts from 2 weeks to 1 month. Orally dissolving tablets of Saphris, Zyprexa, and Risperdal are available and can be invaluable for children who may be hiding medication in their mouth but not swallowing it (cheeking) and who spit it out later. These preparations dissolve in the mouth and cannot be cheeked.

Side Effects

Both the older and the second-generation antipsychotics have many side effects. Common short-term, reversible side effects of antipsychotic drugs are drowsiness, increased appetite, and weight gain. Certain side effects like dizziness, dry mouth, congested nose, and blurred vision are more commonly seen with the low-potency agents such as Thorazine. High-potency agents such as Abilify, Haldol, and Orap are more commonly associated with a set of side effects affecting various muscle groups (*extrapyramidal effects*) leading to muscle tightness and spasm (*dystonia*), rolling eyes, and restlessness leading to the inability to stay seated (*akathisia*). All antipsychotics may also cause a reversible Parkinson-like clinical picture characterized by general slowing, tremor, tenseness, and a masked face. The use of another medication called Cogentin can reverse these problems.

Although visually bothersome to others, and sometimes uncomfortable for the child, many of the short-term side effects of the antipsychotics can be managed. Excessive sedation can be avoided by using less sedating antipsychotics (e.g., Geodon or Abilify instead of Seroquel, Thorazine, or Zyprexa) and managed by prescribing most of the daily dose at night either with dinner or at bedtime. Drowsiness should not be confused with impaired thinking and can usually be corrected by adjusting the dose and timing of administration. In fact, antipsychotics cause little mental confusion or impairment when used in low doses. Certain side effects such as dry mouth, constipation, and blurred vision can be minimized by choosing a medium- or high-potency compound (Abilify, Risperdal, Saphris, Stelazine, Navane, or Haldol, instead of Seroquel, Thorazine, or Mellaril). Muscular spasms (extrapyramidal reactions) can be avoided in most cases by slowly increasing these medications or using a lower-potency, weaker agent such as Navane or Stelazine instead of Haldol or Orap.

In our clinic, outside of tics/Tourette's disorder, we tend to avoid using Haldol or Prolixin in children because of these muscle spasms, which, although not dangerous, are bothersome. If, however, your child *is* responding well to a particular antipsychotic and has the muscular spasms, a class of safe medications (anti-Parkinson agents) can be added just for the side effects. The agents useful for these spasms include over-the-counter Benadryl for the short term, if relief is needed immediately, or prescribed Cogentin or amantadine to be taken daily for the long haul. If your child is on antipsychotics and develops agitation with an inability to sit still, the possibility that this is a side effect of the medication should be considered. Similar to treating muscular spasms, Benadryl, Cogentin, amantadine, the beta blockers (such as propranolol), and the benzodiazepines (Klonopin) may be helpful in eliminating these side effects.

Another very infrequent but severe reaction to antipsychotic agents is *neuroleptic malignant syndrome.* This reaction consists of severe muscle tightness, confusion, sweating, fever, and instability of blood pressure and pulse. *If you see anything resembling these symptoms in your child, contact your physician immediately or take your child to the emergency room.* If neuroleptic malignant syndrome is suspected, blood tests should be completed to help determine if there has been any muscle or kidney damage. Treatment of neuroleptic malignant syndrome requires intensive medical surveillance and consists of immediate stopping of the drug.

As in adults, the long-term use of antipsychotic drugs in children and adolescents may be associated with a feared, often irreversible, side effect called *tardive dyskinesia.* Tardive dyskinesia is a group of movements that the child is not able to stop entirely. It often starts as lip smacking and tongue rolling and may progress to involve other facial muscles, leading to prominent eye blinks and grimacing. Tardive dyskinesia can proceed to involve spasms and dance-like movements of the shoulders, trunk, and limbs. The risk for tardive dyskinesia appears to increase with the dose of the medication and the length of time the child takes it. Generally there is minimal risk in a child who is receiving an agent for 1 month; however, children who are receiving these agents should be monitored for the development of abnormal muscle movements.

The treatment for tardive dyskinesia is usually removal of the antipsychotic drug, but this measure should not be taken lightly. Discontinuing the medication may actually worsen the tardive dyskinesia temporarily and is certainly likely to bring on the return of the behavioral and/or thought problems for which the medication has been prescribed. One patient, William, developed mild lip smacking while on 3 mg of risperidone for his bipolar disorder, and when we discontinued the medication over 2 weeks, Bill's lip smacking progressed to facial grimacing. The grimacing and lip smacking improved over the next 2 months, but stopping the antipsychotic medication had the predictable result of bringing back very disabling behavioral problems and some paranoia. We're happy to report that he is now doing better on olanzapine. Pharmacological treatments may help reduce tardive dyskinesia. To date, these drugs include many of the same agents used in adult neurology for the amelioration of Parkinson's disease. In addition, recent interest has arisen in the use of vitamin E to possibly prevent tardive dyskinesia.

In any case, tardive dyskinesia should be distinguished from the more common, generally benign withdrawal spasms associated with the abrupt cessation of antipsychotic drugs, which tend to subside without treatment after days to weeks of drug discontinuation. In children with cognitive disabilities and ASD, tardive dyskinesia should be differentiated from the commonly occurring stereotypies such as head banging or rocking.

> **stereotypies:** repetitive movements such as head banging or rocking.

Take-Home Point: Because the symptoms treated by antipsychotics can be so disabling, it's important to try to deal with side effects where possible instead of stopping the medication altogether.

The Second-Generation (Atypical) Antipsychotics

The newer antipsychotics—Risperdal, Invega, Seroquel, Zyprexa, Geodon, Abilify, Saphris, Latuda, and, to a lesser extent, Clozaril—are used as first-line drugs of choice for bipolar disorder, schizophrenia and other psychotic illnesses, and pronounced aggression/irritability because side effects are less common, and they improve all aspects of psychosis. These medications are being FDA approved for a number of disorders in kids, including bipolar disorder, schizophrenia, and severe irritability and dangerous behaviors in children with ASD. Symptoms such as withdrawal, loss of interest, ambivalence, and flattening of mood respond to these new antipsychotics. Like the traditional antipsychotics, they affect the dopamine system but appear to influence different subsets of dopamine and serotonin receptors. These newer drugs are being used for psychosis, marked mood swings, severe irritability, and severe tics/Tourette's disorder. Clozaril continues to be a highly effective agent reserved for treatment-refractory (nonresponsive) children and adolescents due to its significant side effects and intense monitoring requirements.

Dosage

Dosing is based on potency. Risperdal is the most potent of the agents. Therefore, the usual daily dose is lower and spans from 0.5 daily to 2 mg three times a day. Invega, related to risperidone (actually a breakdown by-product in the blood of people given risperidone), is slightly less potent and is dosed from 1.5 to 9 mg daily. Abilify is more of a middle-potency agent that is dosed from 2.5 mg to 30 mg daily. Zyprexa is considered a middle-potency agent and is commonly dosed between 5 and 20 mg daily in children and adolescents. Geodon and Latuda are dosed from 20 to 160 mg per day. Seroquel and Clozaril are lower-potency agents, and dosing ranges generally from 100 to 600 mg daily. Often, if a child is tolerating the medication well but responding only partially, higher doses may be used. A number of studies also show that these medications generally work within 2 weeks for managing the aggression and irritability associated with severe disorders such as bipolar disorder, but that it may also take up to 2 or 3 months to see their full effectiveness, particularly with Clozaril.

Side Effects

Side effects of Risperdal, Invega, Zyprexa, Geodon, Abilify, Latuda, Saphris, and Seroquel appear similar to those of the traditional antipsychotics, but the rate of side effects and the risk for long-term tardive dyskinesia appear to be *substantially lower*. A transient increase in prolactin levels has been noted with Risperdal. This elevation is of unclear significance, and data suggest it is largely ameliorated after 6 months of treatment. Many practitioners now routinely monitor for prolactin levels after 6 months to 1 year of exposure to risperidone. If your child is taking risperidone, watch for enlarged breasts in males or discharge in breasts from girls—which is a sign of the prolactin levels being too high (often necessitating a change to another medication). Clozaril needs to be monitored very carefully, since it has been associated with both a dangerous drop in blood cell production and severe seizures. Currently, weekly blood monitoring is necessary for Clozaril to be prescribed. The other agents do not require blood monitoring. In rare cases, a physician may request an ECG (Geodon) or an eye examination (Seroquel only). Because of weight gain associated with these medicines, attention to diet is imperative. In more extreme cases, adding Topamax (topiramate—50 mg twice a day), metformin (a medication to reduce blood sugar in diabetics), and/or stimulants can be helpful in losing weight or keeping weight gain to a minimum.

Probably the most problematic longer-term effects of any of the newest medications used to treat psychiatric disorders in children are weight gain and metabolic problems (involving blood sugar and fats in the blood called lipids and cholesterol) with the atypical antipsychotics. From clinical experience, it appears that Zyprexa and Clozaril have the largest effect and Abilify, Saphris, and Geodon the least effect on weight, with the other agents intermediate in their effect. Invega may cause less weight gain than Risperdal, so some clinicians will prescribe Invega where Risperdal has been helpful but weight gain has been problematic. The most recent data indicate that all of these medications can increase weight very substantially and may also have effects on blood sugar (glucose) levels as well as increasing the normal levels of blood fats (lipids) and cholesterol. These medications have been associated with massive weight gain, diabetes (blood glucose that is too high), and high levels of lipids and cholesterol. Because of these concerns, guidelines have been released for the use of these medications in children and adolescents. In addition to careful monitoring of your child's weight, these guidelines advocate regular monitoring (maybe every 6 months to 1 year) of blood sugar and lipids/cholesterol. In addition, you are strongly encouraged to work on eating and exercise habits with your child if he is taking these medications. These medications appear to increase the child's appetite, especially increasing cravings for foods high in carbohydrate (sugar) and fat. As well as you can, increase your child's physical activity, limit sedentary behavior (watching TV, playing video games, etc.), and provide lower-fat, healthier foods and snacks. Often you will have to model behavior to get your child to follow: take frequent walks or runs together, play basic sports together, walk instead of driving to and from school, and so forth. Eliminate easy-to-eat high-fat foods, keep vegetables cut and available with low-fat dips, encourage your child to eat smaller portions of food, and try not to keep cookies or other dessert items easily available. Every little bit helps in keeping weight off and improving the metabolic status of your child. Your child's doctor may want to use metformin (a diabetes medication) to help keep your child's blood sugar levels and weight under control while your child receives an SGA.

Take-Home Point: While the newer antipsychotics impose a lower risk of side effects, including tardive dyskinesia, weight gain can be a problem.

Use of Antipsychotics

Over the past few years, clinicians have tended to employ the SGAs as first-line agents for the treatment of children and adolescents who have psychosis (hallucinations, delusions, paranoia), severe disruptive disorders, self-injurious behavior, and bipolar disorder.

In children, hallucinations frequently occur with a mood disorder. In these cases, specific treatments for the mood disorder are crucial. It's not uncommon to place a child on lithium for bipolar disorder and Abilify or risperidone for the hallucinations. In cases where a child has disturbances in thought process along with severe agitation or anxiety, anxiety-breaking medications (benzodiazepines), such as lorazepam (Ativan) and clonazepam (Klonopin), can help and may also lead to the use of lower doses of antipsychotics.

One of the most difficult issues to address is treating depression in children with other psychotic or severe behavioral issues. Whereas some of the antipsychotics, such as Seroquel or Latuda, seem better for treating both depression and agitation/mania, sometimes two or more medications may be necessary. For instance, an antidepressant such as bupropion may be used with an antipsychotic such as risperidone. We also use Lamictal, lithium, Tegretol, or Depakote and an antipsychotic agent such as risperidone, Seroquel, and Abilify for complex cases. In these situations, children may be receiving medications two or three times a day to the tune of eight tablets of medication daily.

> A medication that isn't helping should be discontinued—not supplemented with another medication.

The thought of combining agents can be uncomfortable for your child, family, and doctor, but it may be necessary. In using combination treatment, be sure you know what each agent is for and whether another medication is necessary. If one medication is not helping, it should be discontinued instead of another medication being added. Fourteen-year-old Adam had marked mood swings, irritability, anger outbursts, and paranoia, and he recently started hearing voices telling him to harm others. Risperidone was not helpful and was discontinued. Abilify at 5 mg twice a day markedly reduced the hallucinations and paranoia but only modestly helped the mood instability, and he developed muscular spasms requiring Cogentin. Adam's mood finally stabilized after he was also placed on 400 mg of Tegretol twice daily. Adam tolerated the combination well despite receiving three different medications totaling five tablets daily. Attempts to reduce the medications over the ensuing year resulted in recurrence of the moodiness and hallucinations.

18
Medications for Sleep, Bedwetting, and Other Problems

A number of medications are used to treat problems that do not fall under the heading of emotional or behavioral problems yet often affect children with or without psychiatric disorders. These drugs come from different families and typically have more than one use. Clonidine, for one, is a blood-pressure-lowering agent in adults that is also useful for ADHD, tics, and emotional dysregulation and, because of its sedative properties, for children who have trouble sleeping. Benadryl, for another, is used to relieve allergies but also serves as a sleep aid.

Benadryl

Benadryl (diphenhydramine) is an antihistamine used commonly in all age groups for seasonal allergies, medication allergies, nonspecific rashes, and itching. Probably every family should keep a small quantity of Benadryl in the medicine cabinet for its multiplicity of uses. Because of its sedative properties, Benadryl can be useful for assisting with children who are out of control or very anxious and those with occasional sleep problems. Benadryl can also be beneficial in treating reactions to medications such as the skin rashes and muscular spasms associated with some of the antipsychotics (see Chapter 17).

Dosage

Benadryl has a very good track record in children and adolescents and is available in capsules, tablets, liquid (the preferable form because it works faster), and a better-tasting pediatric form. Typical dosing of full-strength Benadryl is 12.5 mg (1/2 teaspoon) for young children and 25–50 mg for older children. Benadryl usually works within 30 minutes, and its effectiveness may last up to 8 hours.

Side Effects

Major side effects are short term and include sedation, morning drowsiness (if used at night), confusion at higher doses, and dry mouth.

> **Take-Home Point:** Benadryl probably should not be used long term since children rapidly develop tolerance to the sleep-inducing characteristics of the medication.

Melatonin

Melatonin, a naturally occurring hormone related to sleep cycles in humans, has also been used in the treatment of sleep problems. During dark phases of the day, when most people are sleeping, melatonin levels naturally rise in the brain. Conversely, during daylight, melatonin levels diminish. Therefore introducing a natural compound prior to the hour of sleep may induce a more natural sleep.

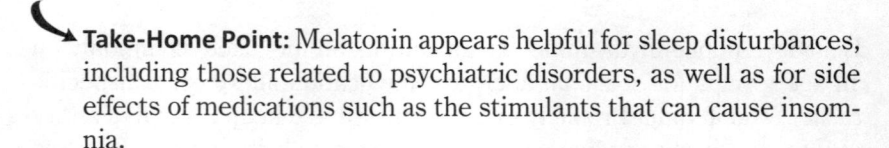

> **Take-Home Point:** Melatonin appears helpful for sleep disturbances, including those related to psychiatric disorders, as well as for side effects of medications such as the stimulants that can cause insomnia.

Dosage

Some parents and a number of recent controlled short- and longer-term studies have indicated that this agent helps children with a sleep disturbance (usually trouble falling asleep) relax and fall asleep naturally. Controlled studies in children suggest that doses of 0.5–3 mg of melatonin at bedtime are helpful and safe. Because melatonin doses differ substantially based on the preparation, it is recommended that you start your child on half the recommended starting adult dose. Also, if you find a preparation of melatonin that works for your child, stick with the same brand to reduce the variance in response related to the differences in the various over-the-counter formulations.

Side Effects

Side effects are not well studied in children but include morning sedation and changes in dream activity. Unlike some of the sleeping medications used in adults, because of its chemical properties, this medication does not appear to have significant addiction potential. No significant interactions between melatonin and psychotropic agents have been reported. It is also heartening to know that some studies have examined the use of this agent over as long as 2 years without any untoward side effects being observed.

Antidiuretic Hormone Desmopressin

Children with bedwetting or enuresis not caused by a medical condition usually respond to nonpharmacological therapies. These treatments, including behavior modification and psychotherapy, should be considered first. A synthetic form of a naturally occurring hormone called *antidiuretic hormone* has been used increasingly for bedwetting. This agent, called desmopressin (ddAVP), comes in a tablet form and can be quite expensive.

Desmopressin safely and effectively suppresses urine production, generally for 7–10 hours.

Take-Home Point: Desmopressin is useful for children who want to sleep over at a friend's house or go to an overnight summer camp.

Dosage

Daily doses are a 0.1–0.2 mg tablet initially prior to bedtime. Since bedwetting generally disappears with age, ddAVP therapy should not be continued indefinitely.

Side Effects

Side effects are minimal with shorter-term use; however, your child's practitioner may want to monitor blood pressure and the level of salt (sodium) in the blood with ongoing use. Long-term use for enuresis is not recommended.

Naltrexone

Naltrexone (Trexan or ReVia) appears helpful for two very different conditions: (1) the treatment of self-abuse, such as self-mutilation and head banging, and (2) the treatment of excessive intake of alcohol and opioids (including narcotic painkillers) in adolescents and adults. It appears that the drug naltrexone, a potent, long-acting agent, may work by partially blocking the effect of the brain's natural pain relief, or opioid, system, called the *endorphin system*. For adolescents and young adults who have an opioid use problem (pain killers, heroin), an intranasal form of naloxone (Narcan), a drug related to naltrexone, is available and advisable to have around in case of an overdose (e.g., unconscious, unresponsive, slowed breathing, blue color).

Dosage

In both children with ASD and those with self-abuse, the drug is used in doses of 25–150 mg daily. It appears that similar dosing may be necessary to reduce consumption of alcohol and opioids (including painkillers and heroin), although at the time of this writing it has not been studied extensively in adolescents.

Side Effects

Although naltrexone is relatively free of serious adverse effects, there have been some rare reports of liver problems in adults, the majority of whom had preexisting liver problems, generally from alcoholism. A once-a-month shot (Vivitrol), shown to produce improved outcomes for both opioid and alcohol use in adults, is available with the added benefit of not worrying about having to take the medication every day. Its main disadvantage is that it is expensive and has to be administered by a professional health provider.

APPENDIX A
Representative Medication Preparations and Sizes Used for the Treatment of Childhood Emotional and Behavioral Disorders

Generic name	Medication Brand name	Sizes and preparation
Stimulants		
Methylphenidate	Ritalin	5, 10, 20 mg; tablets
	Methylin	2.5, 5, 10 mg; tablets (chewable)
		5 mg/1 tsp, 10 mg/1 tsp; solution
	Ritalin SR*	20 mg; tablets
	Ritalin LA*	20, 30, 40 mg; capsules
	Methylin ER*	20 mg; sustained-release tablets
	Focalin	2.5, 5, 10 mg; tablets
	Focalin XR*	10, 15, 20 mg; capsules
	Concerta*	18, 27, 36, 54 mg; capsules
	Metadate CD*	20 mg; capsules
	Daytrana*	10, 15, 20, 30 mg; skin patch
	Quillivant*	5 mg/cc; suspension
	Aptensio	10, 15, 20, 30, 40, 50, 60 mg; capsules
Amphetamine compounds	Adderall	5, 10, 20, 30 mg; tablets
	Adderall XR*	5, 10, 15, 20, 25, 30 mg; capsules

Note. 5 cc = 5 ml = 1 tsp.
*Extended-release preparation (8- to 12-hour duration).

Medication		
Generic name	Brand name	Sizes and preparation

Stimulants (*cont.*)

Dextroamphetamine	Dexedrine	5, 10 mg; tablets
		5, 10, 15 mg; spansules
	Vyvanse*	20, 30, 40, 50, 60, 70 mg; capsules

Nonstimulants (noradrenergic)

Atomoxetine	Strattera	10, 18, 25, 40, 60, 80 mg; capsules

Alpha agonists

Clonidine	Catapres	0.1, 0.2, 0.3 mg; tablets
		1, 2, 3 mg; skin patch
	Kapvay*	0.1, 0.2 mg; tablets
Guanfacine	Tenex	1 mg; tablet
	Intuniv*	1, 2, 3, 4 mg; tablets
Prazosin	Minipress	1, 2, 3 mg; tablets

Antihypertensives (betablockers)

Propranolol	Inderal	10, 20, 40, 60, 80 mg; tablets
		20, 60, 120 mg; sustained-release tablets
Nadolol	Corgard	20, 40, 80, 120, 160 mg; tablets

Antidepressants (selective serotonin reuptake inhibitors)

Fluoxetine	Prozac	10, 20, 40, 60 mg; capsules and tablets
		20 mg/1 tsp; suspension
Sertraline	Zoloft	50, 100 mg; tablets
		20 mg/cc; suspension
Fluvoxamine	Luvox	25, 50, 100 mg; tablets
Paroxetine	Paxil	10, 20, 30, 40 mg; tablets
		20 mg/1 tsp; suspension
Citalopram	Celexa	10, 20, 40 mg; tablets
Escitalopram	Lexapro	10, 20 mg; tablets

Medication		
Generic name	Brand name	Sizes and preparation
Antidepressants (tricyclics)		
Desipramine	Norpramin Pertofrane	10, 25, 50, 75, 100, 150 mg; tablets
Nortriptyline	Pamelor Aventyl	10, 25, 50 mg; capsules 10 mg/1 tsp; suspension
Imipramine	Tofranil	10, 25, 50, 75, 100, 150 mg; tablets and capsules
Amitriptyline	Elavil	10, 25, 50, 75, 100, 150 mg; tablets
Protriptyline	Vivactil	5, 10 mg; capsules
Maprotiline	Ludiomil	25, 50, 75 mg; tablets
Clomipramine	Anafranil	25, 50, 100 mg; tablets
Antidepressants (atypical)		
Venlafaxine	Effexor	25, 37.5, 50, 75 mg; tablets 37.5, 75, 150 mg; extended-release tablets
Duloxetine	Cymbalta	20, 30, 60 mg; capsules
Trazodone	Desyrel	50, 100, 150, 300 mg; tablets
Vilazodone	Viibryd	10, 20, 40 mg; tablets
Nefazodone	Serzone	50, 100, 150, 200, 250 mg; tablets
Bupropion	Wellbutrin	75, 100 mg; tablets 100, 150, 200 mg; sustained-release tablets 150, 300, 450 mg; extended-release tablets
Mirtazapine	Remeron	15, 30 mg; tablets
Doxepin	Sinequan	10, 25, 50, 75, 100, 150 mg; capsules 10 mg/cc; solution
Vortioxetine	Brintellex	5, 10, 20 mg; tablets

Medication		
Generic name	Brand name	Sizes and preparation
Monamine oxidase inhibitors		
Phenelzine	Nardil	15 mg; tablets
Tranylcypromine	Parnate	10 mg; tablets
Antipsychotics (second-generation/atypical)		
Risperidone	Risperdal	0.25, 0.5, 1, 2, 3, mg; tablets
Paliperidone	Invega	1.5, 3, 6, 9 mg; tablets
Olanzapine	Zyprexa	2.5, 5, 7.5, 10, 15 mg; tablets
Quetiapine	Seroquel	25, 100, 200 mg; tablets
Aripiprazole	Abilify	5, 10, 15, 20, 30 mg; tablets
Brexpiprazole	Rexulti	0.25, 0.5, 1, 2, 3, 4 mg; tablets
Vortioxetine	Brintellex	5, 10, 20 mg; tablets
Ziprasidone	Geodon	20, 40, 60, 80 mg; capsules
Asenapine	Saphris	5, 10 mg; sublingual (dissolving) tablets
Lurasidone	Latuda	20, 40, 60, 80, 120 mg; tablets
Clozapine	Clozaril	25, 50, 100 mg; tablets
Antipsychotics (high-potency)		
Haloperidol	Haldol	0.5, 1, 2, 5, 10, 20 mg; tablets 2 mg/cc; suspension
Pimozide	Orap	2 mg; tablets
Fluphenazine	Prolixin	1, 2.5, 5, 10 mg; tablets 5 mg/cc; suspension
Antipsychotics (medium-potency)		
Trifluoperazine	Stelazine	1, 2, 5, 10 mg; tablets
Perphenazine	Trilafon	2, 4, 8, 16 mg; tablets
Thiothixene	Navane	1, 2, 5, 10, 20 mg; tablets 5 mg/cc; suspension
Loxapine	Loxitane	5, 10, 25, 50 mg; tablets 5 mg/1 tsp; suspension

Medication		
Generic name	Brand name	Sizes and preparation
Antipsychotics (low-potency)		
Molindone	Moban	5, 10, 25, 50, 100 mg; tablets 4 mg/1 tsp; suspension
Mesoridazine	Serentil	10, 25, 50, 100 mg; tablets 25 mg/1 tsp; suspension
Thioridazine	Mellaril	10, 15, 25, 50, 100, 200 mg; tablets 5, 6, 20 mg/1 tsp; suspension
Chlorpromazine	Thorazine	10, 25, 50, 100, 200 mg; tablets 5, 6, 20 mg/1 tsp; suspension
Mood stabilizers		
Lithium salts	Lithobid Lithonate Lithotabs Eskalith Cibalith	150, 300, 450 mg; tablets 8 mEq/1 tsp (= 300-mg tablet)
Carbamazepine	Tegretol Carbachol Equetrol	100, 200, 400 mg; tablets 100 mg/1 tsp; suspension
Oxcarbazepine	Trileptal	150, 300, 600 mg; tablets
Valproic acid	Valproate Depakote Depakene sprinkles	125, 250, 500 mg; tablets and capsules 250 mg/1 tsp; suspension
Gabapentin	Neurontin	100, 300, 400 mg; capsules 400, 600, 800 mg; tablets
Lamotrigine	Lamictal	25, 100, 150, 200 mg; tablets
Topiramate	Topamax	25, 100, 200 mg; tablets
Tiagabine	Gabitril	4, 12, 16, 20 mg; tablets

Medication		
Generic name	Brand name	Sizes and preparation

Anxiety-breaking agents (anxiolytics)

Antihistamines

Diphenhydramine	Benadryl	25, 50 mg; tablets 25 mg/1 tsp; suspension
Hydroxyzine	Vistaril, Atarax	25, 50 mg; tablets 2 mg/1 tsp; suspension
Chlorpheniramine maleate	Chlor-Trimeton	2, 4, 8 mg; tablets

Benzodiazepines (partial list)

Clonazepam	Klonopin	0.5, 1, 2 mg; tablets
Alprazolam	Xanax	0.25, 0.5, 1 mg; tablets
Triazolam	Halcion	0.5, 1, 2 mg; tablets
Lorazepam	Ativan	0.5, 1, 2 mg; tablets
Oxazepam	Serax	15, 30 mg; tablets
Diazepam	Valium	2, 5, 10 mg; tablets
Clorazepate	Tranxene	3.75, 7.5, 15 mg; capsules

Atypical

Buspirone	Buspar	5, 10, 15 mg; tablets
Zolpidem	Ambien	5, 10 mg; tablets
Zaleplon	Sonata	5, 10 mg; tablets
Eszopiclone	Lunesta	1, 2 mg; tablets

Miscellaneous

Naltrexone	ReVia, Trexan	25–150 mg; tablets
Naloxone	Narcan	1 mg/cc; intranasal

APPENDIX B
Medication Log

Example of a Completed Medication Log

Start/end date	Medication	Daily dose	Response	Side effect(s)	Comments
11/14–2/15	Concerta	36 mg	Good	Edginess	Good school performance
2/15–3/15	Focalin XR	30 mg	Very good	Edginess	Good school performance
2/15–4/15	Vyvanse	30 mg	Very good	Edginess Moodiness	Good school performance
4/15–7/15	Strattera	60 mg	Good	Tired	Good behavior, attention problems
7/15–	Strattera + Focalin XR	60 mg + 20 mg	Excellent	None	Good school performance and behavior Improved mood

Medication Log

Start/end date	Medication	Daily dose	Response	Side effect(s)	Comments

From *Straight Talk about Psychiatric Medications for Kids, Fourth Edition*, by Timothy E. Wilens and Paul G. Hammerness. Copyright © 2016 Timothy E. Wilens and Paul G. Hammerness. Purchasers of this book can photocopy and/or download enlarged versions of this material (see the box at the end of the table of contents).

Resources

The following are organizations addressing mental health issues in children and adolescents.

General Information

American Academy of Child and Adolescent Psychiatry (AACAP)
3615 Wisconsin Avenue, NW
Washington, DC 20016-3007
Phone: 202-966-7300
Fax: 202-966-2891
Website: *www.aacap.org*

The AACAP is the largest organization of child and adolescent psychiatrists who practice, research, and teach about the myriad mental health problems in youth. AACAP has superb educational materials for families.

American Academy of Pediatrics (AAP)
141 Northwest Point Boulevard
Elk Grove Village, IL 60007-1098
Phone: 847-434-4000
Fax: 847-434-8000
Website: *www.aap.org*

The AAP is the largest national organization of pediatricians. The academy has educational materials on common child psychiatric disorders.

American Foundation for Suicide Prevention (AFSP)
Website: *www.afsp.org*

Established privately in 1987, the foundation funds research, creates educational programs, advocates for public policy, and supports survivors of suicide loss.

American Psychiatric Association
1000 Wilson Boulevard, Suite 1825
Arlington, VA 22209-3901
Phone: 703-907-7300; toll free: 1-888-35-PSYCH (77924)
E-mail: *apa@psych.org*
Website: *www.psych.org*

The American Psychiatric Association is a broad-based organization with more than 36,000 physician members—the oldest medical specialty organization in the United States—that publishes the *Diagnostic and Statistical Manual of Mental Disorders* and many other resources for mental health professionals, establishes psychiatric practice standards, advocates for mental health patients, provides voluminous public information, and supports education and research.

American Psychological Association
Website: *www.apa.org*

The American Psychological Association is the leading scientific and professional organization representing psychology in the United States, with 120,000 members and 54 divisions in subfields of psychology.

American School Counselor Association (ASCA)
Website: *www.schoolcounselor.org*

The ASCA supports school counselors' efforts to help students focus on academic, career, and social/emotional development so they achieve success in school and are prepared to lead fulfilling lives as responsible members of society.

Brain and Behavior Research Foundation
90 Park Avenue, 16th floor
New York, NY 10016
Phone: 646-681-4888; Toll free: 800-829-8289
E-mail: *info@bbrfoundation.org*
Website: *https://bbrfoundation.org*

Mainly research-based, this organization sponsors small grants for studies related to mental illness. Members receive an acclaimed newsletter with timely findings on mental health.

Dana Foundation
E-mail: *dabiinfo@dana.org*
Website: *www.dana.org*

The Dana Foundation is a private philanthropic organization that supports brain research through grants, publications, and educational programs. It is also a source for accessing other sites on the web related to mental health and disabilities, and provides monthly updates on neuroscience content from around the world.

MIND (National Association for Mental Health United Kingdom)
15–19 Broadway
London E15 4BQ
United Kingdom
Phone: 44 (0)20 8519 2122
Website: *www.mind.org.uk*

This is the leading mental health charity in England and Wales, providing advice and support and campaigning to improve services, raise awareness, and promote understanding.

National Alliance on Mental Illness (NAMI)
Colonial Place Three
3803 North Fairfax Drive, Suite 100
Arlington, VA 22203
Phone: 703-524-7600; TDD: 703-516-7227; member services: 888-999-NAMI
Fax: 703-524-9094
Website: *www.nami.org*; *www.StrengthofUs.org*

NAMI is the nation's largest grassroots mental health organization dedicated to building better lives for the millions of Americans affected by mental illness. StrengthofUs.org is NAMI's online resource center and social networking website for young adults living with mental health conditions. It exists to empower young adults to live out their dreams and goals through peer support and resource sharing.

National Association of Social Workers (NASW)
Website: *www.naswdc.org*

The NASW is the largest membership organization of professional social workers in the world, with 132,000 members. NASW works to enhance the professional growth and development of its members, to create and maintain professional standards, and to advance sound social policies.

National Federation of Families for Children's Mental Health
15883A Crabbs Branch Way
Rockville, MD 20855
Phone: 240-403-1901
Fax: 240-403-1909
E-mail: *ffcmh@ffcmh.org*
Website: *www.ffcmh.org*

This is a national family-run organization linking more than 120 chapters and state organizations focused on the issues of children and youth with emotional, behavioral, or mental health needs and their families.

National Institute of Mental Health (NIMH)
Public Inquiries
6001 Executive Boulevard, Room 8184, MSC 9663
Bethesda, MD 20892-9663
Phone: 301-443-4513; Toll free: 866-615-NIMH (6464); TTY: 301-443-8431; Fax: 301-443-4279; FAX 4U: 301-443-5158
E-mail: *nimhinfo@nih.gov*
Website: *www.nimh.nih.gov*

This subsection of the U.S. Public Health Service is the major government agency involved in the research of juvenile behavioral, emotional, and cognitive disorders. The mission of NIMH is to transform the understanding and treatment of mental illnesses through basic and clinical research, paving the way for prevention, recovery, and cure.

National Mental Health Association (Mental Health America)
2000 North Beauregard Street, 6th floor
Alexandria, VA 22311
Phone: 800-969-NMHA, ext. 6642
Fax: 703-684-5968
Website: *www.nmha.org*

Founded in 1909, MHA is the nation's leading community-based nonprofit dedicated to helping all Americans achieve wellness by living mentally healthier lives.

School Psychiatry Program and the Mood & Anxiety Disorders Institute (MADI) Resource Center
Website: *www.schoolpsychiatry.org*

From the Department of Psychiatry at Massachusetts General Hospital (MGH), this website is committed to enhancing the education and mental health of every student in every school. The website has resources for parents, educators, and clinicians to ensure that all groups are working together to support children and teens with mental health conditions.

The Trevor Project
Website: *www.thetrevorproject.org*

Founded in 1998 by the creators of the Academy Award–winning short film *Trevor*, the Trevor Project is the leading national organization providing crisis intervention and suicide prevention services to lesbian, gay, bisexual, transgender, and questioning (LGBTQ) young people ages 13–24.

Anxiety Disorders

Anxiety and Depression Association of America (ADAA)
8701 Georgia Avenue, Suite 412
Silver Spring, MD 20910
Phone: 240-485-1001
Website: *http://www.adaa.org*

The association's mission is to promote the prevention, treatment, and cure of anxiety and mood disorders, OCD, and PTSD through education, practice, and research.

Freedom from Fear
308 Seaview Avenue
Staten Island, NY 10305
Phone: 718-351-1717, ext. 24
Fax: 718-980-5022
E-mail: *help@freedomfromfear.org*
Website: *www.freedomfromfear.org*

Founded in 1984, Freedom from Fear is a national not-for-profit mental health advocacy organization.

Selective Mutism Foundation
P.O. Box 13133
Sissonville, WV 25360-0133
Website: *www.selectivemutismfoundation.org*

This is a nonprofit, public service organization whose mission since 1991 has been to broaden public awareness and understanding of selective mutism.

Attention-Deficit/Hyperactivity Disorder

Attention Deficit Disorder Association (ADDA)
P.O. Box 7557
Wilmington, DE 19803-1019
Phone/Fax: 800-939-1019
E-mail: *info@add.org*
Website: *www.add.org*

ADDA is an international nonprofit organization founded in 1990 to help adults with attention-deficit/hyperactivity disorder (ADHD) lead better lives.

Canadian ADHD Resource Alliance (CADRA)
3950 14th Avenue, Suite 604
Markham, Ontario L3R 0A9, Canada
Phone: 416-637-8583
Fax: 905-475-3232
Website: *www.caddra.ca*

CADDRA is a Canadian nonprofit, multidisciplinary alliance of health care professionals working in the field of ADHD. It produces the Canadian ADHD Practice Guidelines and assessment tool kits. CADDRA provides education, training, and support on ADHD for health care clinicians through annual national conferences and training courses.

Children and Adults with Attention Deficit/Hyperactivity Disorder (CHADD)
8181 Professional Place, Suite 150
Landover, MD 20785
Phone: 800-233-4050
Fax: 301-306-7090
Website: *www.chadd.org*

CHADD is a national nonprofit organization providing education, advocacy, and support for individuals with ADHD. CHADD sponsors an annual conference to provide a comprehensive understanding and update of research on ADHD. The group also provides referrals to local practitioners knowledgeable in the diagnosis and treatment of ADHD as well as local support groups.

Autism Spectrum Disorder

Autism Research Institute (ARI)
4182 Adams Avenue
San Diego, CA 92116
Phone: 866-366-3361
Fax: 619-563-6840
Website: *www.autism.com/ari*

Established in 1967 by Dr. Bernard Rimland, ARI is a pioneer in research, outreach, and cooperative efforts with other organizations worldwide. ARI advocates for the rights of people with ASD.

Autism Society of America
4340 East–West Highway, Suite 350
Bethesda, MD 20814
Phone: 800-3AUTISM
Website: *www.autism-society.org*

Founded in 1965 by Drs. Bernard Rimland and Ruth Sullivan and by parents of children with autism, the Autism Society is a leading source of information about autism. Its Autism Source online resource database contains over 30,000 listings of local autism service providers with a contact center available to take calls, e-mails, and letters.

Autism Speaks
1 East 33rd Street, 4th floor
New York, NY 10016
Phone: 212-252-8584
Fax: 212-252-8676
Website: *https://www.autismspeaks.org*

Autism Speaks was founded in February 2005 by Bob and Suzanne Wright, grandparents of a child with autism. Since then, Autism Speaks has grown into a leading autism science and advocacy organization, dedicated to funding research into the causes, prevention, treatments, and a cure for autism; increasing awareness of autism spectrum disorders; and advocating for the needs of individuals with autism and their families. Autism Response Team (ART) members are available to connect families with information, resources, and opportunities.

The National Autistic Society (United Kingdom)
393 City Road
London EC1V 1NG
United Kingdom
Phone: 44 (0)20 7833 2299
Fax: 44 (0)20 7833 9666
E-mail: *nas@nas.org.uk*
Website: *www.nas.org.uk*

This is the leading U.K. charity for people on the autism spectrum and their families, providing information, support, and pioneering services and campaigns for a better world for people with autism.

Eating Disorders

Beat: Beating Eating Disorders (United Kingdom)
Windsor House, 1st floor
103 Prince of Wales Road
Norwich NR1 1DW, United Kingdom
Phone: 44 (0)16 0361 9090
Helpline: 44 (0)34 5634 1414; Youth Helpline: 44 (0)34 5634 7650
Website: *www.b-eat.co.uk*

Beat is the United Kingdom's leading charity supporting anyone affected by eating disorders or difficulties with food, weight, and shape. Features a self-help network and wide range of resources for getting help.

Eating Disorders Association (Australia)
12 Chatsworth Road
Greenslopes, Queensland 4120, Australia
Phone: (07)3394 3661
Fax: (07)3394 3663
E-mail: *admin@eda.org.au*
Website: *www.eda.org.au*

This is a nonprofit organization dedicated to improving intervention, education, and support for those with eating disorders as well as to improving awareness and promoting prevention.

National Eating Disorders Association (NEDA)
603 Stewart Street, Suite 803
Seattle, WA 98101
Phone: 206-382-3587; Toll free: 800-931-2237
Website: *www.nationaleatingdisorders.org*

NEDA was formed in 2001, when Eating Disorders Awareness & Prevention (EDAP) joined the American Anorexia Bulimia Association (AABA)—merging the largest and longest-standing eating disorders prevention and advocacy organizations in the world. The merger was the most recent in a series of alliances that has also included the National Eating Disorder Organization (NEDO) and Anorexia Nervosa & Related Disorders (ANRED). The organization develops prevention programs, publishes and distributes educational materials, and operates the nation's first toll-free eating disorders information and referral helpline.

Mood Disorders

Bipolar UK (United Kingdom)
11 Belgrave Road
London SW1V 1RB, United Kingdom
Website: *www.bipolaruk.org.uk*

Bipolar UK is the national charity dedicated to supporting individuals with bipolar disorder and their families and carers.

Child and Adolescent Bipolar Foundation
820 Davis Street, Suite 520
Evanston, IL 60201
Phone: 847-492-8519
E-mail: *cabf@bpkids.org*
Website: *www.bpkids.org*

The Child and Adolescent Bipolar Foundation educates families, professionals, and the public about pediatric bipolar disorder; connects families with resources and support; advocates for and empowers affected families; and supports research on pediatric bipolar disorder and its cure.

Depression and Bipolar Support Alliance (DBSA)
730 North Franklin Street, Suite 501
Chicago, IL 60654-7225
Phone: 800-826-3632
Fax: 312-642-7243
Website: *www.dbsalliance.org*

The DBSA is a leading peer-directed national organization that reaches millions of people each year with in-person and online peer support through more than 700 support groups and nearly 300 chapters. The Balanced Mind Parent Network (BMPN) program guides families raising children with mood disorders to the answers, support, and stability they seek.

Depression Alliance (United Kingdom)
212 Spitfire Studios
63-71 Collier Street
London N1 9BE, United Kingdom
Phone: 0845 123 23 20
E-mail: *information@depressionalliance.org*
Website: *www.depressionalliance.org*

Depression Alliance is a leading charity in the United Kingdom for anyone affected by depression and can help people meet and chat with others, join a self-help group, and learn more about depression, treatment, and recovery.

Families for Depression Awareness
Website: *http://familyaware.org*

This is a national nonprofit organization helping families recognize and cope with depression and bipolar disorder to get people well and prevent suicides. It offers depression wellness guides for adults, for teens, and for parents of teens and children with depression.

Obsessive–Compulsive Disorder and Tourette's Disorder

National Institute of Neurological Disorders and Stroke (NINDS)
NIH Neurological Institute
P.O. Box 5801
Bethesda, MD 20824
Phone: 301-496-5751; Toll free: 800-352-9424
Website: *www.ninds.nih.gov*

The NINDS is a national organization that supports and performs basic, translational, and clinical neuroscience research, funds and conducts research training and career development programs, and promotes the dissemination of scientific discoveries and their implications for neurological health to the public, health professionals, researchers, and policy makers.

International OCD Foundation
112 Water Street, Suite 501
Boston, MA 02109
Phone: 617-973-5801
Website: *www.ocfoundation.org*

The International OCD Foundation is a donor-supported nonprofit membership-based organization founded in 1986 by a small group of individuals with OCD. The foundation serves a broad community of individuals with OCD and related disorders, their family members, and mental health professionals and researchers. There are affiliates in 25 states and territories in the United States, in addition to global partnerships with other OCD organizations and mental health nonprofits around the world.

Tourette Association of America
42-40 Bell Boulevard, Suite 205
Bayside, NY 11361-2820
Phone: 718-224-2999
Fax: 718-279-9596
Website: *www.tsa-usa.org*

Founded in 1972, the Tourette Association of America is the only national voluntary nonprofit membership organization in this field. This organization fosters advocacy, education, and research about Tourette. They offer publications, events, conferences, grants, and government outreach.

Trichotillomania Learning Center (TLC)
207 McPherson Street, Suite H
Santa Cruz, CA 95060-5863
Phone: 831-457-1004
Fax: 831-426-4383
E-mail: *info@trich.org*
Website: *www.trich.org*

Founded in 1991, TLC provides education, outreach, and support of research into the cause and treatment of hair-pulling disorder, skin-picking disorder, and related body-focused repetitive behaviors.

Psychosis

International Early Psychosis Association (Australia)
P.O. Box 143
Parkville, Victoria 3052, Australia
Phone: 61 3 8346 8256
E-mail: *secretariat@iepa.org.au*
Website: *www.iepa.org.au*

This international organization based in Australia provides a forum for international collaboration and communication on psychosis in young people by facilitating research and optimal diagnostic and treatment practices, arranging conferences, and advocating public policies that will improve services to patients.

National Schizophrenic Fellowship (Rethink) (United Kingdom)
89 Albert Embankment
London SE1 7TP, United Kingdom
Phone: 44 (0)84 5456 0455; National advice hotline: 44 (0)20 7840 3188
E-mail: *info@rethink.org*
Website: *www.rethink.org*

The United Kingdom's largest nonprofit organization devoted to severe mental illness provides a wide range of community services aimed at allowing patients to take greater control of their lives and also advocates for policies and practices that will support that goal and the goals of increasing awareness and reducing stigma.

Sleep Disorders

American Academy of Sleep Medicine
One Westbrook Corporate Center, Suite 920
Westchester, IL 60154
Phone: 708-492-0930
Fax: 708-492-0943
Website: *www.aasmnet.org*

This national professional organization provides patient resources, from a sleep quiz to locations of sleep centers across the United States to links to related sites.

National Center on Sleep Disorders Research
National Heart, Lung, and Blood Institute
6701 Rockledge Drive
Bethesda, MD 20892-7993
Phone: 301-435-0199
Fax: 301-480-3451
Website: *www.nhlbi.nih.gov/about/ncsdr*

This is a government-funded organization that has information available about sleep-related problems.

Substance Abuse

Canadian Centre on Substance Abuse
75 Albert Street, Suite 500
Ottawa ON K1P 5E7, Canada
Phone: 613-235-4048
Fax: 613-235-8101
E-mail: *info@ccsa.ca*
Website: *www.ccsa.ca*

The Canadian Centre on Substance Abuse, Canada's 15-year-old national addictions agency, provides helplines, toolkits, directories, news archives, informational databases, prevention activities, and links to other sites.

National Addiction Centre (United Kingdom)
Institute of Psychiatry, Addictions Research Unit
King's College London
P.O. Box 48
4 Windsor Walk
London SE5 8BB, United Kingdom
Phone: 44 (0)20 7848 0438
E-mail: *d.mellors@iop.kcl.ac.uk*
Website: *www.iop.kcl.ac.uk/Departments/?Locator=346*

The National Addiction Centre is a network of clinicians, researchers, and clinical teachers sharing a commitment to excellence in work directed at the prevention and treatment of substance misuse, and to the support and strengthening of national and international endeavors in this field.

National Institute on Alcohol Abuse and Alcoholism (NIAAA)
5635 Fishers Lane, MSC 9304
Bethesda, MD 20892-9304
Phone: 301-443-3860
E-mail: *niaaaweb-r@exchange.nih.gov*
Website: *www.niaaa.nih.gov*

National Institute on Drug Abuse (NIDA)
6001 Executive Boulevard, Room 5213
Bethesda, MD 20892-9561
Phone: 800-729-6686 (for information on drug abuse); Toll-free: 800-662-4357 (for information on counselors and treatment facilities)
Website: *www.nida.nih.gov*

These subsections of the U.S. Public Health Service are the major government agencies involved in the research of juvenile and adult drug and alcohol use, misuse, abuse, and dependence. In addition to providing funding for a variety of research activities, NIDA and NIAAA are involved in conferences and public policy. NIDA has an incredibly informative and user-friendly website—one of the best we have seen.

Network of Alcohol and Other Drugs Agencies (Australia)
P.O. Box 2345
Strawberry Hills, New South Wales 2012, Australia
Phone: 61(02) 9698 8669
Fax: 61(02) 9690 0727
E-mail: *admin@nada.org.au*
Website: *www.nada.org.au*

This is the principal organization for the public alcohol and drug sector throughout New South Wales, funded by NSW Health, with a membership made up of over 100 agencies. It is a good source of information on policy issues and advocacy.

Pharmaceutical Companies

Most of the medications listed in this book have a dedicated website sponsored by the respective pharmaceutical company. Many of these are accessed by typing the medication (usually the brand name) into your search engine or by using *www.[drugname].com*. These sites often contain detailed information about side effects and FDA-approved use of these compounds. Some of the websites have links to other websites of interest, many of which are maintained by nonprofit organizations.

Bibliography

General

Baldessarini, R. J. (2013). *Chemotherapy in Psychiatry: Pharmacologic Basis of Treatments for Major Mental Illness* (3rd ed.). Springer, New York.

Brown, R. T., Carpenter, L. A., & Simerly, E. (2005). *Mental Health Medications for Children: A Primer*. Guilford Press, New York.

Dulcan, M. (2010). *Textbook of Child and Adolescent Psychiatry*. American Psychiatric Press, Washington, DC.

Gleason M. M., Egger, H. L., Emslie, G. J., Greenhill, L. L., Kowatch, R. A., Lieberman, A. F., et al. (2007). Psychopharmacological treatment for very young children: Contexts and guidelines. *Journal of the American Academy of Child and Adolescent Psychiatry, 46*(12), 1532–1572.

Greene, R. W. (1998). *The Explosive Child: A New Approach for Understanding and Parenting Easily Frustrated, "Chronically Inflexible" Children*. HarperCollins, New York.

Klykylo, W., Bowers, R., Jackson, J., & Weston, C. (2013). *Green's Child and Adolescent Clinical Psychopharmacology* (5th ed.). Lippincott Williams & Wilkins, Philadelphia.

Martin, A., Scahill, L., & Kratchovil, C. (2013). *Pediatric Psychopharmacology* (2nd ed.). Oxford University Press, New York.

Merikangas, K. (2010). Lifetime prevalence of mental disorders in US adolescents: Results from the National Comorbidity Study—Adolescent Supplement (NCS-A). *Journal of the American Academy of Child and Adolescent Psychiatry, 49*(10), 980–989.

Plizka, S. R. (2003). *Neuroscience for the Mental Health Clinician*. Guilford Press, New York.

Rosenberg, D. R., Hottum, J., & Gershon, S. (Eds.). (2012). *Pharmacotherapy of Child and Adolescent Psychiatric Disorders*. Wiley, Chichester, UK.

Rutter, M., & Rutter, M. (1993). *Developing Minds*. HarperCollins, New York.

Stahl, S. M. (2013). *Essential Psychopharmacology: Neuroscientific Basis and Practical Applications*. Cambridge University Press, Cambridge, UK.

Swedo, S., & Leonard, H. (1996). *It's Not All in Your Head*. HarperCollins, San Francisco.

Wilens, T., & Kratchovil, C. (2015). Pharmacotherapy. In B. Sadock, V. Sadock, & P. Ruiz. (Eds.), *Kaplan and Sadock's Synopsis of Psychiatry* (11th ed., pp. 1295–1300). Wolters Kluwer, New York.

Anxiety Disorders

Barlow, D. H. (2002). *Anxiety and Its Disorders: The Nature and Treatment of Anxiety and Panic* (2nd ed.). Guilford Press, New York.

Beck, A. (1990). *Anxiety Disorders and Phobias: A Cognitive Perspective* (rev. ed.). Basic Books, New York.

Birmaher, B., Waterman, G. S., Ryan, N., Cully, M., Balach, L., Ingram, J., et al. (1994). Fluoxetine for childhood anxiety disorders. *Journal of the American Academy of Child and Adolescent Psychiatry, 33*(7), 993–999.

Clark, D. B., Smith, M. G., Neighbors, B. D., Skerlec, L. M., & Randall, J. (1994). Anxiety disorders in adolescence: Characteristics, prevalence, and comorbidities. *Clinical Psychology Review, 14*(2), 113–137.

Connolly, S. D., Bernstein, G. A., & the Work Group on Quality Issues. (2007). Practice parameter for the assessment and treatment of children and adolescents with anxiety disorders. *Journal of the American Academy of Child and Adolescent Psychiatry, 46*(2), 267–283.

Davidson, J. (2003). *The Anxiety Book: Developing Strength in the Face of Fear*. Riverhead Books, New York.

Klein, R. G., & Last, C. G. (1989). *Developmental Clinical Psychology and Psychiatry: Vol. 20. Anxiety Disorders in Children*. Sage, Newbury Park, CA.

Last, C. G. (2006). *Help for Worried Kids: How Your Child Can Conquer Anxiety and Fear*. Guilford Press, New York.

Last, C. G., Perrin, S., Hersen, M., & Kazdin, A. E. (1996). A prospective study of childhood anxiety disorders. *Journal of the American Academy of Child and Adolescent Psychiatry, 35*(11), 1502–1510.

Pediatric OCD Treatment Study (POTS) Team. (2004). Cognitive-behavior therapy, sertraline, and their combination for children and adolescents with obsessive-compulsive disorder: The Pediatric OCD Treatment Study (POTS) randomized controlled trial. *Journal of the American Medical Association, 292*(16), 1969–1976.

Piacentini, J., Bennett, S., Compton, S. N., Kendall, P. C., Birmaher, B., Albano, A. M., et al. (2014). 24- and 36-week outcomes for the Child/Adolescent Anxiety Multimodal Study (CAMS). *Journal of the American Academy of Child and Adolescent Psychiatry, 53*(3), 297–310.

Pine, D. S. (2002). Treating children and adolescents with selective serotonin reuptake inhibitors: How long is appropriate? *Journal of Child and Adolescent Psychopharmacology, 12*(3), 189–203.

Strawn, J. R., Welge, J. A., Wehry, A. M., Keeshin, B., & Rynn, M. A. (2014). Efficacy and tolerability of antidepressants in pediatric anxiety disorders: A systematic review and meta-analysis. *Depression and Anxiety, 32*(3), 149–157.

Swedo, S. E., Fleeter, J. D., Richter, D. M., Hoffman, C. L., Allen, A. J., Hamburger, S. D., et al. (1995). Rates of seasonal affective disorder in children and adolescents. *American Journal of Psychiatry, 152*(7), 1016–1019.

Walkup, J., Albano, A., Piacentini, J., Birmaher, B., Compton, S., Sherrill, J., et al. (2008). Cognitive behavioral therapy, sertraline, or a combination in childhood anxiety. *New England Journal of Medicine, 359*(26), 2753–2766.

Walkup, J., Labellarte, M. J., Riddle, M., Pine, D. S., Greenhill, L., Klein, R., et al. (2001). Fluvoxamine for the treatment of anxiety disorders in children and adolescents: The Research Unit on Pediatric Psychopharmacology Anxiety Study Group. *New England Journal of Medicine, 344*(17), 1279–1285.

Attention-Deficit/Hyperactivity Disorder

Abikoff, H., Hechtman, L., Klein, R. G., Weiss, G., Fleiss, K., Etcovitch, J., et al. Symptomatic improvement in children with ADHD treated with long-term methylphenidate and multimodal psychosocial treatment. *Journal of the American Academy of Child and Adolescent Psychiatry, 43*(7), 802–811.

Adler, L., Spencer, T., & Wilens, T. (2015). *ADHD in Adults and Children*. Cambridge University Press, Cambridge, UK.

Barkley, R. A. (1997). *ADHD and the Nature of Self-Control*. Guilford Press, New York.

Barkley, R. A. (Ed.). (2015). *Attention-Deficit Hyperactivity Disorder: A Handbook for Diagnosis and Treatment* (4th ed.). Guilford Press, New York.

Barkley, R. A., Edwards, G., Laneri, M., Fletcher, K., & Metevia, L. (2001). Executive functioning, temporal discounting, and sense of time in adolescents with attention deficit hyperactivity disorder (ADHD) and oppositional defiant disorder (ODD). *Journal of Abnormal Child Psychology, 29*(6), 541–555.

Biederman, J., Faraone, S. V., & Mick, E. (2000). Age dependent decline of ADHD symptoms revisited: Impact of remission definition and symptom subtype. *American Journal of Psychiatry, 157,* 816–817.

Biederman, J., Melmed, R., Patel, A., McBurnett, K., Konow, J., Lyne, A., et al. (2008). A randomized, double blind, placebo controlled study of guanfacine extended release in children and adolescents with ADHD. *Pediatrics, 121,* 373–384.

Biederman, J., Newcorn, J., & Sprich, S. (1991). Comorbidity of attention deficit hyperactivity disorder with conduct, depressive, anxiety, and other disorders. *American Journal of Psychiatry, 148,* 564–577.

Biederman, J., & Spencer, T. (1999). Attention deficit hyperactivity disorder (ADHD) as a noradrenergic disorder. *Biological Psychiatry, 46*(9), 1234–1242.

Brown, T. (1999). *Subtypes of Attention Deficit Disorders in Children, Adolescents, and Adults*. American Psychiatric Press, Washington, DC.

Conners, C., & Jett, J. (1999). *Attention Deficit Hyperactivity Disorder (in Adults and Children): The Latest Assessment and Treatment Strategies*. Compact Clinicals, Salt Lake City.

Connor, D. (1993). Beta-blockers for aggression: The pediatric experience. *Journal of Child and Adolescent Psychopharmacology, 3*(2), 99–114.

Geller, D., Donnelly, C., Lopez, F., Rubin, R., Newcorn, J., Sutton, V., et al. (2007). Atomoxetine treatment for pediatric patients with attention-deficit/hyperactivity disorder with comorbid anxiety disorder. *Journal of the American Academy of Child and Adolescent Psychiatry, 46*(9), 1119–1127.

Goldman, L., Genel, M., Bezman, R., & Slanetz, P. (1998). Diagnosis and treatment of attention-deficit/hyperactivity disorder in children and adolescents. *Journal of the American Medical Association, 279*(4), 1100–1107.

Greenhill, L. L., Kollins, S., Abikoff, H., McCracken, J., Riddle, M., Swanson, J., et al. (2006). Efficacy and safety of immediate-release methylphenidate treatment for preschoolers with ADHD. *Journal of the American Academy of Child and Adolescent Psychiatry, 45*(11), 1284–1293.

Greenhill, L. L., & Osman, B. B. (1991). *Ritalin: Theory and Patient Management.* Liebert, New York.

Greenhill, L. L., & Osman, B. B. (Eds.). (1999). *Ritalin: Theory and Practice.* Liebert, New York.

Greenhill, L. L., Pliszka, S., Dulcan, M. K., Bernet, W., Arnold, V., Beitchman, J., et al. (2002). Practice parameter for the use of stimulant medications in the treatment of children, adolescents, and adults. *Journal of the American Academy of Child and Adolescent Psychiatry, 41*(Suppl. 2), 26S–49S.

Hammerness, P., & Moore, M. (2011). *Organize Your Mind, Organize Your Life: Train Your Brain to Get More Done in Less Time.* Harlequin Press, New York.

Hammerness, P., Perrin, J., Shelley-Abrahamson, R., & Wilens, T. E. (2011). Cardiovascular risk of stimulant treatment in pediatric attention deficit hyperactivity disorder: Update and clinical recommendations. *Journal of the American Academy of Child and Adolescent Psychiatry, 50*(10), 978–990.

Hunt, R. D., Minderaa, R. B., & Cohen, D. J. (1985). Clonidine benefits children with attention deficit disorder and hyperactivity: Report of a double-blind placebo-crossover therapeutic trial. *Journal of the American Academy of Child and Adolescent Psychiatry, 24*(5), 617–629.

Jensen, P. S., Arnold, E. L., Swanson, J. M., Vitiello, B., Abikoff, H. B., Greenhill, L. L., et al. (2007). 3-year follow-up of the NIMH MTA Study. *Journal of the American Academy of Child and Adolescent Psychiatry, 46*(8), 989–1002.

Kolberg, J., & Nadeau, K. (2002). *ADD-Friendly Ways to Organize Your Life.* Brunner-Routledge, New York.

Mannuzza, S., Klein, R. G., Bessler, A., Malloy, P., & LaPadula, M. (1993). Adult outcome of hyperactive boys: Educational achievement, occupational rank, and psychiatric status. *Archives of General Psychiatry, 50*(7), 565–576.

Mannuzza, S., Klein, R. G., Bonagura, N., Malloy, P., Giampino, T. L., & Addalli, K. A. (1991). Hyperactive boys almost grown up: V. Replication of psychiatric status. *Archives of General Psychiatry, 48*(1), 77–83.

MTA Cooperative Group. (1999). A 14-month randomized clinical trial of treatment strategies for attention-deficit/hyperactivity disorder. *Archives of General Psychiatry, 56*(12), 1073–1086.

Pelham, W. E., Greenslade, K. E., Vodde-Hamilton, M., Murphy, D. A., Greenstein, J. J., Gnagy, E. M., et al. (1990). Relative efficacy of long-acting stimulants on children with attention-deficit/hyperactivity disorder: A comparison of standard methylphenidate, sustained-release methylphenidate, sustained-release dextroamphetamine, and pemoline. *Pediatrics, 86,* 226–237.

Pliszka, S., & the AACAP Work Group on Quality Issues. (2007). Practice parameter for the assessment and treatment of children and adolescents with attention-deficit/hyperactivity disorder. *Journal of the American Academy of Child and Adolescent Psychiatry, 46*(7), 894–921.

Safer, D. J., & Allen, R. P. (1989). Absence of tolerance to the behavioral effects of methylphenidate in hyperactive and inattentive children. *Journal of Pediatrics, 115*(6), 1003–1008.

Safer, D. J., & Zito, J. M. (1996). Increased methylphenidate usage for ADHD. *Pediatrics, 98*(6), 1084–1088.

Safer, D., & Zito, J. M. (1999). Pharmacoepidemiology of methylphenidate and other stimulants for the treatment of ADHD. In L. Greenhill & B. Osman (Eds.), *Ritalin: Theory and Practice* (pp. 7–26). Liebert, New York.

Spencer, T. J., Biederman, J., Faraone, S., Mick, E., Coffey, B., Geller, D., et al. (2001). Impact of tic disorders on ADHD outcome across the life cycle: Findings from a large group of adults with and without ADHD. *American Journal of Psychiatry, 158*(4), 611–617.

Spencer, T. J., Abikoff, H. B., Connor, D. F., Biederman, J., Pliszka, S. R., Boellner, S., et al. (2006). Efficacy and safety of mixed amphetamine salts extended release (Adderall XR) in the management of oppositional defiant disorder with or without comorbid attention-deficit/hyperactivity disorder in school-aged children and adolescents: A 4-week, multicenter, randomized, double-blind, parallel-group, placebo-controlled, forced-dose-escalation study. *Clinical Therapeutics, 28*(3), 402–418.

Swanson, J., Lerner, M., Gupta, S., Shoulson, I., & Wigal, S. (2003). Development of a new once-a-day formulation of methylphenidate for the treatment of ADHD: Proof of concept and proof of product studies. *Archives of General Psychiatry, 60*(2), 204–211.

Umansky, W. (2003). *AD/HD: Helping Your Child: A Comprehensive Program to Treat Attention Deficit/Hyperactivity Disorders at Home and in School.* Warner Books, New York.

Weiss, G. (1992). *Attention-Deficit Hyperactivity Disorder.* Saunders, Philadelphia.

Weiss, G., & Hechtman, L. T. (1993). *Hyperactive Children Grown Up: ADHD in Children, Adolescents, and Adults* (2nd ed.). Guilford Press, New York.

Wender, P. (1987). *The Hyperactive Child, Adolescent, and Adult: Attention Deficit Disorder through the Lifespan.* Oxford University Press, New York.

Wilens, T., Biederman, J., & Spencer, T. (2002). Attention deficit/hyperactivity disorder across the lifespan. *Annual Review of Medicine, 53,* 113–131.

Wilens, T., Hammerness, P., Utzinger, L., Schillinger, M., Georgiopoulos, A., Doyle, R., et al. (2009). An open study of adjunct OROS methylphenidate in children and adolescents who are atomoxetine partial responders: Efficacy. *Journal of Child and Adolescent Psychopharmacology, 19*(5), 485–492.

Wilens, T. E., Bukstein, O., Brams, M., Cutler, A., Childress, A. Rugino, T., et al. (2012). A controlled trial of extended-release guanfacine and psychostimulants for attention-deficit/hyperactivity disorder. *Journal of the American Academy of Child and Adolescent Psychiatry, 51*(1), 74–85.

Wolraich, M. L., Lindgren, S. D., Stumbo, P. J., Stegink, L. D., Appelbaum, M. I., & Kiritsy, M. C. (1994). Effects of diets high in sucrose or aspartame on the behavior and cognitive performance of children. *New England Journal of Medicine, 330,* 301–307.

Autism Spectrum Disorder

Aman, M. G., De Smedt, G., Derivan, A., Lyons, B., & Findling, R. L. (2002). Double-blind, placebo-controlled study of risperidone for the treatment of disruptive behaviors in children with subaverage intelligence. *American Journal of Psychiatry, 159*(8), 1337–1346.

Attwood, T. (1998). *Asperger's Syndrome: A Guide for Parents and Professionals.* Kingsley, Philadelphia.
Campbell, M. (1984). Fenfluramine treatment of autism. *Journal of Child Psychology and Psychiatry and Allied Disciplines, 29,* 1–10.
Campbell, M., Small, A., & Green, W. (1984). Behavioral efficacy of haloperidol and lithium carbonate. *Archives of General Psychiatry, 41*(7), 650–656.
Feldman, H. M., Kolmen, B. K., & Gonzaga, A. M. (1999). Naltrexone and communication skills in young children with autism. *Journal of the American Academy of Child and Adolescent Psychiatry, 38*(5), 587–593.
McCracken, J. T., McGough, J., Shah, B., Cronin, P., Hong, D., Aman, M. G., et al. (2002). Risperidone in children with autism and serious behavioral problems. *New England Journal of Medicine, 347*(5), 314–321.
McDougle, C. J., Scahill, L., Aman, M. G., McCracken, J. T., Tierney, E., Davies, M., et al. (2005). Risperidone for the core symptom domains of autism: Results from the study by the autism network of the research units on pediatric psychopharmacology. *American Journal of Psychiatry, 162*(6), 1142–1148.
Ozonoff, S., Dawson, G., & McPartland, J. (2002). *A Parent's Guide to Asperger Syndrome and High-Functioning Autism: How to Meet the Challenges and Help Your Child Thrive.* Guilford Press, New York.
Research Units on Pediatric Psychopharmacology Autism Network. (2005). Randomized, controlled crossover trial of methylphenidate in pervasive developmental disorders with hyperactivity. *Archives of General Psychiatry, 62*(11), 1266–1274.
Ritvo, E. R., Freeman, B. J., Yuwiler, A., Geller, E., Yokota, A., Schroth, P., et al. (1984). Study of fenfluramine in outpatients with the syndrome of autism. *Journal of Pediatrics, 105*(5), 823–828.
Siegel, B. (2008). *Getting the Best for Your Child with Autism: An Expert's Guide to Treatment.* Guilford Press, New York.
Snyder, R., Turgay, A., Aman, M., Binder, C., Fisman, S., & Carroll, A. (2002). Effects of risperidone on conduct and disruptive behavior disorders in children with subaverage IQs. *Journal of the American Academy of Child and Adolescent Psychiatry, 41*(9), 1026–1036.
Szatmari, P. (2004). *A Mind Apart: Understanding Children with Autism and Asperger Syndrome.* Guilford Press, New York.
Unis, A. S., Munson, J. A., Rogers, S. J., Goldson, E., Osterling, J., Gabriels, R., et al. (2002). A randomized, double-blind, placebo-controlled trial of porcine versus synthetic secretion for reducing symptoms of autism. *Journal of the American Academy of Child and Adolescent Psychiatry, 41*(11), 1315–1321.
Waltz, M. (2002). *Autistic Spectrum Disorders: Understanding the Diagnosis and Getting Help* (2nd ed.). O'Reilly, Sebastopol, CA.
Yapko, D. (2003). *Understanding Autism Spectrum Disorders: Frequently Asked Questions.* Kingsley, London.

Bipolar Disorder

Biederman, J., Mick, E., Faraone, S. V., Spencer, T., Wilens, T. E., & Wozniak, J. (2000). Pediatric mania: A developmental subtype of bipolar disorder? *Biological Psychiatry, 48*(6), 458–466.
Correll, C. U. (2007). Weight gain and metabolic effects of mood stabilizers and anti-

psychotics in pediatric bipolar disorder: A systematic review and pooled analysis of short-term trials. *Journal of the American Academy of Child and Adolescent Psychiatry, 46*(6), 687–700.

DelBello, M. P., Kowatch, R. A., Warner, J., Schwiers, M. L., Rappaport, K. B., Daniels, J. P., et al. (2000). Adjunctive topiramate treatment for pediatric bipolar disorder: A retrospective chart review. *Journal of Child and Adolescent Psychopharmacology, 12*(4), 323–330.

Findling, R., Kowatch, R., & Post, R. (2003). *Pediatric Bipolar Disorder.* Dunitz, London.

Geller, B., Cooper, T. B., Sun, K., Zimerman, B., Frazier, J., Williams, M., et al. (1998). Double-blind and placebo-controlled study of lithium for adolescent bipolar disorders with secondary substance dependency. *Journal of the American Academy of Child and Adolescent Psychiatry, 37*(2), 171–178.

Geller, B., Craney, J. L., Bolhofner, K., Nickelsburg, M. J., Williams, M., & Zimerman, B. (2002). Two-year prospective follow-up of children with a prepubertal and early adolescent bipolar disorder phenotype. *American Journal of Psychiatry, 159*(6), 927–933.

Geller, B., & DelBello, M. (2011). *Treatment of Bipolar Disorder in Children and Adolescents.* Guilford Press, New York.

Kowatch, R. A., Fristad, M., Birmaher, B., Wagner, K. D., Findling, R. L., & Hellander, M. (2005). Treatment guidelines for children and adolescents with bipolar disorder. *Journal of the American Academy of Child and Adolescent Psychiatry, 44*(3), 213–235.

Kowatch, R. A., Suppes, T., Carmody, T. J., Bucci, J. P., Hume, J. H., Kromelis, M., et al. (2000). Effect size of lithium, divalproex sodium, and carbamazepine in children and adolescents with bipolar disorder. *Journal of the American Academy of Child and Adolescent Psychiatry, 39*(6), 713–720.

McClellan, J., Kowatch, R., Findling, R. L., & Work Group on Quality Issues. (2007). Practice parameter for the assessment and treatment of children and adolescents with bipolar disorder. *Journal of the American Academy of Child and Adolescent Psychiatry, 46*(1), 107–125.

McElroy, S., Strakowski, S., West, S., Keck, P., & McConville, B. (1997). Phenomenology of adolescent and adult mania in hospitalized patients with bipolar disorder. *American Journal of Psychiatry, 154*(1), 44–49.

Miklowitz, D. J. (2011). *The Bipolar Disorder Survival Guide: What You and Your Family Need to Know* (2nd ed.). Guilford Press, New York.

Miklowitz, D. J., & George, E. L. (2008). *The Bipolar Teen: What You Can Do to Help Your Child and Your Family.* Guilford Press, New York.

Papolos, D. (2002). *The Bipolar Child: The Definitive and Reassuring Guide to Childhood's Most Misunderstood Disorder* (rev. and exp. ed.). Broadway Books, New York.

Pavuluri, M. (2008). *What Works for Bipolar Kids: Help and Hope for Parents.* Guilford Press, New York.

Strakowski, S., DelBello, M., & Adler, C. (Eds.). (2015). *Bipolar Disorder in Youth: Presentation, Treatment, and Neurobiology.* Oxford University Press, New York.

Strober, M., Morrell, W., Lampert, C., & Burroughs, J. (1990). Relapse following discontinuation of lithium maintenance therapy in adolescents with bipolar I illness: A naturalistic study. *American Journal of Psychiatry, 147*(4), 457–461.

Tohen, M., Kryzhanovskaya, L., Carlson, G., DelBello, M., Wozniak, J., Kowatch, R., et al. (2007). Olanzapine versus placebo in the treatment of adolescents with bipolar mania. *American Journal of Psychiatry, 164*(10), 1547–1156.

Weller, E. B., Weller, R. A., & Fristad, M. A. (1995). Bipolar disorder in children: Misdiagnosis, underdiagnosis, and future directions. *Journal of the American Academy of Child and Adolescent Psychiatry, 34,* 709–714.

Wilens, T. E., Biederman, J., Martelon, M., Zulauf, C., Anderson, J., Yule, A., et al. (in press). A five-year follow-up of the development of substance use disorders in adolescents with bipolar disorder. *Journal of Clinical Psychiatry.*

Wozniak, J., & Biederman, J. (1996). A pharmacological approach to the quagmire of comorbidity in juvenile mania. *Journal of the American Academy of Child and Adolescent Psychiatry, 35*(6), 826–829.

Wozniak, J., Biederman, J., Faraone, S. V., Frazier, J., Kim, J., Millstein, R., et al. (1997). Mania in children with pervasive developmental disorder revisited. *Journal of the American Academy of Child and Adolescent Psychiatry, 36*(11), 1552–1559.

Depression

Birmaher, B., Brent, D. A., Kolko, D., Baugher, M., Bridge, J., Holder, D., et al. (2000). Clinical outcome after short-term psychotherapy for adolescents with major depressive disorder. *Archives of General Psychiatry, 57*(1), 29–36.

Birmaher, B., Brent, D., & Work Group on Quality Issues. (2007). Practice parameter for the assessment and treatment of children and adolescents with depressive disorders. *Journal of the American Academy of Child and Adolescent Psychiatry, 46*(11), 1503–1526.

Brent, D. A., Baugher, M., Bridge, J., Chen, T., & Chiappetta, L. (1999). Age- and sex-related risk factors for adolescent suicide. *Journal of the American Academy of Child and Adolescent Psychiatry, 38*(12), 1497–1505.

Brent, D., Emslie, G., Clarke, G., Wagner, K. D., Asarnow, J. R., Keller, M., et al. (2008). Switching to another SSRI or to Venlafaxine with or without cognitive behavioral therapy for adolescents with SSRI-resistant depression: The TORDIA randomized controlled trial. *Journal of the American Medical Association, 299*(8), 901-913.

Bridge, J. A., Iyengar, S., Salary, C. B., Barbe, R. P., Birmaher, B., Pincus, H. A., et al. (2007). Clinical response and risk for reported suicidal ideation and suicide attempts in pediatric antidepressant treatment: A meta-analysis of randomized controlled trials. *Journal of the American Medical Association, 297*(15), 1683–1696.

Copeland, M. E. (2001). *Depression Workbook: A Guide to Living with Depression and Manic Depression* (2nd ed.). New Harbinger, Oakland, CA.

Emslie, G. J., Heiligenstein, J. H., Wagner, K. D., Hoog, S. L., Ernest, D. E., Brown, E., et al. (2002). Fluoxetine for acute treatment of depression in children and adolescents: A placebo-controlled, randomized clinical trial. *Journal of the American Academy of Child and Adolescent Psychiatry, 41*(10), 1205–1215.

Emslie, G. J., Kratochvil, C., Vitiello, B., Silva, S., Mayes, T., McNulty, S., et al. (2006). Treatment for Adolescents with Depression Study (TADS): Safety results. *Journal of the American Academy of Child and Adolescent Psychiatry, 45*(12), 1440–1455.

Fristad, M. A., & Arnold, J. S. (2004). *Raising a Moody Child: How to Cope with Depression and Bipolar Disorder.* Guilford Press, New York.

Goode, E. (2003, December 11). British warning on antidepressant use for youth. *New York Times,* p. A1.

Gotlib, I. H., & Hammen, C. L. (Eds.). (2014). *Handbook of Depression* (3rd ed.). Guilford Press, New York.

Kovacs, M., Akiskal, H. S., Gatsonis, C., & Parrone, P. L. (1994). Childhood-onset dysthymic disorder: Clinical features and prospective naturalistic outcome. *Archives of General Psychiatry, 51*(5), 365–374.

Kovacs, M., Feinberg, T. L., Crouse-Novak, M. A., Paulauskas, S. L., & Finkelstein, R. (1984). Depressive disorders in childhood: I. A longitudinal prospective study of characteristics and recovery. *Archives of General Psychiatry, 41*(3), 229–237.

Kratochvil, C. J., Vitiello, B., Walkup, J., Emslie, G., Waslick, B. D., Weller, E. B., et al. (2006). Selective serotonin reuptake inhibitors in pediatric depression: Is the balance between benefits and risks favorable? *Journal of Child and Adolescent Psychopharmacology, 16*(1–2), 11–24.

March, J. S., Silva, S., Petrycki, S., Curry, J., Wells, K., Fairbank, J., et al. (2004). Fluoxetine, cognitive-behavioral therapy, and their combination for adolescents with depression: Treatment for Adolescents with Depression Study (TADS) randomized controlled trial. *Journal of the American Medical Association, 292*(7), 807–820.

March, J. S., Silva, S., Petrycki, S., Curry, J., Wells, K., Fairbank, J., et al. (2007). The Treatment of Adolescents with Depression Study (TADS): Long-term effectiveness and safety outcomes. *Archives of General Psychiatry, 64*(10), 1132–1143.

Riggs, P., Mikulich, S. K., Davies, R. D., Lohman, M., Klein, C., & Stover, S. (2007). A randomized controlled trial of fluoxetine and cognitive-behavioral therapy in adolescents with major depression, behavior problems, and substance use disorders. *Archives of Pediatrics and Adolescent Medicine, 161*(11), 1026–1034.

Shafii, M., & Shafii, S. L. (1992). *Clinical Guide to Depression in Children and Adolescents.* American Psychiatric Press, Washington, DC.

Wagner, A., & Vitiello, B. (2002). Teen angst from psychopathology. *Current Psychiatry, 1*(7), 41–50.

Obsessive–Compulsive Disorder

Fitzgibbons, L., & Pedrick, C. (2003). *Helping Your Child with OCD: A Workbook for Parents of Children with Obsessive–Compulsive Disorder.* New Harbinger, Oakland, CA.

Francis, G. (1996). *Childhood Obsessive Compulsive Disorder.* Sage, Thousand Oaks, CA.

Franklin, M. E., Sapyta, J., Freeman, J. B., Khanna, M., Compton, S., Almirall, D., et al. (2011). Cognitive behavior therapy augmentation of pharmacotherapy in pediatric obsessive-compulsive disorder: The Pediatric OCD Treatment Study II (POTS II) randomized controlled trial. *Journal of the American Medical Association, 306*(11), 1224–1232.

Geller, D. (2003). Special issue on obsessive compulsive disorder. *Journal of Child and Adolescent Psychopharmacology, 13*(Suppl.).

Leonard, H. L., & Rapoport, J. L. (1989). Pharmacotherapy of childhood obsessive–compulsive disorder. *Psychiatric Clinics of North America, 12*(4), 963–970.

March, J. S., with Benton, C. M. (2007). *Talking Back to OCD: The Program That Helps Kids and Teens Say "No Way"—and Parents Say "Way to Go."* Guilford Press, New York.

March, J. S., Biederman, J., Wolkow, R., Safferman, A., Mardekian, J., Cook, E. H., et al. (1998). Sertraline in children and adolescents with obsessive–compulsive disorder: A multicenter randomized controlled trial. *Journal of the American Medical Association, 280*(20), 1752–1756.

Pediatric OCD Treatment Study (POTS) Team. (2004). Cognitive-behavioral therapy, sertraline, and their combination for children and adolescents with obsessive-compulsive disorder: The pediatric OCD treatment study (POTS) randomized controlled trial. *Journal of the American Medical Association, 292*(16), 1969–1976.

Rapoport, J. (1994). *The Boy Who Couldn't Stop Washing.* Dutton, New York.

Riddle, M. A., Reeve, E. A., Yaryura-Tobias, J. A., Yang, H. M., Claghorn, J. L., Gaffney, G., et al. (2001). Fluvoxamine for children and adolescents with obsessive-compulsive disorder: A randomized, controlled, multicenter trial. *Journal of the American Academy of Child and Adolescent Psychiatry, 40*(2), 222–229.

Swedo, S. E., Leonard, H. L., Garvey, M., Mittleman, B., Allen, A. J., Perlmutter, S., et al. (1998). Pediatric autoimmune neuropsychiatric disorders associated with streptococcal infections: Clinical description of the first 50 cases. *American Journal of Psychiatry, 155*(2), 264–271.

Thomsen, P. H. (1999). *From Thoughts to Obsessions: Obsessive–Compulsive Disorder in Children and Adolescents.* Kingsley, London.

Wagner, K. D., Cook, E. H., Chung, H., & Messig, M. (2003). Remission status after long-term sertraline treatment of pediatric obsessive–compulsive disorder. *Journal of Child and Adolescent Psychopharmacology, 13*(Suppl. 1), S53–S60.

Psychosis

Amminger, G. P., Schafer, M. R., Papageorgiou, K., Clier, C. M., Cotton, S. M., Harrington, S. M., et al. (2010). Long-chain omega-3 fatty acids for indicated prevention of psychotic disorders: A randomized, placebo-controlled trial. *Archives of General Psychiatry, 67*(2),146–154.

Berke, J. (2001). *Beyond Madness: Psychosocial Interventions in Psychosis.* Kingsley, London.

Birchwood, M. J. (2001). *Early Intervention in Psychosis: A Guide to Concepts, Evidence and Interventions.* Wiley, New York.

Boer, J. A. (Ed.). (1996). *Advances in the Neurobiology of Schizophrenia.* Wiley, New York.

Cantor, S. (1988). *Childhood Schizophrenia.* Guilford Press, New York.

Frazier, J. A., Spencer, T., Wilens, T., Wozniak, J., & Biederman, J. (1997). Childhood-onset schizophrenia as the prototypic disorder of childhood. In D. L. Dunner & J. F. Rosenbaum (Eds.), *Psychiatric Clinics of North America: Annual of Drug Therapy 1997* (pp. 167–193). Saunders, Philadelphia.

Kumra, S., Jacobsen, L. K., Lenane, M., Karp, B. I., Frazier, J. A., Smith, A. K., et al. (1998). Childhood-onset schizophrenia: An open-label study of olanzapine in adolescents. *Journal of the American Academy of Child and Adolescent Psychiatry, 37*(4), 377–385.

McClellan, J. M., & Werry, J. S. (1992). Schizophrenia. *Psychiatric Clinics of North America, 15,* 131–148.

Mueser, K. T., & Gingerich, S. (2006). *The Complete Family Guide to Schizophrenia: Helping Your Loved One Get the Most Out of Life.* Guilford Press, New York.

Pappadopulos, E., MacIntyre, J. C., Crismon, M. L., Findling, R. L., Malone, R. P., Derivan, A., et al. (2003). Treatment recommendations for the use of antipsychotics for aggressive youth (TRAAY). Part II. *Journal of the American Academy of Child and Adolescent Psychiatry, 42*(2), 145–161.

Rapoport, J., Giedd, J., Blumenthal, J., Hamburger, S., Jeffries, N., Fernandez, T., et al. (1999). Progressive cortical change during adolescence in childhood-onset schizophrenia. *Archives of General Psychiatry, 56*(7), 649–654.

Rapoport, J. L., Giedd, J., Kumra, S., Jacobsen, L., Smith, A., Lee, P., et al. (1997). Childhood-onset schizophrenia. *Archives of General Psychiatry, 54*(10), 897–903.

Robbins, M. D. (1993). *Experiences of Schizophrenia: An Integration of the Personal, Scientific, and Therapeutic.* Guilford Press, New York.

Volkmar, F. R. (1996). *Psychoses and Pervasive Developmental Disorder in Children and Adolescents.* American Psychiatric Press, Washington, DC.

Substance Abuse

Bukstein, O.G., Bernet, W., Arnold, V., Beitchman, J., Shaw, J., Benson, R. S., et al. (2005). Practice parameter for the assessment and treatment of children and adolescents with substance use disorders. *Journal of the American Academy of Child and Adolescent Psychiatry, 44*(6), 609–621.

Crowley, T. J., Macdonald, M. J., Whitmore, E. A., & Mikulich, S. K. (1998). Cannabis dependence, withdrawal, and reinforcing effects among adolescents with conduct symptoms and substance use disorders. *Drug and Alcohol Dependency, 50*(1), 27–37.

Galanter, M., & Kleber, H. D. (Eds.). (2014). *American Psychiatric Press Textbook of Substance Abuse Treatment.* American Psychiatric Press, Arlington, VA.

Gignac, M., Waxmonsky, J., & Wilens, T. E. (2010). Psychopharmacology and substance use disorders: A pediatric approach. In A. Martin, L. Scahill, & C. Kratochvil (Eds.), *Pediatric Psychopharmacology: Principles and Practice* (2nd ed., pp. 587–599). Oxford University Press, New York.

Kaminer, Y. (Ed.). (2016). *Youth Substance Abuse and Co-Occurring Disorders.* American Psychiatric Press, Arlington, VA.

Marlatt, G. A., Larimer, M. E., & Witkiewitz, K. (Eds.). (2012). *Harm Reduction: Pragmatic Strategies for Managing High-Risk Behaviors* (2nd ed.). Guilford Press, New York.

Riggs, P. D., & Davies, R. D. (2002). A clinical approach to integrating treatment for adolescent depression and substance abuse. *Journal of the American Academy of Child and Adolescent Psychiatry, 41*(10), 1253–1255.

Volpicelli, J. (2000). *Recovery Options: The Complete Guide.* Wiley, New York.

Waldron, H. B., Slesnick, N., Brody, J., Turner, C. W., & Peterson, T. R. (2001). Treatment outcomes for adolescent substance abuse at 4- and 7-month assessments. *Journal of Consulting and Clinical Psychology, 69*(5), 802–813.

Yule, A., & Wilens, T. (2015) Substance use disorders in adolescents with psychiatric comorbidity: When to screen and how to treat. *Current Psychiatry, 14*(4), 802–813.

Tic and Tourette's Disorders

Chappell, P., Riddle, M., Scahill, L., Lynch, K., Schultz, R., Arnsten, A., et al. (1995). Guanfacine treatment of comorbid attention-deficit hyperactivity disorder and

Tourette's syndrome. *Journal of the American Academy of Child and Adolescent Psychiatry, 34*(9), 1140–1146.
Cohen, D. J., Bruun, R. D., & Leckman, J. F. (Eds.). (1988). *Tourette's Syndrome and Tic Disorders: Clinical Understanding and Treatment.* Wiley, New York.
Cohen, D. J., Detlor, J., Young, J. G., & Shaywitz, B. A. (1980). Clonidine ameliorates Gilles de la Tourette syndrome. *Archives of General Psychiatry, 37*(12), 1350–1357.
Haerle, T. (2003). *Children with Tourette Syndrome: A Parent's Guide.* Woodbine House, Bethesda, MD.
Kurlan, R. (2002). Treatment of ADHD in children with tics: A randomized controlled trial. *Neurology, 58*(4), 527–536.
Leckman, J. (2001). *Tourette's Syndrome: Tics, Obsessions, Compulsions: Developmental Psychopathology and Clinical Care.* John Wiley, New York.
Leckman, J. F., Hardin, M. T., Riddle, M. A., Stevenson, J., Ort, S. I., & Cohen, D. J. (1991). Clonidine treatment of Gilles de la Tourette's syndrome. *Archives of General Psychiatry, 48*(4), 324–328.
Robertson, M. (1998). *Tourette Syndrome: The Facts.* Oxford University Press, London.
Scahill, L. (2000). Controlled clinical trial of guanfacine in ADHD youth with tic disorders. NCDEU, Boca Raton, FL.
Spencer, T., Biederman, J., Coffey, B., Geller, D., Wilens, T., & Faraone, S. (1999). The 4-year course of tic disorders in boys with attention-deficit/hyperactivity disorder. *Archives of General Psychiatry, 56*(9), 842–847.
Woods, D. W., Piacentini, J. C., & Walkup, J. T. (2007). *Treating Tourette Syndrome and Tic Disorders: A Guide for Practitioners.* Guilford Press, New York.

Miscellaneous

Braaten, E., & Felopolous, G. (2003). *Straight Talk about Psychological Testing for Kids.* Guilford Press, New York.
Chokroverty, S. (2001). *100 Questions about Sleep and Sleep Disorders.* Blackwell, Malden, MA.
Costin, C. (1999). *The Eating Disorder Sourcebook: A Comprehensive Guide to the Causes, Treatments, and Prevention of Eating Disorders.* McGraw-Hill, New York.
Dahl, R. E., & Puig-Antich, J. (1990). Sleep disturbances in child and adolescent psychiatric disorders. *Pediatrician, 17*(1), 32–37.
Fairburn, C. G., & Brownell, K. D. (Eds.). (2001). *Eating Disorders and Obesity: A Comprehensive Handbook* (2nd ed.). Guilford Press, New York.
Jimmerson, D. C., Herzog, D. B., & Brotman, A. W. (1993). Pharmacological approaches in the treatment of eating disorders. *Harvard Review of Psychiatry, 1*(2), 82–93.
Lock, J., & Le Grange, D. (2015). *Help Your Teenager Beat an Eating Disorder* (2nd ed.). Guilford Press, New York.
Loney, J. (1988). Substance abuse in adolescents: Diagnostic issues derived from studies of attention deficit disorder with hyperactivity. *NIDA Research Monograph, 77,* 19–26.
Neumark-Sztainer, D. (2005). *"I'm, Like, So Fat!": Helping Your Teen Make Healthy Choices about Eating and Exercise in a Weight-Obsessed World.* Guilford Press, New York.
Owens, J. (2014). Behavioral aspects of sleep problems in childhood and adolescence [Special issue]. *Sleep Medicine Clinics, 9*(2).

Palm, L., Blennow, G., & Wetterberg, L. (1997). Long-term melatonin treatment in blind children and young adults with circadian sleep-wake disturbances. *Developmental Medicine and Child Neurology, 39*(5), 319–325.

Prince, J., Wilens, T., Biederman, J., Spencer, T., & Wozniak, J. (1996). Clonidine for sleep disturbances associated with attention-deficit hyperactivity disorder: A systematic chart review of 62 cases. *Journal of the American Academy of Child and Adolescent Psychiatry, 35*(5), 599–605.

Reite, M. (1997). *Concise Guide to Evaluation and Management of Sleep Disorders* (2nd ed.). American Psychiatric Press, Arlington, VA.

Robins, L. N. (1966). *Deviant Children Grown Up: A Sociological and Psychiatric Study of Sociopathic Personality.* Williams & Wilkins, Baltimore.

Thomas, J. (2013). *Almost Anorectic: Is My (Or My Loved One's) Relationship with Food a Problem?* Hazelden, Center City, MN.

Thompson, K. J. (Ed.). (2001). *Body Image, Eating Disorders, and Obesity in Youth: Assessment, Prevention, and Treatment.* American Psychological Association, Washington, DC.

Wilhelm, S. (2006). *Feeling Good about the Way You Look: A Program for Overcoming Body Image Problems.* Guilford Press, New York.

Index

Note: *f* or *t* following a page number indicates a figure or a table.

Abilify. *See also* Aripiprazole; Second-generation antipsychotic (SGAs)
antipsychotics and, 280
autism spectrum disorders and, 169, 170, 172*t*
bipolar disorder and, 162, 165*t*
conduct disorder and, 138, 140*t*
depression and, 158, 165*t*
DMDD and, 164
dosage determination and, 93*t*, 272*t*, 273, 277, 288
obsessive–compulsive disorder and, 152*t*
oppositional defiant disorder and, 137, 140*t*
overview, 269, 270, 276–277, 279
psychosis and, 175, 176, 177*t*
PTSD and, 148
side effects, 274, 275, 277–278
tics and Tourette's disorder and, 181
Abuse of medications, 28, 29–30, 189, 205. *See also* Substance abuse
Academic functioning, 60–61, 66, 88, 130. *See also* School functioning
Adderall and Adderall XR. *See also* Amphetamines
abuse of, 189
ADHD and, 133, 139*t*
clonidine and, 262
diagnosis and, 212
dosage determination and, 211, 211*t*, 212–213, 285
drug scheduling by the DEA and, 205
overview, 19
prescription and dosing of, 218
Addiction, 28–29, 259
Adherence, 107, 112–113, 117–121, 222, 248
Adolescents
bipolar disorder and, 160–161
depression and, 156, 158
discussing treatment and medication with, 37–38
monitoring without hovering and, 107
mood disorders and, 153–154
preparing for the psychopharmacology evaluation, 63–66
role of in treatment, 61–62, 117–121
Aggression
ADHD and, 133
anticonvulsants and, 253
antipsychotics and, 269, 270
autism spectrum disorders and, 172*t*
clonidine and, 261, 264
conduct disorder and, 137, 138, 140*t*
depression and, 156
effectiveness of medications and, 19
guanfacine and, 265
mental disorders due to medical conditions and, 185
oppositional defiant disorder and, 136, 140*t*
second-generation antipsychotics and, 277
as a side effect, 108–109
Strattera and, 226
Agitation. *See also* Side effects
anticonvulsants and, 253
antipsychotics and, 269, 280
benzodiazepines and, 258
bipolar disorder and, 162
depression and, 156
SSRIs and, 234–235, 236
stimulants and, 216*t*
Agoraphobia, 143. *See also* Anxiety disorders
Akathisia, 274. *See also* Side effects
Alcohol abuse, 23*t*, 189–191, 191–194, 284, 308–310. *See also* Substance abuse
Alcoholism, 23*t*, 189. *See also* Alcohol abuse; Substance abuse
Alpha agonists. *See also* Antihypertensives; Clonidine; Guanfacine; Psychotropic medications
ADHD and, 227–228
autism spectrum disorders and, 170, 171

321

Alpha agonists (*cont.*)
  conduct disorder and, 140*t*
  DMDD and, 164
  dosage determination and, 262*t*, 263, 286
  mental disorders due to medical conditions and, 185
  oppositional defiant disorder and, 140*t*
  overview, 200, 261
  PTSD and, 148, 151*t*
  substance abuse and, 193
  tics and Tourette's disorder and, 180
Alprazolam, 256*t*, 257, 290. *See also* Xanax
Alternatives to medication, 114–115
Alzheimer's medications, 134, 135, 171
Amantadine, 275
Ambien, 197, 256*t*, 290. *See also* Zolpidem
American Academy of Child and Adolescent Psychiatry (AACAP), 39
American Psychiatric Association (APA), 62
Americans with Disabilities Act Amendments Act, 63
Amitriptyline. *See also* Elavil
  depression and, 158, 165*t*
  dosage determination and, 92*t*, 232*t*, 287
  eating disorders and, 188
  overview, 240–243
  sleep problems and, 197
  tics and Tourette's disorder and, 180–181
Amphetamines. *See also* Adderall and Adderall XR; Dexedrine; Stimulants; Vyvanse
  dosage determination and, 92*t*, 209–214, 211*t*, 285
  how stimulants work and, 204–206, 207*t*–208*t*
  long-term use of, 221–224
  overview, 19
  side effects, 213–219, 215*t*–216*t*, 221–224
Anafranil. *See also* Clomipramine
  autism spectrum disorders and, 170, 172*t*
  dosage determination and, 232*t*, 287
  obsessive–compulsive disorder and, 150, 152*t*

overview, 240–243
tics and Tourette's disorder and, 181
Anger, 136, 155
Anorexia nervosa, 186–188. *See also* Eating disorders
Antibiotics, 220*t*, 237
Anticonvulsants. *See also* Carbachol; Psychotropic medications; Tegretol
  autism spectrum disorders and, 171, 172*t*
  bipolar disorder and, 161, 165*t*
  conduct disorder and, 140*t*
  dosage determination and, 249
  mood stabilizers and, 252–254
  oppositional defiant disorder and, 140*t*
  overview, 248
  psychosis and, 177*t*
  side effects, 249
  stimulants and, 220*t*
  temporal lobe epilepsy and, 183
  valproic acid, 251–252
Antidepressants. *See also* Atypical antidepressants; Monoamine oxidase inhibitors (MAOIs); Psychotropic medications; SSRIs (selective serotonin reuptake inhibitor); Tricyclics antidepressants (TCAs)
  ADHD and, 133–135, 228
  antipsychotics and, 280
  anxiety disorders and, 145, 151*t*
  anxiety-breaking medications and, 255, 257
  autism spectrum disorders and, 171
  conduct disorder and, 140*t*
  depression and, 157–158, 165*t*
  dosage determination and, 91, 92*t*, 232*t*–233*t*, 286–288
  eating disorders and, 188
  new options that aren't tested in children, 240
  obsessive–compulsive disorder and, 150
  oppositional defiant disorder and, 140*t*

overview, 21*f*, 84, 200, 230
psychosis and, 175
PTSD and, 148, 151*t*
sleep problems and, 197
stimulants and, 220*t*
substance abuse and, 194
tics and Tourette's disorder and, 185*t*
Antidiuretic hormone desmopressin (ddAVP), 94*t*, 198, 283, 284
Antihistamines
  anxiety and, 260
  anxiety disorders and, 145, 146
  dosage determination and, 256*t*, 290
  overview, 102, 281–282
  sleep problems and, 196
  SSRIs and, 237
  stimulants and, 220*t*
Antihypertensives. *See also* Alpha agonists; Blood pressure medications; Clonidine; Guanfacine; Psychotropic medications
  ADHD and, 133, 227–228
  dosage determination and, 94*t*, 262*t*, 286
  overview, 200, 261
  PTSD and, 148
Anti-Parkinson agents, 275
Antipsychotics. *See also* Atypical antipsychotics; Psychotropic medications; Second-generation antipsychotic (SGAs)
  anxiety and, 255
  Benadryl and, 281
  bipolar disorder and, 161, 162, 165*t*
  conduct disorder and, 138, 140*t*
  decisions regarding medications to prescribe, 84
  depression and, 165*t*
  dosage determination and, 93*t*, 271, 272*t*–273*t*, 273–274, 288–289
  eating disorders and, 188
  effectiveness of, 19
  FDA approval and, 82
  oppositional defiant disorder and, 140*t*
  overview, 21*f*, 200, 269–273, 272*t*–273*t*, 279–280

Index

psychosis and, 175–176, 177*t*
PTSD and, 148, 151*t*
side effects, 110, 274–276
sleep problems and, 197
stimulants and, 220*t*
substance abuse and, 194
temporal lobe epilepsy and, 183
tics and Tourette's disorder and, 185*t*
Topamax and, 253
Anxiety. *See also* Anxiety disorders; Mood disorders
antipsychotics and, 279
autism spectrum disorders and, 168, 170, 172*t*
benzodiazepines and, 257–259
bipolar disorder and, 165*t*
decisions regarding medications to prescribe, 84
depression and, 154, 159, 165*t*
DMDD and, 164
eating disorders and, 187, 188
effectiveness of medications and, 18
family history and, 54–55
monitoring the effects of a medication and, 106
multiple disorders and, 17
multiple medications and, 86–87
neurotransmitters and, 23*t*
psychopharmacology evaluation and, 46
PTSD and, 147
recommendations regarding medications and, 11
sleep problems and, 197
SSRIs and, 18, 234–235, 236–237
Strattera and, 225
temporal lobe epilepsy and, 183
tics and Tourette's disorder and, 179
Anxiety disorders. *See also* Anxiety; Generalized anxiety disorder; Obsessive–compulsive disorder (OCD); Panic disorders; Posttraumatic stress disorder (PTSD)
ADHD and, 134
antidepressants and, 230

overview, 141–144
PTSD and, 148–149
resources regarding, 300
substance abuse and, 190
tics and Tourette's disorder and, 179
treatment and, 144–147, 151*t*–152*t*
Anxiety-breaking medications. *See also* Psychotropic medications; SSRIs (selective serotonin reuptake inhibitor)
antipsychotics and, 279
dosage determination and, 93*t*, 256*t*, 290
effectiveness of, 18
overview, 21*f*, 200, 255, 257
stimulants and, 220*t*
Anxiolytics, 200, 255
Appetite effects. *See also* Side effects
antipsychotics and, 274
buproprion and, 238
depression and, 156
monitoring the effects of a medication and, 109
overview, 101–102
second-generation antipsychotics and, 278–279
stimulants and, 215*t*, 217, 223
Strattera and, 226
Topamax and, 253–254
valproic acid, 252
Aptensio and Aptensio XR, 133, 210*t*, 285. *See also* Methylphenidate
Aricept, 134
Aripiprazole, 169, 170, 272*t*, 288. *See also* Abilify
Asenapine, 272*t*, 288. *See also* Saphris
Asperger's syndrome, 167–168. *See also* Autism spectrum disorders
Assessment. *See also* Psychopharmacology evaluation
ADHD and, 131
depression and, 156–157
overview, 41
sleep problems and, 195–196
what to expect from, 49–56, 50*t*
Atarax, 145, 256*t*, 290. *See also* Hydroxyzine

Atenolo, 266
Ativan. *See also* Lorazepam
abuse of, 189
antipsychotics and, 279
anxiety and, 145, 145–146, 151*t*, 257
autism spectrum disorders and, 171
conduct disorder and, 140*t*
depression and, 165*t*
dosage determination and, 93*t*, 256*t*, 257, 290
oppositional defiant disorder and, 140*t*
psychosis and, 177*t*
PTSD and, 148, 151*t*
sleep problems and, 197
Atomoxetine. *See also* Strattera
ADHD and, 139*t*, 220
anxiety disorders and, 145
bipolar disorder and, 163
dosage determination and, 92*t*, 286
overview, 224–227
stimulants and, 220*t*
tics and Tourette's disorder and, 185*t*
Attention-deficit/hyperactivity disorder (ADHD)
antidepressants and, 230, 241
antipsychotics and, 270
autism spectrum disorders and, 168, 170, 171, 172*t*
bipolar disorder and, 163, 165*t*
clonidine and, 261, 262, 264, 267, 281
conduct disorder and, 138
depression and, 154, 159
diagnosis and, 67
DMDD and, 164
dosage determination and, 91
DSM and, 62
effectiveness of medications and, 18
executive functions and, 30
family history and, 54–55
guanfacine and, 265, 265–266, 267
improving without treatment, 16
mania and, 160
monitoring the effects of a medication and, 106
multiple disorders and, 16–17
multiple medications and, 86–87, 87

Attention-deficit/
hyperactivity disorder
(ADHD) (cont.)
neurotransmitters and, 23t
nonstimulant medications
and, 224–229
normalizing, 120
overview, 129–132
Provigil, 229
psychopharmacology
evaluation and, 66
psychosis and, 174
recommendations
regarding medications
and, 12
resources regarding, 301
sleep problems and, 195,
196, 197
stimulants and, 203–224,
207t–208t, 210t–211t,
215t–216t, 220t
Strattera and, 224–227
substance abuse and,
190–191, 192, 193–194
symptoms of, 129–130
tics and Tourette's disorder
and, 178, 179, 180
treatment and, 132–136,
139t–140t, 200
Wellbutrin and, 238
Atypical antidepressants. See
also Antidepressants
depression and, 165t
dosage determination and,
232t, 287
overview, 230–231,
237–240
PTSD and, 151t
Atypical antipsychotics. See
also Antipsychotics;
Second-generation
antipsychotic (SGAs)
autism spectrum disorders
and, 170
bipolar disorder and, 162
DMDD and, 164
dosage determination and,
92t
effectiveness of, 19
mental disorders due to
medical conditions and,
185
obsessive–compulsive
disorder and, 152t
overview, 269
psychosis and, 177t
substance abuse and, 194
tics and Tourette's disorder
and, 181
Auditory hallucinations, 51,
156

Autism spectrum disorders
clonidine and, 261
DSM and, 62
effectiveness of
medications and, 19
overview, 166–169
resources regarding,
302–303
symptoms of, 166–168
treatment and, 169–171,
172t
Aventyl, 228–229, 232t, 287.
See also Nortriptyline
Avoidance, 141, 144, 147

Barbiturates, 257
BEAMs (brain electrical
activity mapping), 131
Bedwetting. See Enuresis
Behavioral modification, 144,
180, 185
Behavioral symptoms, 109,
167, 172t, 174, 195, 270
Behavioral treatment, 138,
144, 169
Benadryl. See also
Diphenhydramine
antipsychotics and, 275
anxiety and, 145, 260
dosage determination and,
256t, 282, 290
monitoring the effects of a
medication and, 111
overview, 281–282
side effects, 282
sleep problems and, 196
stimulants and, 220t
Benzodiazepines
abuse of, 189
addiction and, 28
antipsychotics and, 275,
279
anxiety and, 255, 257,
257–259
anxiety disorders and,
145–146, 151t
autism spectrum disorders
and, 171, 172t
conduct disorder and, 140t
depression and, 165t
dosage determination and,
93t–94t, 256t, 257–258,
290
eating disorders and, 188
mental disorders due to
medical conditions and,
185
obsessive–compulsive
disorder and, 150, 152t
oppositional defiant
disorder and, 140t

overview, 257
psychosis and, 177t
PTSD and, 148
side effects and, 110, 146,
258
substance abuse and, 194
temporal lobe epilepsy
and, 183
tics and Tourette's disorder
and, 185t
Best Pharmaceuticals for
Children Act, 25
Beta blockers. See also
Propranolol
antipsychotics and, 275
autism spectrum disorders
and, 170, 172t
clonidine and, 264
conduct disorder and, 140t
dosage determination and,
286
oppositional defiant
disorder and, 140t
Binge-eating disorder,
186–188. See also Eating
disorders
Bingeing, 51
Biochemical testing, 60
Biological factors. See also
Neurological factors
how medications work,
19–24, 19f, 21f, 23t
overview, 12, 24
psychopharmacology
evaluation and, 56–58
Bipolar disorder. See also
Mood disorders
ADHD and, 130, 135
anticonvulsants and, 253
antipsychotics and, 269,
270, 279
appetite and, 102
autism spectrum disorders
and, 168
compared to depression,
154–155
conduct disorder and, 137,
138
decisions regarding
medications to
prescribe, 84
diagnosis and, 66–67
effectiveness of
medications and, 19
family history and, 54–55
monitoring the effects of a
medication and, 106
multiple disorders and,
16–17, 17
multiple medications and,
86–87

outcomes associated with, 2–3
overview, 154, 160–161
psychosis and, 174–175
resources regarding, 304–305
second-generation antipsychotics and, 277
sleep problems and, 195, 196, 197
substance abuse and, 190, 192–193, 194
symptoms of, 162
treatment and, 161–164, 165t
Blood level testing
ADHD and, 131
anticonvulsants and, 249
bipolar disorder and, 161
Depakote and, 251–252
depression and, 156–157
dosage determination and, 95–96
lithium and, 246
monitoring the effects of a medication and, 111
over-the-counter medications and, 102
overview, 95–96
psychopharmacology evaluation and, 59–60
temporal lobe epilepsy and, 183
Topamax and, 254
Blood pressure, 264, 266, 268
Blood pressure medications, 151t, 185. *See also* Antihypertensives
Blurred or double vision, 249, 251, 274–275. *See also* Side effects
Brain imaging, 56–57, 131, 182–183
Brain structures. *See also* Biological factors
anxiety disorders and, 142
brain damage/injury, 183–185
eating disorders and, 187
how medications work, 19–23, 19f, 21f, 23t
psychosis and, 173–174
resources regarding, 297
temporal lobe epilepsy and, 182
Brand-name medications, 103–104
Breathing difficulties, 109, 268. *See also* Side effects
Brintellix, 233t, 240, 288. *See also* Vortioxetine

Bulimia nervosa, 186–188. *See also* Eating disorders
Buproprion. *See also* Wellbutrin; Zyban
ADHD and, 228
antipsychotics and, 280
dosage determination and, 92t, 233t, 287
nicotine use and, 191
overview, 237–238
psychosis and, 177t
stimulants and, 220t
Buspar. *See also* Buspirone
anxiety and, 145, 146, 151t, 257, 259
dosage determination and, 256t, 290
substance abuse and, 194
Buspirone. *See also* Buspar
anxiety and, 145, 257, 259
depression and, 159
dosage determination and, 93t, 256t, 290

Callousness, 147
Carbachol, 165t, 245t, 248, 249, 289. *See also* Anticonvulsants; Carbamazepine
Carbamazepine. *See also* Carbachol; Equetro; Tegretol
bipolar disorder and, 165t
dosage determination and, 93t, 245t, 289
overview, 253
temporal lobe epilepsy and, 183
Cardiovascular problems. *See* Heart symptoms
Catapres. *See also* Clonidine
ADHD and, 133, 139t, 227–228
dosage determination and, 262t, 286
overview, 261–263
PTSD and, 148–149
tics and Tourette's disorder and, 185t
Causes of disorders, 11–13, 157, 168, 174, 184
Celexa. *See also* Citalopram; SSRIs (selective serotonin reuptake inhibitor)
anxiety disorders and, 145, 151t
autism spectrum disorders and, 170, 172t
bipolar disorder and, 163

depression and, 157, 158, 165t
dosage determination and, 232t, 235, 286
eating disorders and, 188
obsessive–compulsive disorder and, 152t
PTSD and, 148
side effects, 236
substance abuse and, 194
Central nervous symptoms, 247. *See also* Side effects
Ceruloplasmin (copper-containing protein) test, 59–60
Cessation of medication. *See* Stopping medications
Chantix, 191
Chemical signals (neurotransmitters), 21–23, 21f, 23t, 28
Children
antidepressants and, 230
bipolar disorder and, 160–161
depression and, 156, 157–158
discussing treatment and medication with, 35–37
involving in the psychopharmacology evaluation, 61–62
mood disorders and, 153–154
preparing for the psychopharmacology evaluation, 63–66
role of in treatment, 117–121
Chlordiazepoxide, 257. *See also* Librium
Chlorpheniramine maleate, 256t, 290. *See also* Chlor-trimeton
Chlorpromazine, 271, 273t, 289. *See also* Thorazine
Chlor-trimeton, 256t, 290. *See also* Chlorpheniramine maleate
Cholinesterase inhibitors, 134, 169
Cibalith, 244, 245t, 289. *See also* Lithium
Cigarette use, 190, 191–192. *See also* Substance abuse
Citalopram, 92t, 232t, 286. *See also* Celexa; SSRIs (selective serotonin reuptake inhibitor)

Clinic settings, 13–14, 31–32, 61–62. *See also* Treatment
Clinical trials, 82–84
Clinicians. *See* Mental health professionals
Clomipramine, 92*t*, 165*t*, 232*t*, 240–243, 287. *See also* Anafranil
Clonazepam, 185*t*, 256*t*, 257, 279, 290. *See also* Klonopin
Clonidine. *See also* Alpha agonists; Antihypertensives; Catapres; Kapvay
 ADHD and, 134, 220
 autism spectrum disorders and, 169, 170, 172*t*
 bipolar disorder and, 163, 165*t*
 conduct disorder and, 140*t*
 DMDD and, 164
 dosage determination and, 94*t*, 262*t*, 263, 286
 guanfacine and, 267
 mental disorders due to medical conditions and, 185
 multiple medications and, 87
 oppositional defiant disorder and, 137, 140*t*
 overview, 200, 261–263, 281
 PTSD and, 148, 151*t*
 side effects, 110, 263–264
 sleep problems and, 197
 tics and Tourette's disorder and, 180, 181, 185*t*
Clonidine XR, 94*t*
Clorazepate, 256*t*, 290. *See also* Tranxene
Clozapine, 272*t*, 288. *See also* Clozaril
Clozaril. *See also* Clozapine
 dosage determination and, 93*t*, 272*t*, 273, 277, 288
 monitoring the effects of a medication and, 111
 overview, 276–277
 psychosis and, 175, 177*t*
 side effects, 278
Cogentin, 274, 275, 280
Cognitive functions, 19–20, 30, 170–171. *See also* Thinking processes
Cognitive-behavioral therapy (CBT). *See also* Psychotherapy; Treatment
 anxiety disorders and, 144

eating disorders and, 187–188
effectiveness of medications along with, 18
executive functions and, 30
obsessive–compulsive disorder and, 150
overview, 14, 18
substance abuse and, 191
tics and Tourette's disorder and, 180
Collaborating in your child's care. *See* Parent–practitioner collaboration
College, 118
Combined pharmacotherapy, 85–88, 280. *See also* Multiple medications
Communication skills, 72, 167
Comorbidity. *See also* Disorders
 ADHD, 130, 134
 anxiety disorders and, 146–147
 autism spectrum disorders and, 168, 169
 bipolar disorder and, 163
 clonidine and, 264
 DMDD and, 164
 eating disorders and, 187, 188
 multiple medications and, 86–87
 overview, 16–17, 86
 psychopharmacology evaluation and, 42
 PTSD and, 147, 148–149
 stimulants and, 219–221
 substance abuse and, 190, 192–193
 tics and Tourette's disorder and, 178, 179–180
Complex partial seizures, 181–183, 183. *See also* Seizures
Compulsions, 149, 170
Concerta. *See also* Methylphenidate
 ADHD and, 133, 134, 139*t*
 bipolar disorder and, 163
 clonidine and, 262
 dosage determination and, 209, 210*t*, 212, 285
 drug scheduling by the DEA and, 205
 prescription and dosing of, 218

substance abuse and, 194
tics and Tourette's disorder and, 185*t*
Conduct disorder
 ADHD and, 130
 depressive disorders and, 154
 family history and, 54–55
 mania and, 160
 overview, 137
 substance abuse and, 190
 treatment and, 138, 140*t*
Confidentiality, 60–61
Constipation, 268, 274–275. *See also* Gastrointestinal problems; Side effects
Copayments, 38–39, 88, 192. *See also* Financial concerns
Corgard, 262*t*, 286. *See also* Nadolol
Costs of medications, 38–39, 88. *See also* Financial concerns
Counseling. *See* Psychotherapy; Treatment
CPT (Continuous Performance Test), 131
CT (computed tomography) scan, 57–58
Cymbalta. *See also* Atypical antidepressants; Duloxetine
 anxiety disorders and, 145, 151*t*
 depression and, 158, 165*t*
 dosage determination and, 233*t*, 287
 overview, 240
 PTSD and, 148

Daily routines, 101, 104–105, 107, 167, 195–196
Day treatment facilities, 123–126
Daytrana. *See also* Methylphenidate
 ADHD and, 133, 139*t*
 autism spectrum disorders and, 167
 dosage determination and, 210*t*, 212, 285
 prescription and dosing of, 218
Decanoate, 274
Decongestants, 220*t*
Dehydration, 247, 253. *See also* Side effects
Delusions, 173, 279–280. *See also* Psychosis

Demoralization, 16, 29–30, 168
Depakene sprinkles, 165t, 245t, 251, 289. See also Valproic acid
Depakote. See also Valproic acid
  antipsychotics and, 280
  autism spectrum disorders and, 169, 171
  bipolar disorder and, 161, 165t
  conduct disorder and, 138
  dosage determination and, 95, 245t, 250, 251–252, 289
  eating disorders and, 188
  mental disorders due to medical conditions and, 185
  monitoring the effects of a medication and, 111
  overview, 251
  temporal lobe epilepsy and, 183
Depakote ER, 245t. See also Valproic acid
Dependency, 28–29, 259
Depression. See also Mood disorders
  ADHD and, 130, 134–135
  antidepressants and, 230
  antipsychotics and, 269, 280
  anxiety disorders and, 145
  autism spectrum disorders and, 168, 171, 172t
  bipolar disorder and, 161, 162–163
  clonidine and, 264
  compared to bipolar disorder, 154–155
  conduct disorder and, 137, 138
  diagnosis and, 67
  DSM and, 62
  eating disorders and, 187, 188
  effectiveness of medications and, 18
  family history and, 54–55
  guanfacine and, 266
  mania and, 160
  monitoring the effects of a medication and, 106
  multiple disorders and, 16–17
  multiple medications and, 86–87
  neurotransmitters and, 23t
  normalizing, 120
  overview, 155–157
  propranolol, 268
  psychosis and, 174–175
  PTSD and, 147, 148–149
  resources regarding, 300, 304–305
  sleep problems and, 195
  SSRIs and, 18, 231, 234–235
  substance abuse and, 190, 192, 194
  symptoms of, 156
  treatment and, 157–160, 165t
Desipramine. See also Norpramin; Pertofrane; Tricyclics antidepressants (TCAs)
  ADHD and, 133–135, 139t, 228–229
  depression and, 158, 165t
  dosage determination and, 92t, 232t, 287
  eating disorders and, 188
  monitoring the effects of a medication and, 111
  overview, 240–243
  side effects, 241–242
  tics and Tourette's disorder and, 180–181, 181, 185t
Desmopressin (ddAVP), 94t, 198, 283, 284
Desvenlafaxine, 233t. See also Pristiq
Desyrel, 233t, 287. See also Trazodone
Developmental disorders, 166, 262. See also Autism spectrum disorders; individual disorders
Developmental history, 52–53
Dexedrine. See also Amphetamines
  ADHD and, 133, 139t
  dosage determination and, 209, 210t, 211, 212–213, 286
  drug scheduling by the DEA and, 205
  overview, 19
  prescription and dosing of, 218
  side effects and, 241
Dextroamphetamine, 92t, 286
Diagnosis
  ADHD and, 131–132
  advances in, 2
  autism spectrum disorders and, 166–167, 168–169
  challenges related to, 66–68
  depression and, 156–157
  disagreements regarding, 33–34
  DSM and, 62
  early diagnosis, 3–4
  executive functions and, 30
  mood disorders and, 153–154
  overview, 5, 10, 69–70
  physicians and, 31
  psychiatric history of, 53
  psychopharmacology evaluation and, 42–43
  role of your child in treatment and, 117
  safety of medications and, 26
  schools and, 60–61, 88–89
  seeking treatment and, 31–32
  treatment and, 70–71, 80, 271
  trying alternatives to medication and, 114
Diagnostic and Statistical Manual of Mental Disorders (DSM), 62, 131–132
Diarrhea, 236, 268. See also Gastrointestinal problems
Diazepam, 256t, 257, 290. See also Valium
Diet changes, 101–102. See also Appetite effects
Differential diagnosis, 66–67. See also Diagnosis
Dimetapp, 196, 220t
Diphenhydramine, 256t, 281–282, 290. See also Benadryl
Disability, 63
Discipline needs, 75–77
Discontinuing medications. See Stopping medications
Disinhibition, 146, 258
Disorders. See also Comorbidity; individual disorders
  causes of, 11–13
  multiple disorders and, 16–17
  multiple medications and, 86–87
  neurotransmitters and, 23t
  normalizing, 119–120
  overview, 9, 62, 127–128

Disorders (cont.)
  psychopharmacology
    evaluation and, 62
  return or worsening of
    symptoms and, 112–116
Disruptive mood
  dysregulation disorder
  (DMDD), 155, 164. See
  also Mood disorders
Dissociation, 147, 148
Distractibility, 129. See
  also Attention-deficit/
  hyperactivity disorder
  (ADHD)
Divorced parents, 68
Dizziness. See also Side
  effects
  anticonvulsants and, 249
  antipsychotics and, 274
  guanfacine and, 266
  stimulants and, 215t
  Topamax and, 254
  Trileptal and, 253
  valproic acid, 252
d-Methylphenidate, 92t, 210t
Doctors. See Mental health
  professionals; Physicians
Dopamine system, 21, 23t,
  187, 228, 238
Dosage determination
  alpha agonists, 262t
  anticonvulsants, 249
  antidepressants, 91, 92t,
    232t–233t
  antidiuretic hormone
    desmopressin (ddAVP),
    283
  antihistamines, 256t
  antihypertensives, 94t, 262t
  antipsychotics, 93t,
    272t–273t, 273–274, 277
  anxiety-breaking
    medications, 93t, 256t
  atypical antidepressants,
    232t
  atypical antipsychotics, 92t
  Benadryl and, 282
  benzodiazepines, 256t,
    257–258
  Buspar and, 259
  clonidine and, 263, 267
  complete list of, 285–290
  depression and, 159–160
  Desyrel, 239
  Effexor, 239
  guanfacine, 265, 267
  Lamictal, 250
  lithium, 246
  melatonin, 282–283
  methylphenidate, 92t,
    209–214, 210t

mood stabilizers, 245t
naltrexone, 284
Neurontin, 254
nonstimulants, 92t
overview, 90–96, 92t–94t
propranolol, 268
Remeron, 239
second-generation
  antipsychotics and, 277
sleep problems and,
  196–197
SNRIs, 93t
SSRIs, 92t, 232t, 234–236
stimulants, 91, 92t,
  209–214, 210t–211t
Strattera, 225–226
tics and Tourette's disorder
  and, 180–181
tricyclic antidepressants,
  92t, 232t, 241
Trileptal, 253
valproic acid, 251–252
Wellbutrin, 238
Doxepin, 233t, 240–243, 287.
  See also Sinequan
Drug abuse, 23t, 189–191,
  191–194, 308–310. See
  also Substance abuse
Drug Enforcement
  Administration (DEA),
  205
Drug holiday, 122, 223.
  See also Stopping
  medications
Drug interactions. See also
  Multiple medications;
  Over-the-counter (OTC)
  medications
  buproprion and, 238
  clonidine and, 264
  dosage determination and,
    95–96
  Gabitril, 254
  SSRIs and, 237
  stimulants and, 219, 220t
  Strattera and, 226
  Topamax, 253, 254
  Trileptal and, 253
Drug scheduling by the DEA,
  205
Drug testing, 191
Dry mouth, 241, 242, 274–275.
  See also Side effects
DSM, 62
Duloxetine, 93t, 145, 233t,
  240, 287. See also
  Cymbalta
Dyanavel XR, 211t. See also
  Amphetamines
Dynamic-oriented
  therapies, 14. See

also Psychotherapy;
  Treatment
Dysthymia, 155, 158, 165t
Dystonia, 274. See also Side
  effects

Eating disorders, 123,
  186–188, 303–304
EEG (electroencephalogram),
  58, 111, 131, 138,
  182–183
Effectiveness of medications.
  See also Monitoring the
  effects of a medication;
  Side effects
  conflicting reports
    regarding, 24–25
  dosage determination and,
    90–91, 94–95
  FDA approval and, 82–84
  noticing, 105–112
  overview, 18–19
  return or worsening of
    symptoms and, 112–116
  safety and, 25–30
  stimulants and, 206,
    208–209
Effexor and Effexor XR.
  See also Atypical
  antidepressants; Pristiq;
  Venlafaxine
  ADHD and, 135
  anxiety disorders and, 145,
    151t
  bipolar disorder and, 163
  depression and, 158, 159,
    165t
  dosage determination and,
    233t, 287
  eating disorders and, 188
  overview, 238–239
  PTSD and, 148
  substance abuse and, 193,
    194
Efficacy. See Effectiveness of
  medications
Elavil, 232t, 240–243, 287.
  See also Amitriptyline
Electroconvulsive therapy
  (ECT), 165t
Emergency situations, 112,
  113, 123–126
Emotional control, 30, 67,
  281
Emotional problems. See
  Mood disorders
Enuresis, 197, 198, 230
Environmental factors, 12,
  24, 113, 147–148, 168
Epilepsy. See Temporal lobe
  epilepsy

Index

Equetrol, 165*t*, 171, 183, 245*t*, 289. *See also* Carbamazepine
Escitalopram, 92*t*, 232*t*, 286. *See also* Lexapro; SSRIs (selective serotonin reuptake inhibitor)
Eskalith, 165*t*, 244, 245*t*, 289. *See also* Lithium
Eszopiclone, 256*t*, 290. *See also* Lunesta
Etiology, 11–12
Evaluation, 26, 31–32
Executive functions, 30, 134, 170–171
Exelon, 134
Exposure techniques, 150
Extended-release preparation, 88, 94*t*, 108, 212–213
Externalizing symptoms, 64, 185
Extrapyramidal effects, 274, 275. *See also* Side effects

Family and Medical Leave Act (FMLA), 123
Family evaluation, 50*t*. *See also* Psychopharmacology evaluation
Family factors, 53–55, 68, 198
Family therapy, 14, 138, 187–188, 191. *See also* Psychotherapy; Treatment
Fatigue, 156
Fear, 64, 143
Financial concerns, 38–39, 88, 124–125, 192
Fish oil. *See* Supplements
Fluoxetine, 92*t*, 232*t*, 286. *See also* Prozac; SSRIs (selective serotonin reuptake inhibitor)
Fluphenazine, 272*t*, 288. *See also* Prolixin
Fluvoxamine, 92*t*, 145, 232*t*, 286. *See also* Luvox; SSRIs (selective serotonin reuptake inhibitor)
Focalin and Focalin XR. *See also* Methylphenidate
ADHD and, 133, 134, 139*t*
dosage determination and, 210*t*, 211, 212, 285
prescription and dosing of, 218

Food and Drug Administration (FDA) approval
bipolar disorder and, 162
decisions regarding medications to prescribe and, 81–88
dosage determination and, 90, 91
generics instead of brand name medications, 103
multiple medications and, 87
overview, 2, 5, 24–25
researching specific medications and, 74
safety of medications and, 25–26
schizophrenia in children and, 175
tics and Tourette's disorder and, 181
Friendships. *See* Peer relationships

GABA (gamma-aminobutyric acid), 21, 23*t*, 257
Gabapentin. *See also* Neurontin
bipolar disorder and, 161, 253
dosage determination and, 93*t*, 245*t*, 289
psychosis and, 177*t*
temporal lobe epilepsy and, 183
Gabitril, 161, 165*t*, 254, 289
Gastrointestinal problems. *See also* Diarrhea; Nausea; Side effects; Stomachaches; Vomiting
anticonvulsants and, 249
autism spectrum disorders and, 168–169
lithium and, 247
propranolol, 268
SSRIs, 236
valproic acid, 252
Generalized anxiety disorder, 143, 151*t*. *See also* Anxiety disorders
Generic medications, 103–104
Genetic factors, 11, 54–55, 160, 174, 179
Genetic testing, 60
Geodon. *See also* Second-generation antipsychotic (SGAs); Ziprasidone
autism spectrum disorders and, 170

bipolar disorder and, 162, 165*t*
conduct disorder and, 138
dosage determination and, 93*t*, 272*t*, 273, 274, 277, 288
overview, 269, 276–277
psychosis and, 176, 177*t*
side effects, 274, 277–278, 278
tics and Tourette's disorder and, 181
Glutamate, 204
Glutamine, 21, 23*t*
Goals in treatment, 14, 105–112
Growth problems, 216*t*, 221–223. *See also* Side effects
Guanfacine. *See also* Alpha agonists; Antihypertensives; Intuniv; Tenex
ADHD and, 139*t*, 220, 227–228
autism spectrum disorders and, 170, 172*t*
bipolar disorder and, 163, 165*t*
clonidine and, 267
conduct disorder and, 140*t*
DMDD and, 164
dosage determination and, 94*t*, 262*t*, 265, 286
mental disorders due to medical conditions and, 185
multiple medications and, 87
oppositional defiant disorder and, 137, 140*t*
overview, 200
PTSD and, 151*t*
side effects, 265–266
tics and Tourette's disorder and, 180, 185*t*
Guilt, 156

Hair pulling (trichotillomania), 149, 150, 307
Halcion, 256*t*, 290. *See also* Triazolam
Haldol. *See also* Haloperidol
autism spectrum disorders and, 170
dosage determination and, 93*t*, 271, 272*t*, 273, 274, 288
psychosis and, 175, 177*t*
side effects, 274, 275

Haldol (cont.)
 tics and Tourette's disorder and, 181, 185t
Hallucinations. See also Psychosis
 antipsychotics and, 270, 279–280
 bipolar disorder and, 162
 depression and, 156, 165t
 overview, 173
 propranolol, 268
 SSRIs and, 234–235
 temporal lobe epilepsy and, 183
 when to seek help, 51
Haloperidol, 271, 272t, 288. See also Haldol
Harm to others, 107, 123–126
Headaches, 109, 218–219, 226, 236. See also Side effects
Health issues, 102–103. See also Medical factors
Heart symptoms, 216t, 223–224, 241–242, 266, 268. See also Side effects
Hepatitis, 226. See also Side effects
Hospitalization, 48, 107, 123–126
Hydroxyzine, 256t, 290. See also Atarax; Vistaril
Hyperactivity, 129, 130, 264. See also Attention-deficit/hyperactivity disorder (ADHD)

Imipramine. See also Tofranil; Tricyclics antidepressants (TCAs)
 ADHD and, 133–135, 139t, 228–229
 anxiety disorders and, 151t
 depression and, 158, 165t
 dosage determination and, 92t, 232t, 287
 eating disorders and, 188
 enuresis and, 198
 monitoring the effects of a medication and, 111
 overview, 240–243
 PTSD and, 148
 sleep problems and, 197
 substance abuse and, 194
 tics and Tourette's disorder and, 180–181, 185t
Improvement without treatment, 15–16
Impulsivity, 12, 129, 130, 149, 264. See also Attention-deficit/hyperactivity disorder (ADHD)

Inattentiveness, 129, 130. See also Attention-deficit/hyperactivity disorder (ADHD)
Inderal, 169, 262t, 286. See also Propranolol
Individualized educational plans (IEPs), 63
Individuals with Disabilities Education Act (IDEA), 63
Inflexibility, 136, 167, 170
In-patient care. See Hospitalization
Insomnia. See Sleep problems
Insurance, 38–39, 88, 124–125, 192. See also Financial concerns
Intuniv. See also Alpha agonists; Guanfacine
 ADHD and, 133, 134, 139t, 220, 227–228
 autism spectrum disorders and, 170, 172t
 bipolar disorder and, 165t
 DMDD and, 164
 dosage determination and, 262t, 265, 286
 multiple medications and, 87
 oppositional defiant disorder and, 137
 overview, 265, 267
 PTSD and, 149
 side effects, 265–266
 tics and Tourette's disorder and, 180, 185t
Invega. See also Paliperidone; Second-generation antipsychotic (SGAs)
 bipolar disorder and, 162, 165t
 dosage determination and, 93t, 272t, 273, 277, 288
 overview, 269–270, 276–277
 psychosis and, 177t
 side effects, 277–278, 278
Irritability. See also Side effects
 autism spectrum disorders and, 170, 171, 172t
 bipolar disorder and, 155
 buproprion and, 238
 clonidine and, 264
 depression and, 155, 156
 guanfacine and, 266
 second-generation antipsychotics and, 277
 SSRIs, 236

 stimulants and, 216t, 217–218
 Strattera and, 226
Isolation, 51, 156

Kapvay. See also Clonidine
 ADHD and, 133, 220, 227–228
 autism spectrum disorders and, 170, 172t
 DMDD and, 164
 dosage determination and, 262t, 263, 286
 multiple medications and, 87
 oppositional defiant disorder and, 137
 overview, 261–263, 267
 tics and Tourette's disorder and, 180, 185t
Ketamine, 242–243
Kidney functioning, 111, 247
Klonopin. See also Clonazepam
 abuse of, 189
 antipsychotics and, 275, 279
 anxiety and, 146, 151t, 257
 autism spectrum disorders and, 169, 171, 172t
 conduct disorder and, 140t
 dosage determination and, 93t, 256t, 257, 290
 mental disorders due to medical conditions and, 185
 obsessive–compulsive disorder and, 150
 oppositional defiant disorder and, 140t
 psychosis and, 177t
 PTSD and, 151t
 sleep problems and, 197
 temporal lobe epilepsy and, 183
 tics and Tourette's disorder and, 185t

Lamictal. See also Lamotrigine; Mood stabilizers
 antipsychotics and, 280
 autism spectrum disorders and, 171
 bipolar disorder and, 161, 163, 165t
 depression and, 159, 165t
 dosage determination and, 245t, 250, 289
 overview, 250
 psychosis and, 177t

side effects, 242–243, 251
temporal lobe epilepsy
 and, 183
Lamotrigine. *See also*
 Lamictal
 bipolar disorder and, 161,
  163
 depression and, 165*t*
 dosage determination and,
  93*t*, 245*t*, 289
 psychosis and, 177*t*
 side effects, 110, 242–243
 temporal lobe epilepsy
  and, 183
Latuda. *See also* Lurasidone;
 Second-generation
 antipsychotic (SGAs)
 antipsychotics and, 279–280
 dosage determination and,
  272*t*, 273, 277, 288
 overview, 269, 276–277
 psychosis and, 177*t*
 side effects, 277–278
Lead level test, 59–60
Learning disabilities, 120, 135
Lexapro. *See also*
 Escitalopram; SSRIs
 (selective serotonin
 reuptake inhibitor)
 anxiety disorders and, 145,
  151*t*
 autism spectrum disorders
  and, 170, 172*t*
 bipolar disorder and, 163
 depression and, 157–158,
  159, 165*t*
 DMDD and, 164
 dosage determination and,
  232*t*, 235, 286
 obsessive–compulsive
  disorder and, 152*t*
 overview, 231
 PTSD and, 148
 substance abuse and, 194
Librium, 257. *See also*
 Chlordiazepoxide
Limbic structures, 20
Lithium. *See also* Mood
 stabilizers
 antipsychotics and, 279,
  280
 autism spectrum disorders
  and, 171, 172*t*
 bipolar disorder and, 161,
  165*t*
 conduct disorder and, 140*t*
 depression and, 159
 dosage determination and,
  93*t*, 95, 245*t*, 246, 289
 eating disorders and, 188
 mental disorders due to
  medical conditions and,
   185
 monitoring the effects of a
  medication and, 111
 oppositional defiant
  disorder and, 140*t*
 overview, 244–248
 psychosis and, 177*t*
 side effects, 246–248
Lithobid, 165*t*, 244, 245*t*, 289.
 See also Lithium
Lithonate, 244, 245*t*, 289. *See
 also* Lithium
Lithotabs, 244, 245*t*, 289. *See
 also* Lithium
Liver functioning, 111, 249
Long-term effects of
 psychiatric medication,
 2–3, 27–30, 258, 268
Lorazepam, 256*t*, 257, 279,
 290. *See also* Ativan
Loxapine, 271, 272*t*, 288. *See
 also* Loxitane
Loxitane, 271, 272*t*, 288. *See
 also* Loxapine
Ludiomil, 232*t*, 287. *See also*
 Maprotiline
Lunesta, 256*t*, 290. *See also*
 Eszopiclone
Lurasidone, 272*t*, 288. *See
 also* Latuda
Luvox. *See also* Fluvoxamine;
 SSRIs (selective
 serotonin reuptake
 inhibitor)
 anxiety and, 145, 151*t*, 255
 autism spectrum disorders
  and, 170, 172*t*
 bipolar disorder and, 163
 depression and, 157, 158,
  165*t*
 dosage determination and,
  232*t*, 235–236, 286
 eating disorders and, 188
 obsessive–compulsive
  disorder and, 150, 152*t*
 PTSD and, 148
 substance abuse and, 194
 tics and Tourette's disorder
  and, 181

Major depression, 154,
 165*t*, 174–175. *See also*
 Depression; Mood
 disorders
Major tranquilizers, 175, 269.
 See also Antipsychotics
Mania. *See also* Bipolar
 disorder
 antipsychotics and, 280
 overview, 155, 160
 psychosis and, 174–175
 sleep problems and, 195,
  196
 SSRIs and, 234–235
 treatment and, 162–163
Manic–depression. *See*
 Bipolar disorder
Maprotiline, 232*t*, 287. *See
 also* Ludiomil
Medical factors
 blood tests and, 59–60
 dosage timing and, 105
 medications prescribed in
  addition to psychotropic
  meds, 102–103
 overview, 12
 psychopharmacology
  evaluation and, 52–53,
  56–58
Medical problems, 223–224,
 252
Medical testing, 56–58,
 59–60, 111, 175–176
Medicating process. *See
 also* Psychotropic
 medications
 ADHD and, 132–136,
  139*t*–140*t*, 218
 anxiety disorders and,
  145–147, 151*t*–152*t*
 autism spectrum disorders
  and, 169–171, 172*t*
 bipolar disorder and,
  161–164
 decisions regarding
  medications to
  prescribe, 80–88
 depression and, 157–160
 discussing with your child
  or teenager, 35–38
 DMDD and, 164
 dosage determination and,
  90–96, 92*t*–94*t*
 doubts regarding the
  treatment plan and,
  73–75
 eating disorders and,
  187–188
 effectiveness of
  medications and, 18–19
 enuresis and, 198
 generics instead of brand
  name medications,
  103–104
 how medications work,
  19–24, 19*f*, 21*f*, 23*t*
 monitoring the effects and,
  96–97
 mood disorders and, 165*t*
 multiple disorders and,
  16–17

Index

Medicating process (*cont.*)
  obsessive–compulsive
    disorder and, 150
  overview, 1, 4–5, 17, 39–40
  prescribing multiple
    medications, 85–88
  psychosis and, 175–176,
    177*t*
  recommendations from
    your doctor regarding,
    10–13
  safety and, 25–30
  second opinions regarding,
    77–79
  sleep problems and,
    196–198
  starting and stopping, 34
  stigmatization regarding,
    34–35
  substance abuse and,
    192–194
  temporal lobe epilepsy
    and, 183
  tics and Tourette's disorder
    and, 185*t*
  treatment planning and,
    70–71
  trying alternatives to
    medication, 114–115
  waiting and watching
    approach and, 74–75
  when to seek help, 51
Medication evaluation,
  50*t*. *See also* Psychopharmacology evaluation
Medication history, 52,
  98–99, 100*f*, 200–201.
  See also Medication Log
Medication holidays, 122,
  223. *See also* Stopping
  medications
Medication interaction. *See*
  Drug interactions
Medication Log, 99, 100*f*,
  200–201, 293–294. *See
  also* Medication history;
  Record keeping
Medication trials, 82–85, 86,
  88–90, 96–97, 125
Medications. *See* Psychotropic
  medications
Melatonin, 196–197, 282–283
Mellaril. *See also*
  Thioridazine
  bipolar disorder and, 165*t*
  dosage determination and,
    93*t*, 271, 273, 273*t*, 289
  overview, 270, 273
  psychosis and, 175
  side effects, 275
Memantine, 134, 135, 171

Memory impairment, 247. *See
  also* Side effects
Mental disorders due to
  medical conditions,
  183–185
Mental health professionals.
  See also Parent–
  practitioner
  collaboration; Physicians
  differing options for
    treatment and diagnosis
    and, 33–34
  overview, 6
  psychopharmacology
    evaluation and, 41–49,
    50*t*
  relationships with, 115–116
  resources regarding,
    297–300
  second opinions and, 77–79
  seeking treatment and,
    31–32
  tics and Tourette's disorder
    and, 178
  treatment planning and,
    71–72
  when to seek help, 51
Mental status update, 55–56
Meridia, 188
Mesoridazine, 273*t*, 289. *See
  also* Serentil
Metabolic testing, 60
Metabolism functioning, 247,
  278. *See also* Side effects
Metadate CD. *See also*
  Methylphenidate
  ADHD and, 133, 135, 139*t*
  dosage determination and,
    210*t*, 212, 285
  drug scheduling by the
    DEA and, 205
  prescription and dosing
    of, 218
  side effects and, 241
  substance abuse and, 194
Metformin, 176
Methylin, 210*t*, 285. *See also*
  Methylphenidate
Methylphenidate. *See also*
  Concerta; Daytrana;
  Focalin and Focalin XR;
  Metadate CD; Ritalin,
  Ritalin LA, and Ritalin
  SR; Stimulants
  ADHD and, 133
  clonidine and, 262
  conduct disorder and, 138
  dosage determination and,
    92*t*, 209–214, 210*t*, 285
  generics instead of brand
    name medications, 103

  how stimulants work and,
    204–206, 207*t*–208*t*
  long-term use of, 221–224
  overview, 19
  side effects, 213–219,
    215*t*–216*t*, 221–224
  tics and Tourette's disorder
    and, 185*t*
Methylphenidate patch. *See*
  Daytrana
Mindfulness, 144
Minipress, 197, 262*t*, 286. *See
  also* Prazosin
Mirtazapine, 233*t*, 239, 287.
  See also Remeron
Missing a dose of medication,
  104–105
Moban, 273*t*, 289. *See also*
  Molindone
Modafinil, 165*t*, 229. *See also*
  Provigil; Sparlon
Molindone, 273*t*, 289. *See also*
  Moban
Monitoring the effects of a
  medication, 91, 94–95,
  96–97, 105–116. *See
  also* Effectiveness of
  medications; Side effects
Monoamine oxidase
  inhibitors (MAOIs),
  101–102, 231, 233*t*, 288.
  See also Antidepressants
Mood disorders. *See also*
  Anxiety; Bipolar
  disorder; Depression;
  Major depression
  conduct disorder and, 137
  decisions regarding
    medications to
    prescribe, 84
  diagnosis and, 66–67
  multiple medications and,
    86–87
  overview, 153–154
  psychosis and, 174–175
  resources regarding,
    304–305
  symptoms of, 153
  treatment and, 165*t*
Mood stabilizers. *See also*
  Lithium; Psychotropic
  medications
  anticonvulsants and,
    248–249, 252–254
  appetite and, 101–102
  autism spectrum disorders
    and, 171
  bipolar disorder and, 161,
    162, 163, 165*t*
  conduct disorder and, 138
  DMDD and, 164

dosage determination and, 245t, 289
eating disorders and, 188
Lamictal, 250–251
mental disorders due to medical conditions and, 185
overview, 200, 244
psychosis and, 177t
substance abuse and, 194
valproic acid, 251–252
Moodiness, 171, 216t, 235, 269, 277. *See also* Side effects
Motor functions, 19–20, 20, 178–179. *See also* Tic disorders
MRI (magnetic resonance imaging), 57–58
Multiple medications, 95–96, 102–103, 219, 220t, 226. *See also* Combined pharmacotherapy; Drug interactions
Muscle spasms, 146
Muscle-related symptoms, 274, 275, 281. *See also* Side effects

N-acetylcysteine, 192
Nadolol, 262t, 266, 286. *See also* Corgard
Naloxone. *See* Naltrexone
Naltrexone. *See also* ReVia
autism spectrum disorders and, 170, 172t
conduct disorder and, 140t
dosage determination and, 94t, 284
mental disorders due to medical conditions and, 185
oppositional defiant disorder and, 140t
overview, 284
side effects, 284
substance abuse and, 192
Namenda, 171
Narcan. *See* Naltrexone
Nardil, 233t, 288. *See also* Phenelzine
National Institute of Mental Health (NIMH), 62
Nausea. *See also* Gastrointestinal problems; Side effects
anticonvulsants and, 249
lithium and, 247
propranolol, 268
Strattera and, 226

Trileptal and, 253
valproic acid, 252
Navane, 177t, 271, 272t, 275, 288. *See also* Thiothixene
Nefazodone, 233t, 287. *See also* Serzone
Nerve cells, 21, 21f
Neurobehavioral disorders, 131. *See also* Attention-deficit/hyperactivity disorder (ADHD); Disorders
Neuroleptic malignant syndrome, 275. *See also* Side effects
Neuroleptics, 175, 269. *See also* Antipsychotics
Neurological factors, 178, 187. *See also* Biological factors
Neurological testing, 57–58, 173–174, 182–183. *See also* Psychopharmacology evaluation
Neurontin. *See also* Gabapentin
autism spectrum disorders and, 171, 172t
bipolar disorder and, 161, 165t, 253
conduct disorder and, 140t
dosage determination and, 245t, 289
eating disorders and, 188
oppositional defiant disorder and, 140t
overview, 254
psychosis and, 177t
temporal lobe epilepsy and, 183
Neuropsychological testing, 50t, 58–59. *See also* Psychopharmacology evaluation
Neurotransmitters
ADHD and, 134
overview, 21–23, 21f, 23t, 28
Wellbutrin and, 238
Nicotine use, 190, 191–192. *See also* Substance abuse
Nonstimulants, 92t, 224–229, 286. *See also* Atomoxetine; Psychotropic medications
Noradrenergic effects, 228, 238
Norepinephrine
ADHD and, 133
alpha agonists and, 227

autism spectrum disorders and, 170
clonidine and, 262–263
overview, 21, 23t
Normalizing the disorder, 119–120
Norpramin, 228–229, 232t, 240–243, 287. *See also* Desipramine
Nortriptyline. *See also* Aventyl; Pamelor; Tricyclics antidepressants (TCAs)
ADHD and, 133–134, 139t, 228–229
anxiety disorders and, 146
depression and, 165t
dosage determination and, 92t, 232t, 287
overview, 240–243
psychosis and, 175
PTSD and, 148
side effects and, 241
stimulants and, 223
substance abuse and, 194
tics and Tourette's disorder and, 180–181, 185t
Numbing, 147, 148–149
Nurse practitioners (NPs), 48, 49. *See also* Mental health professionals
Nutritional counseling, 187–188

Obsessions, 149, 168, 170
Obsessive–compulsive disorder (OCD). *See also* Anxiety disorders
antidepressants and, 230
antipsychotics and, 270
anxiety disorders and, 145, 146–147
DSM and, 62
FDA approval and, 82
monitoring the effects of a medication and, 106
multiple disorders and, 16–17
neurotransmitters and, 23t
normalizing, 120
overview, 149–150
recommendations regarding medications and, 11
resources regarding, 306–307
SSRIs and, 234–235, 236–237
substance abuse and, 193
tics and Tourette's disorder and, 178, 179, 181

Index

Obsessive–compulsive disorder (*cont.*)
  treatment and, 15, 150, 152*t*
Occupational therapy, 168
Off-label use, 87, 88
Olanzapine, 161, 176, 272*t*, 276, 288. *See also* Zyprexa
Omega-3 fatty acids. *See* Supplements
Opioid system, 23*t*, 187
Oppositional defiant disorder (ODD)
  ADHD and, 130
  DMDD and, 164
  overview, 136
  substance abuse and, 190
  treatment and, 137, 140*t*
Orap. *See also* Pimozide
  dosage determination and, 93*t*, 271, 272*t*, 288
  side effects, 274, 275
  tics and Tourette's disorder and, 181, 185*t*
Overdose, 26, 109–111, 242. *See also* Safety of medications
Over-the-counter (OTC) medications. *See also* Drug interactions
  buproprion and, 238
  lithium and, 248
  multiple medications and, 88
  overview, 102
  sleep problems and, 196
  SSRIs and, 237
  stimulants and, 220*t*
  using along side prescriptions, 102
Oxazepam, 256*t*, 290. *See also* Serax
Oxcarbazepine, 245*t*, 253, 289. *See also* Trileptal
OxyContin, 189

Painkillers, 189, 248
Paliperidone, 162
Paliperidone, 272*t*, 288. *See also* Invega
Pamelor, 228–229, 232*t*, 240–243, 287. *See also* Nortriptyline
Panic disorders, 143–144, 151*t*, 190. *See also* Anxiety disorders
Paranoia, 279–280
Parental relationship, 68, 75–77

Parenting styles, 15, 24, 29–30, 75–77, 168
Parent–practitioner collaboration. *See also* Mental health professionals
  daily routines, 101
  diagnosis and, 67
  diet changes and, 101–102
  dosage timing, 104–105
  doubts regarding the treatment plan and, 33–34, 73–75
  generics instead of brand name medications, 103–104
  giving over-the-counter medications to your child, 102
  hospitalization and, 123–126
  Medication Log, 99, 100*f*
  medications prescribed in addition to psychotropic meds, 102–103
  mental health professionals involved in treatment and, 71–72
  monitoring the effects and, 105–112
  overview, 4, 7–8, 98–99
  psychopharmacology evaluation and, 42
  relationships with your provider, 115–116
  return or worsening of symptoms and, 112–116
  second opinions and, 79
  tapering off of medications and, 121–122
Parnate, 233*t*, 288. *See also* Tranylcypromine
Paroxetine, 92*t*, 232*t*, 286. *See also* Paxil; SSRIs (selective serotonin reuptake inhibitor)
Paxil. *See also* Paroxetine; SSRIs (selective serotonin reuptake inhibitor)
  anxiety and, 145, 151*t*, 255
  autism spectrum disorders and, 170, 172*t*
  bipolar disorder and, 163
  dosage determination and, 232*t*, 286
  eating disorders and, 188
  obsessive–compulsive disorder and, 150, 152*t*
  overview, 238

PTSD and, 148
  substance abuse and, 194
Pediatric acute-onset neuropsychiatric syndrome (PANS), 149–150
Pediatric autoimmune neuropsychiatric disorders (PANDAS), 149–150
Pediatric Research Equity Act, 25
Pediatricians. *See* Physicians
Peer relationships, 60–61, 168
Perfectionism, 143
Perfenazine, 271. *See also* Prolixin
Perphenazine, 271, 272*t*, 288. *See also* Trilafon
Personality changes, 37, 187. *See also* Side effects
Pertofrane, 232*t*, 287. *See also* Desipramine
Pharmacotherapy, 14, 90–96, 92*t*–94*t*. *See also* Medicating process; Treatment
Phenelzine, 233*t*, 288. *See also* Nardil
Phenothiazines, 93*t*
Phobias, 141. *See also* Anxiety disorders
Phonic tics, 178–179. *See also* Tic disorders
Physical side effects, 109, 156
Physical testing, 56–58, 59–60
Physicians. *See also* Mental health professionals
  differing options for treatment and diagnosis and, 33–34
  overview, 31
  psychopharmacology evaluation and, 41–49
  recommendations regarding medications from, 10–13
  relationships with, 115–116
  seeking treatment and, 31–32
Pimozide, 271, 272*t*, 288. *See also* Orap
Pindolol, 266
Placebo, 82, 83
Planning skills, 30
Positive effect, 105. *See also* Monitoring the effects of a medication

Positive symptoms, 175
Posttraumatic stress disorder (PTSD), 147–149, 151t, 187. See also Anxiety disorders
Potency, 91
Prazosin, 148, 197, 262t, 286. See also Minipress
Prescription drug abuse, 28, 29–30, 189, 205. See also Substance abuse
Primary-care clinicians. See Physicians
Pristiq, 233t, 238. See also Desvenlafaxine; Effexor and Effexor XR
Private practice, 13, 31–32, 61–62, 71–72, 125. See also Treatment
Problems taking the medication, 118–119
Process of choosing or implementing a medication. See Medicating process
Prolixin, 93t, 271, 272t, 273, 274, 275, 288. See also Fluphenazine; Perfenazine
Propranolol. See also Beta blockers; Inderal
 antipsychotics and, 275
 autism spectrum disorders and, 172t
 clonidine and, 264
 conduct disorder and, 140t
 dosage determination and, 262t, 268, 286
 oppositional defiant disorder and, 140t
 overview, 266
 psychosis and, 177t
 PTSD and, 151t
 side effects, 268
Protriptyline, 232t, 240–243, 287. See also Vivactil
Provigil, 134, 140t, 229. See also Modafinil
Prozac. See also Fluoxetine; SSRIs (selective serotonin reuptake inhibitor)
 ADHD and, 135
 anxiety disorders and, 145, 146, 151t
 autism spectrum disorders and, 170, 172t
 bipolar disorder and, 163
 depression and, 157–158, 159, 165t

dosage determination and, 232t, 234–235, 286
 eating disorders and, 188
 obsessive–compulsive disorder and, 152t
 overview, 231
 psychosis and, 175
 PTSD and, 148, 148–149
 side effects, 236
 stimulants and, 220t
 substance abuse and, 194
 tics and Tourette's disorder and, 181
Psychiatric evaluation. See Assessment; Psychopharmacology evaluation
Psychiatric history, 49–52, 50t
Psychiatric hospitalization. See Hospitalization
Psychiatrists, 31, 41–49. See also Mental health professionals; Physicians
Psychic, 182
Psychological testing, 50t, 58–59, 156–157. See also Psychopharmacology evaluation
Psychologists, 31. See also Mental health professionals
Psychopharmacology evaluation. See also Process of choosing or implementing a medication
 challenges in diagnosing and, 66–68
 medical or physical testing and, 56–58
 overview, 41–43
 preparing your child for, 63–66
 second opinions and, 77–79
 selecting a doctor for, 43–47
 what to expect from, 49–56, 50t
 what to take to, 62–63
 when to seek help, 51
Psychopharmacology, 24. See also Medicating process; Psychotropic medications
Psychosis. See also Psychotic disorders; Schizophrenia
 antipsychotics and, 269, 279–280
 autism spectrum disorders and, 168

 depression and, 156, 165t
 mania and, 160
 neurotransmitters and, 23t
 overview, 107, 173–175
 resources regarding, 307
 second-generation antipsychotics and, 277
 SSRIs and, 234–235
 treatment and, 175–176, 177t
Psychotherapy, 13–15, 157, 187–188, 191. See also Treatment
Psychotic disorders, 173–176, 177t, 197. See also Psychosis; Schizophrenia
Psychotropic medications. See also Alpha agonists; Anticonvulsants; Antidepressants; Antihypertensives; Antipsychotics; Anxiety-breaking medications; Medicating process; Medication Log; Medications; Mood stabilizers; Nonstimulants; SSRIs (selective serotonin reuptake inhibitor); Stimulants; Tricyclics antidepressants (TCAs)
 ADHD and, 132–136, 139t–140t
 anxiety disorders and, 145–147, 151t–152t
 autism spectrum disorders and, 169–171, 172t
 bipolar disorder and, 161–164
 conflicting reports regarding, 24–25
 decisions regarding medications to prescribe, 80–88
 depression and, 157–160
 discussing with your child or teenager, 35–38
 DMDD and, 164
 dosage determination and, 90–96, 92t–94t
 eating disorders and, 187–188
 effectiveness of, 18–19
 enuresis and, 198
 generics instead of brand name medications, 103–104
 how medications work, 19–24, 19f, 21f, 23t

Psychotropic medications (*cont.*)
  learning about, 98–99
  monitoring the effects and, 96–97
  mood disorders and, 165*t*
  not responding to, 112–116
  obsessive–compulsive disorder and, 150
  overview, 5–6, 17, 39–40, 199–201
  prescribing multiple medications, 85–88
  psychosis and, 175–176, 177*t*
  research regarding using with children and adolescents, 2
  researching specific medications and, 73–74
  resources regarding, 310
  safety and, 25–30
  sleep problems and, 196–198
  stigmatization regarding, 34–35
  substance abuse and, 192–194
  temporal lobe epilepsy and, 183
  tics and Tourette's disorder and, 185*t*
  trying alternatives to, 114–115

Quetiapine, 272*t*, 288. *See also* Seroquel
Quillivant/Quillichew and Quillivant XR, 133, 139*t*, 167–168, 210*t*, 212, 285. *See also* Methylphenidate

Rashes, 108–109, 110, 229, 249, 251, 264, 281. *See also* Side effects
Reality awareness. *See* Psychosis
Rebound, 207*t*, 215*t*, 217–218, 268. *See also* Side effects
Record keeping, 98–99, 100*f*, 293–294. *See also* Medication Log
Reducing medications, 118, 121–122, 122. *See also* Stopping medications
Rehabilitation Act of 1973, Section 504, 63
Relaxation techniques, 144
Remeron. *See also* Atypical antidepressants; Mirtazapine
  anxiety disorders and, 151*t*
  depression and, 158, 165*t*
  dosage determination and, 233*t*, 287
  overview, 239
  PTSD and, 148
  sleep problems and, 197
  substance abuse and, 194
Reminyl, 134
Repetitive behaviors, 167, 172*t*
Resources, 295–310
Response prevention, 150
Responsibility, 120–121
ReVia, 185, 284. *See also* Naltrexone
Rigidity, 170
Risk factors, 29–30
Risperdal. *See also* Risperidone; Second-generation antipsychotic (SGAs)
  autism spectrum disorders and, 169, 170, 172*t*
  bipolar disorder and, 162, 163, 165*t*
  conduct disorder and, 138, 140*t*
  dosage determination and, 93*t*, 250, 272*t*, 273, 274, 277, 288
  oppositional defiant disorder and, 137, 140*t*
  overview, 269–270, 276–277
  psychosis and, 175, 177*t*
  PTSD and, 148
  side effects, 275, 277–278
  sleep problems and, 197
  tics and Tourette's disorder and, 181, 185*t*
Risperidone. *See also* Risperdal
  antipsychotics and, 280
  autism spectrum disorders and, 169, 170
  bipolar disorder and, 162
  dosage determination and, 272*t*, 277, 288
  overview, 269–270, 279, 280
  psychosis and, 176
  tics and Tourette's disorder and, 185*t*
Ritalin, Ritalin LA, and Ritalin SR. *See also* Methylphenidate
  abuse of, 189
  ADHD and, 133, 139*t*
  dosage determination and, 209, 210*t*, 211, 212–213, 285

  drug scheduling by the DEA and, 205
  generics instead of brand name medications, 103
  overview, 19
  prescription and dosing of, 218
  substance abuse and, 194
Routines. *See* Daily routines

Sadness, 155, 216*t*, 217–218. *See also* Side effects
Safety of medications
  dosage determination and, 90–91, 95
  FDA approval and, 82–84
  monitoring the effects of a medication and, 107, 109–111
  overdose and, 109
  overview, 25–30
  substance abuse and, 194
Saphris. *See also* Asenapine
  autism spectrum disorders and, 170
  bipolar disorder and, 161, 165*t*
  dosage determination and, 272*t*, 273, 274, 288
  overview, 269, 276–277
  psychosis and, 177*t*
  side effects, 275, 277–278
Saphris trilafon, 93*t*
Scheduling appointments, 47–48
Schizophrenia. *See also* Psychosis; Psychotic disorders
  antipsychotics and, 269, 279–280
  obsessive–compulsive disorder and, 149
  overview, 173–175
  resources regarding, 307
  second-generation antipsychotics and, 277
  sleep problems and, 197
  substance abuse and, 192–193
  treatment and, 175–176, 177*t*
School assessment, 50*t*, 59. *See also* Psychopharmacology evaluation
School functioning, 88, 130, 156, 219. *See also* Academic functioning
School history, 52–54
Schools, 60–61, 63, 88–90, 108

Index

Second opinions, 77–79
Second-generation antipsychotic (SGAs). *See also* Antipsychotics; Atypical antipsychotics
  autism spectrum disorders and, 169, 172*t*
  bipolar disorder and, 161, 162, 163, 165*t*
  dosage determination and, 272*t*, 277, 288
  overview, 269, 271, 276–277, 279–280
  psychosis and, 175, 177*t*
  side effects, 274–276
  tics and Tourette's disorder and, 181
Section 504 of the Rehabilitation Act of 1973, 63
Sedation. *See also* Side effects
  antipsychotics and, 274
  Benadryl and, 281
  benzodiazepines and, 258
  clonidine and, 263–264, 281
  guanfacine and, 265–266
  monitoring the effects of a medication and, 110
  Topamax and, 254
  valproic acid, 252
Sedatives, 80, 257
Seizures, 58, 146, 171, 181–183, 219–221
Self-harm
  anticonvulsants and, 253
  antipsychotics and, 270
  autism spectrum disorders and, 170, 172*t*
  bipolar disorder and, 162
  conduct disorder and, 140*t*
  hospitalization and day treatment options and, 123–126
  monitoring the effects of a medication and, 107
  naltrexone and, 284
  oppositional defiant disorder and, 140*t*
  psychopharmacology evaluation and, 65–66
  when to seek help, 51
Self-regulation, 30, 67
Separated parents, 68
Separation anxiety, 15–16, 141, 142, 151*t*. *See also* Anxiety disorders
Serax, 146, 256*t*, 257, 290. *See also* Oxazepam
Serentil, 273*t*, 289. *See also* Mesoridazine

Seroquel. *See also* Quetiapine; Second-generation antipsychotic (SGAs)
  antipsychotics and, 279–280
  bipolar disorder and, 162, 165*t*
  conduct disorder and, 140*t*
  dosage determination and, 93*t*, 272*t*, 273, 277, 288
  oppositional defiant disorder and, 140*t*
  overview, 269, 270, 276–277
  psychosis and, 177*t*
  side effects, 274, 275, 277–278
  sleep problems and, 196, 197
  tics and Tourette's disorder and, 181
Serotonin
  autism spectrum disorders and, 168
  conduct disorder and, 138
  eating disorders and, 187
  obsessive–compulsive disorder and, 150
  oppositional defiant disorder and, 136
  overview, 21, 23*t*
  tics and Tourette's disorder and, 181
Sertraline, 92*t*, 169–170, 232*t*, 286. *See also* SSRIs (selective serotonin reuptake inhibitor); Zoloft (sertraline)
Serzone, 148, 194, 233*t*, 240, 287. *See also* Nefazodone
Shyness, 141
Sibutramine, 188
Side effects. *See also* Effectiveness of medications; Monitoring the effects of a medication
  anticonvulsants and, 249
  antidiuretic hormone desmopressin (ddAVP), 284
  antipsychotics and, 269, 271, 274–276
  appetite and, 101–102
  Benadryl, 282
  benzodiazepines and, 146, 258
  buproprion and, 238
  Buspar and, 259
  clonidine and, 263–264, 267

decisions regarding medications to prescribe, 85
Depakote and, 252
discussion with the doctor, 37
dosage timing and, 104–105
enuresis and, 198
guanfacine and, 265–266, 267
Lamictal, 251
lithium and, 246–248
melatonin, 283
monitoring without hovering and, 107
multiple medications and, 87
naltrexone, 284
neurotransmitters and, 23
nonstimulant medications and, 228–229
overview, 40, 105
propranolol, 268
Provigil, 229
Remeron, 239
safety of medications and, 25
second-generation antipsychotics and, 277–279
sleep problems and, 197
SSRIs, 236–237
SSRIs and, 231, 234–235
stimulants and, 207*t*, 215*t*–216*t*, 221–224
Strattera and, 226–227
Topamax and, 253–254
tricyclic antidepressants, 241–242
Trileptal and, 253
trying alternatives to medication and, 115
types of, 108–111
valproic acid, 252
Sinequan, 233*t*, 287. *See also* Doxepin
Skin disorders, 249. *See also* Rashes
Sleep problems. *See also* Side effects
  anticonvulsants and, 249
  antipsychotics and, 274
  benzodiazepines and, 258
  buproprion and, 238
  clonidine and, 261, 263–264, 281
  depression and, 156
  guanfacine and, 265–266
  lithium and, 247
  melatonin and, 282–283

338 Index

Sleep problems (*cont.*)
  monitoring the effects of a
    medication and, 109
  overview, 195
  resources regarding, 308
  SSRIs, 236
  stimulants and, 215*t*, 217
  Strattera and, 226
  treatment and, 195–198
  tricyclic antidepressants
    and, 241
  Trileptal and, 253
Sleepiness, 110
SNRIs (serotonin-
    norepinephrine reuptake
    inhibitors). *See also*
    Effexor and Effexor XR;
    Venlafaxine
  anxiety and, 145, 255
  depression and, 159, 165*t*
  dosage determination and,
    93*t*
  PTSD and, 148, 151*t*
Social anxiety disorder, 16
Social history, 52–54
Social phobia, 144. *See also*
    Anxiety disorders
Social skills, 14, 167
Social withdrawal, 51, 156,
    258, 264
Social workers. *See* Mental
    health professionals
Sonata, 256*t*, 290. *See also*
    Zaleplon
Sparlon, 229. *See also*
    Modafinil
Specialists, 31–32, 44, 79.
    See also Mental health
    professionals
SPECT (single-photon-
    emission space
    tomography), 131
SSRIs (selective serotonin
    reuptake inhibitor). *See
    also* Antidepressants;
    Anxiety-breaking
    medications;
    Psychotropic
    medications
  ADHD and, 135
  anxiety and, 145, 151*t*, 255
  autism spectrum disorders
    and, 170, 172*t*
  bipolar disorder and,
    162–163
  Buspar and, 259
  decisions regarding
    medications to
    prescribe, 84
  depression and, 157–158,
    159, 165*t*

DMDD and, 164
dosage determination and,
  92*t*, 232*t*, 234–236, 286
eating disorders and, 188
effectiveness of, 18
FDA approval and, 82
obsessive–compulsive
  disorder and, 150, 152*t*
overview, 18, 200,
  230–237, 232*t*–233*t*
psychosis and, 177*t*
PTSD and, 148, 151*t*
side effects, 231, 236–237
substance abuse and, 192,
  193, 194
tics and Tourette's disorder
  and, 181
Stelazine. *See also*
    Trifluoperazine
  dosage determination and,
    271, 272*t*, 273, 288
  psychosis and, 175, 177*t*
  side effects, 275
Stereotypic behaviors, 167,
  276
Stimulants. *See also*
    Amphetamines;
    Methylphenidate;
    Psychotropic
    medications
  addiction and, 28
  ADHD and, 133, 134, 139*t*
  appetite and, 101
  autism spectrum disorders
    and, 167–168, 171
  bipolar disorder and, 163,
    165*t*
  buproprion and, 238
  clonidine and, 262
  conduct disorder and, 140*t*
  depression and, 159
  dosage determination and,
    91, 92*t*, 285–286
  effectiveness of, 18, 206,
    208–209
  failure to respond to, 206,
    207*t*–208*t*
  how stimulants work,
    204–206, 207*t*–208*t*
  long-term use of, 221–224
  mental disorders due to
    medical conditions and,
    184–185
  multiple medications and,
    219, 220*t*
  nonstimulant medications
    and, 227–228
  oppositional defiant
    disorder and, 137, 140*t*
  overview, 19, 21*f*, 200,
    203–204

prescription and dosing of,
  209–214, 210*t*–211*t*
side effects, 207*t*, 213–219,
  215*t*–216*t*, 221–224
sleep problems and, 197
substance abuse and, 193
tics and Tourette's disorder
  and, 181, 185*t*
tricyclic antidepressants
  and, 241
Stomachaches, 109, 218–219,
  226, 236, 247. *See
  also* Gastrointestinal
  problems; Side effects
Stopping medications. *See
  also* Medicating process
  benzodiazepines and, 258
  child's desire to, 222
  depression and, 159–160
  medication holidays, 122
  overview, 34, 121–122
  role of your child in
    treatment and, 118
  tapering off of medications,
    121–122
Strattera. *See also*
    Atomoxetine
  ADHD and, 133, 134, 135,
    139*t*, 140*t*, 220
  anxiety disorders and, 145,
    146–147, 151*t*
  conduct disorder and, 140*t*
  dosage determination and,
    225–226, 286
  long-term use of, 221
  oppositional defiant
    disorder and, 137, 140*t*
  overview, 224–227
  side effects, 226–227
  stimulants and, 220*t*
  substance abuse and, 193
  tics and Tourette's disorder
    and, 181, 185*t*
Striatum, 20
Stroop Test, 131
Structured interviews, 50*t*,
  61–62, 65–66. *See also*
  Psychopharmacology
  evaluation
Substance abuse. *See also*
    Abuse of medications;
    Alcohol abuse; Drug
    abuse
  depression and, 154
  family history and, 54–55
  monitoring the effects of a
    medication and, 107
  multiple disorders and, 17
  naltrexone and, 284
  overview, 17, 29–30,
    189–191

psychosis and, 174
resources regarding,
  308–310
role of your child in
  treatment and, 121
Strattera and, 225
treatment and, 191–194
when to seek help, 51
Suicidality. *See also* Side
  effects
depression and, 156, 158
hospitalization and day
  treatment options and,
  123–126
monitoring the effects of a
  medication and, 107, 109
psychopharmacology
  evaluation and, 65–66
resources regarding, 296
as a side effect, 108–109
SSRIs and, 231, 236–237
Strattera and, 226–227
treatment and, 157
when to seek help, 51
Supplements, 88, 159, 161
Swallowing pills, 118–119,
  248
Symptoms. *See also*
  Disorders; *individual
  disorders*; *individual
  symptoms*
ADHD, 129–130
anxiety disorders, 141, 143
autism spectrum disorders
  and, 166–168
bipolar disorder and,
  154–155, 160–161, 162
challenges in diagnosing
  and, 66–68
conduct disorder and, 137
depression, 154–155, 156
diagnosis and, 66–68
DMDD and, 164
DSM and, 62
eating disorders, 186–187
family history and, 54–55
monitoring the effects of a
  medication and, 105–112
mood disorders, 153
neurotransmitters and,
  22–23, 23t
obsessive–compulsive
  disorder, 149–150
oppositional defiant
  disorder and, 136
overview, 5, 9, 127–128
preparing your child for
  the psychopharmacology
  evaluation and, 64
psychopharmacology
  evaluation and, 66

psychosis and, 173–174
PTSD, 147
recommendations
  regarding medications
  and, 10–13, 40
return or worsening of,
  112–116
second-generation
  antipsychotics and, 277
stimulants and,
  207t–208t
substance abuse and,
  29–30, 189–190
temporal lobe epilepsy and,
  181–182
tics and Tourette's
  disorder, 178
treatment planning and,
  70–71, 80
when to seek help, 51

Tapering off of medications,
  121–122, 159–160,
  264, 266, 268. *See also*
  Stopping medications
Tardive dyskinesia, 176,
  275–276, 278
Tegretol. *See also*
  Anticonvulsants;
  Carbamazepine
antipsychotics and, 280
autism spectrum disorders
  and, 171, 172t
bipolar disorder and, 161,
  165t
conduct disorder and, 138,
  140t
dosage determination and,
  245t, 249, 289
mental disorders due to
  medical conditions and,
  185
monitoring the effects of a
  medication and, 111
oppositional defiant
  disorder and, 140t
overview, 248, 253
side effects, 249
temporal lobe epilepsy
  and, 183
Temper, 136
Temperament, 156
Temporal lobe epilepsy,
  181–183. *See also*
  Seizures
Tenex. *See also* Alpha
  agonists; Guanfacine
ADHD and, 133, 139t,
  227–228
autism spectrum disorders
  and, 172t

dosage determination and,
  262t, 265, 286
oppositional defiant
  disorder and, 137
overview, 265
side effects, 265–266
tics and Tourette's disorder
  and, 185t
Therapists. *See* Mental health
  professionals
Therapy. *See* Psychotherapy;
  Treatment
Thinking processes, 149, 156,
  253, 274–275. *See also*
  Cognitive functions
Thioridazine, 271, 273t, 289.
  See also Mellaril
Thiothixene, 271, 272t, 288.
  See also Navane
Thirst, 247. *See also* Side
  effects
Thorazine. *See also*
  Chlorpromazine
bipolar disorder and, 162,
  165t
dosage determination and,
  93t, 271, 273, 273t, 274,
  289
overview, 270
psychosis and, 175, 177t
side effects, 274, 275
sleep problems and, 197
Threatening harm, 51, 107,
  123–126
Thyroid functioning, 59–60,
  247. *See also* Side effects
Tiagabine, 289. *See also*
  Gabitril
Tic disorders
antidepressants and, 230,
  241
antihypertensives and, 261
antipsychotics and, 269,
  275
bipolar disorder and, 162
buproprion and, 238
clonidine and, 261, 262,
  281
guanfacine and, 265
neurotransmitters and, 23t
overview, 178–180
second-generation
  antipsychotics and, 277
stimulants and, 208t,
  219–221
Strattera and, 225
treatment and, 180–181,
  185t, 200
Timing of doses, 104–105.
  See also Dosage
  determination

Index

Tofranil, 228–229, 232t, 240–243, 287. *See also* Imipramine
Tolerance, 258
Topamax
  bipolar disorder and, 161, 165t, 253
  dosage determination and, 93t, 245t, 289
  eating disorders and, 188
  overview, 253–254
Topiramate, 245t, 253–254, 289. *See also* Topamax
Tourette's disorder
  antihypertensives and, 261
  antipsychotics and, 269, 270, 275
  clonidine and, 261, 262
  family history and, 54–55
  guanfacine and, 265
  multiple disorders and, 17
  neurotransmitters and, 23t
  overview, 178–180
  resources regarding, 306–307
  second-generation antipsychotics and, 277
  stimulants and, 208t
  treatment and, 180–181, 185t
TOVA, 131
Tranxene. *See also* Clorazepate
  anxiety disorders and, 146, 151t
  autism spectrum disorders and, 172t
  dosage determination and, 94t, 256t, 257–258, 290
  PTSD and, 151t
Tranylcypromine, 233t, 288. *See also* Parnate
Trazodone. *See also* Atypical antidepressants; Desyrel
  depression and, 158, 159
  dosage determination and, 233t, 287
  overview, 240
  PTSD and, 148
  substance abuse and, 194
Treatment. *See also* Psychotherapy; Treatment plan
  ADHD and, 132–136, 139t–140t
  anxiety disorders, 144–147
  autism spectrum disorders and, 169–171, 172t
  bipolar disorder and, 161–164, 165t

conduct disorder and, 138, 140t
decisions regarding medications to prescribe, 80–88
depression and, 157–160, 165t
diagnosis and, 271
disagreements regarding, 33–34
discussing with your child or teenager, 35–38
DMDD and, 164
early treatment, 3–4
eating disorders and, 187–188
enuresis and, 198
executive functions and, 30
improving without, 15–16
mental health professionals involved in, 71–72
multiple disorders and, 16–17
not responding to, 112–116
obsessive–compulsive disorder and, 150
oppositional defiant disorder and, 137, 140t
options for, 31–32, 33–34, 70–71
other than medication, 13–15
psychopharmacology evaluation and, 45, 47–48
psychosis and, 175–176, 177t
PTSD and, 147–149
safety of medications and, 25–30
schools and, 60–61
second opinions regarding, 77–79
sleep problems and, 195–198
stigmatization regarding, 34–35
substance abuse and, 191–194
temporal lobe epilepsy and, 183
tics and Tourette's disorder and, 180–181
Treatment histories, 98–99, 100f, 114–115, 293–294
Treatment plan. *See also* Treatment
  comprehensive treatment plan, 70–71
  decisions regarding

medications to prescribe, 80–88
disagreements regarding, 75–77
dosage determination and, 90–96, 92t–94t
doubts regarding, 73–80
hospitalization and day treatment options, 123–126
mental health professionals involved in, 71–72
monitoring the effects of a medication and, 96–97, 105–112
not responding to treatment and, 112–116
overview, 69–70
prescribing multiple medications, 85–88
second opinions regarding, 77–79
Treatment teams, 71–72. *See also* Mental health professionals
Tremors, 247, 274. *See also* Side effects
Trexan, 185, 284
Triazolam, 256t, 290. *See also* Halcion
Tricyclics antidepressants (TCAs). *See also* Antidepressants; Psychotropic medications
  ADHD and, 133–135, 139t, 220, 228–229
  autism spectrum disorders and, 170
  bipolar disorder and, 163
  depression and, 158, 159, 165t
  dosage determination and, 92t, 232t, 241, 287
  eating disorders and, 188
  enuresis and, 198
  monitoring the effects of a medication and, 111
  oppositional defiant disorder and, 137
  overview, 200, 231, 240–243
  PTSD and, 148, 151t
  side effects, 241–242
  stimulants and, 220t
  substance abuse and, 193, 194
  tics and Tourette's disorder and, 180–181, 185t
Trifluoperazine, 271, 272t, 288. *See also* Stelazine

Trilafon. *See also*
    Perphenazine
  bipolar disorder and, 165*t*
  dosage determination and,
    271, 272*t*, 273, 288
  overview, 270
  psychosis and, 175, 177*t*
Trileptal. *See also*
    Oxcarbazepine
  autism spectrum disorders
    and, 171, 172*t*
  bipolar disorder and, 161,
    165*t*, 253
  conduct disorder and,
    140*t*
  dosage determination and,
    93*t*, 245*t*, 289
  eating disorders and, 188
  oppositional defiant
    disorder and, 140*t*
  overview, 253
  temporal lobe epilepsy
    and, 183

Valium. *See also* Diazepam
  anxiety and, 145, 146,
    257
  dosage determination
    and, 94*t*, 256*t*, 257–258,
    290
  eating disorders and, 188
  mental disorders due to
    medical conditions and,
    185
  PTSD and, 148
  sleep problems and, 197
  substance abuse and, 194
Valproate. *See also* Valproic
    acid
  autism spectrum disorders
    and, 172*t*
  bipolar disorder and, 165*t*
  conduct disorder and, 140*t*
  dosage determination and,
    93*t*, 245*t*, 289
  oppositional defiant
    disorder and, 140*t*
  overview, 251
Valproic acid. *See also*
    Depakene sprinkles;
    Depakote; Depakote ER;
    Valproate
  bipolar disorder and, 165*t*
  dosage determination and,
    245*t*, 251–252, 289
  overview, 251
  side effects, 252
  temporal lobe epilepsy
    and, 183

Varenicline. *See* Chantix
Venlafaxine, 93*t*, 233*t*,
    238–239, 240, 287. *See
    also* Effexor and Effexor
    XR
Vicodin, 189
Viibryd, 151*t*, 233*t*, 240, 287.
    See also Vilazodone
Vilazodone, 233*t*, 240, 287.
    See also Viibryd
Vistaril, 256*t*, 290. *See also*
    Hydroxyzine
Visual hallucinations, 51
Vivactil, 232*t*, 240–243, 287.
    See also Protriptyline
Vivitrol, 192
Vomiting, 226, 247, 249, 268.
    See also Gastrointestinal
    problems; Side effects
Vortioxetine, 158, 233*t*, 240.
    See also Brintellix
Vyvanse. *See also*
    Amphetamines
  ADHD and, 133, 139*t*
  dosage determination and,
    210*t*, 211, 212, 286
  eating disorders and, 188
  prescription and dosing
    of, 218
  substance abuse and, 194

Weight changes. *See also*
    Side effects
  antipsychotics and,
    269–270, 271, 274
  monitoring the effects of a
    medication and, 109
  second-generation
    antipsychotics and,
    278–279
  Strattera and, 226
  Topamax and, 253–254
  valproic acid, 252
  when to seek help, 51
Wellbutrin. *See also* Atypical
    antidepressants;
    Buproprion
  ADHD and, 133–135, 140*t*,
    228
  bipolar disorder and, 163,
    165*t*
  depression and, 158, 159,
    165*t*
  dosage determination and,
    233*t*, 287
  oppositional defiant
    disorder and, 137
  overview, 237–238
  psychosis and, 177*t*

  stimulants and, 220*t*
  substance abuse and, 192,
    193, 194
Wisconsin Card Sort, 131
Withdrawal, 51, 156, 258, 264
Worry, 141, 143
Worthlessness, 156

Xanax. *See also* Alprazolam
  anxiety and, 146, 151*t*, 257
  dosage determination and,
    93*t*, 256*t*, 257, 290
  psychosis and, 177*t*

Zaleplon, 256*t*, 290. *See also*
    Sonata
Ziprasidone, 170, 272*t*, 288.
    See also Geodon
Zoloft. *See also* Sertraline;
    SSRIs (selective
    serotonin reuptake
    inhibitor)
  anxiety and, 145, 146, 151*t*,
    255
  autism spectrum disorders
    and, 169–170, 170, 172*t*
  bipolar disorder and, 163
  depression and, 157, 158,
    165*t*
  dosage determination and,
    232*t*, 235
  eating disorders and, 188
  FDA approval and, 82
  obsessive–compulsive
    disorder and, 150, 152*t*
  PTSD and, 148
  side effects, 236
  substance abuse and, 194
  tics and Tourette's disorder
    and, 185*t*
Zoloft (sertraline), 286
Zolpidem, 256*t*, 290. *See also*
    Ambien
Zyban, 191, 228, 238. *See also*
    Buproprion
Zyprexa. *See also* Olanzapine;
    Second-generation
    antipsychotic (SGAs)
  bipolar disorder and, 162,
    165*t*
  dosage determination and,
    93*t*, 272*t*, 273, 274, 277,
    288
  overview, 269, 276–277
  psychosis and, 175, 177*t*
  side effects, 274, 277–278
  sleep problems and, 197
  tics and Tourette's disorder
    and, 181

About the Authors

Timothy E. Wilens, MD, is Associate Professor of Psychiatry at Harvard Medical School and Chief of the Division of Child and Adolescent Psychiatry at Massachusetts General Hospital. Board certified in child, adolescent, adult, and addiction psychiatry, Dr. Wilens conducts research, lectures, and publishes widely on child and adolescent psychiatric issues.

Paul G. Hammerness, MD, is Assistant Professor of Psychiatry at Harvard Medical School and Medical Director of Outpatient Psychiatry at Boston Children's Hospital. Board certified in child and adolescent psychiatry, Dr. Hammerness is an experienced clinician, educator, and researcher.